"This book is great for the highly educated reader and/or the medical professional."

-Robert Muller M.D.

DEATH IN SMALL DOSES?

Antioxidant Vitamins A, C, and E in the Twenty-first Century

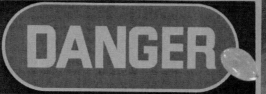

DANGER

CRUCIAL OXYGEN IN USE

LIMIT

ANTIOXIDANTS

Prof. Hon. Randolph M. Howes, M.D., Ph.D.

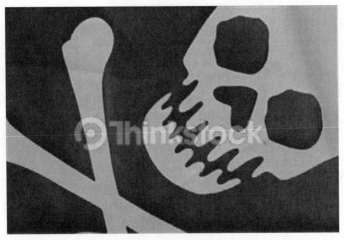

A SELECTIVE REVIEW

Antioxidant Vitamins A, C & E in the 21st Century

Vitamins A, C and E
Negligible Results, Half Truths and Potential Harm
As Demonstrated by Failed Intervention Trials

BOOK ONE: ANTIOXIDANT VITAMIN STUDIES FOR THE LAYMAN

BY

PROF. HON. RANDOLPH M. HOWES, M.D., Ph.D.
Orthomolecular Surgical Scientist and Biochemist

Antioxidant Vitamins A, C & E in the 21st Century:

Vitamins A, C and E
Negligible Results, Half Truths and Potential Harm
As Demonstrated by Failed Intervention Trials

A Selective Review

BY

PROF. HON. RANDOLPH M. HOWES, M.D., Ph.D.

Orthomolecular Surgical Scientist and Biochemist

Adjunct Assistant Professor of Plastic Surgery, The Johns Hopkins Hospital, Baltimore, Md., U.S.A., Espaldon Professor of Plastic and Reconstructive Surgery, University of Santo Tomas, Manila, Philippines. Adjunct Professor of Biological Sciences, Southeastern Louisiana University, Hammond, La., U.S.A.

Founder, Director and Chairman of the Scientific Advisory Board; U.S. Medical and Scientific Research Foundation, Inc.

Address for communication: 27439 Highway 441, Kentwood, Louisiana 70444-8152, USA. *Email:rhowesmd@hughes.net*

It is understood that medicine is an ever-changing science. As new research and clinical experience broaden our
knowledge, changes in treatment and drug therapy are required. The author and the publisher of this work have
checked with sources believed to be reliable in their efforts to provide information that is complete and generally in
accord with the standards accepted at the time of publication. However in view of the possibility of human error or
changes in the medical sciences, neither the authors nor the publisher nor any other party who has been involved in
the preparation of publication of this work warrants that the information contained herein is in every respect accurate
or complete, and they disclaim all responsibility to any errors or omissions or for the results obtained from use of the
information contained in the work. Readers are encouraged to confirm the information contained herein with other
sources. For example and in particular, readers are advised to check the product information sheet included in the
package of each drug they plan to administer to be certain that the information contained in this work is accurate
and that changes have not been made in the recommended dose or in the contraindications for administration. This
recommendation is of particular importance in connection with new or infrequently used drugs.

Financial disclosure: Dr. Howes has no financial conflicts of interest and is not involved in the sale of dietary
supplements or fitness equipment. The author holds no stocks or interests in companies in the supplement business.
Printed in the United States of America.

ISBN: 978-1-4269-3798-9 (SC)
ISBN: 978-1-4269-3799-6 (HC)
ISBN: 978-1-4269-3800-9 (E-BOOK)

Library of Congress Control Number: 2010909592

*Our mission is to efficiently provide the world's finest, most comprehensive book publishing
service, enabling every author to experience success. To find out how to publish your book,
your way, and have it available worldwide, visit us online at www.trafford.com*

Trafford rev. 8/2/2010

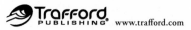 www.trafford.com

North America & international
toll-free: 1 888 232 4444 (USA & Canada)
phone: 250 383 6864 ♦ fax: 812 355 4082

ABOUT THE AUTHOR

Biographical sketch:

Professor Randolph M. Howes M.D., Ph.D. was born on August 17, 1943 in a small rural hospital in Madisonville, Louisiana. While at the hospital, an accidental hip burn from a heating pad introduced Dr. Howes to the harsh realities of life. Raised on a small bucolic strawberry farm in Ponchatoula, Louisiana, Dr. Howes learned ethics, morality, hard work and respect for his fellow man at a young age. Humble beginnings launched his lifetime trek of achievement as a scientist, surgeon, writer, visionary, philanthropist, international lecturer, singer, songwriter, business entrepreneur, broadcaster, inventor, corporate executive and rancher.

He attended St. Joseph's elementary school for eight years, served as an altar boy and sang in the choir. Next, he attended Ponchatoula High School where he finished as President of the Student Council by winning an election over the school's quarterback of the football team. He attributed this hard-fought win to his guitar playing and singing abilities. Dr. Howes began playing self-taught guitar professionally at 13 years of age. In 1961, Dr. Howes entered Southeastern Louisiana College (now Southeastern Louisiana University), where he took premed courses, made the Dean's list, made the honors chemistry class, worked 40 hours/ week at the Psychology Research Laboratory under Dr. John R. Nichols, played music in his 3 piece combo, named The Three Blind Mice, and was elected as president of the Catholic Youth Organization, the Inter-fraternity Council and the Junior class. He was featured in his college newspaper for his versatility and industriousness and he presented his first scientific paper to the Southwestern Psychological Association on interspecies intelligence, while still in his junior year. He has since been honored as an Outstanding SLU Alumnus, along with Robin Roberts of ABC's Good Morning America. Later SLU articles would refer to him as "the da Vinci in cowboy boots." He has served as an Adjunct Professor of Biological Sciences for many years at SLU. His Southeastern Louisiana University education opened the doors of academia for him and he next matriculated to Tulane School of Medicine in New Orleans, Louisiana.

While working on double doctorate degrees, Dr. Howes worked as a technician on the isolation of thyrotropin releasing factor with Nobel Laureate, Dr. Andrew V. Schally, studied under Dr. Richard Steele, whose mentor was Nobel Laureate, Dr. Albert Szent Gyorgii, met Nobel Laureates, George Wald and Dr. Linus Pauling, who felt that Dr. Howes could help bridge the gap between physicians and scientists, served as president of the Biochemistry graduate students, graduated in the top 10, received the 1971 Pathology Association Award, was elected to Sigma Xi honor fraternity and was the first in the history of Tulane School of Medicine to receive double doctorate degrees in medicine and biochemistry simultaneously. He was the first to be designated by the late Dr. Theodore Drapanas as a trained "surgical scientist" at Tulane Medical School.

He matched with his first choice at the prestigious Johns Hopkins Hospital for internship and residency training. He chose it over other top notch programs because Dr. George Zuidema, Chief and Blalock Professor of Surgery, gave him permission to conduct research studies concurrent with his surgical training in the highly sought after William Stewart Halstead program.

Even during his internship year, he was permitted lab space by Dr. John Cameron, past president of the American Surgical Association, co-wrote papers with Dr. Zuidema and Cameron, and he secured his own grants, trained his own lab technicians and later wrote many papers on surgical and oxygen free radical subjects during his residency training. He played music and sang for many of the surgery resident's functions and broke an ankle in a resident's football game and sustained significant trauma from a motorcycle accident. He was the first to complete board eligibility in both general and plastic surgery at The Johns Hopkins Hospital, while doing basic research on oxygen metabolism, all in a six-year period. He had the opportunity to work with the pioneer of mitochondrial biochemical function, Dr. Albert L. Lehninger, and rubbed elbows with many of the greats of science, surgery and medicine. He trained with Dr. Edward Luce and Dr. James Wells, both of whom have served as president of the American Society of Plastic and Reconstructive Surgeons. He trained under Dr. John E. Hoopes, past president of the American Association of Plastic Surgeons. He served as Dr. Paul Manson's chief resident and the distinguished Dr. Manson has also served as president of the American Association of Plastic Surgeons. He received many grants, honors and awards from 1971-1977 during his years at Hopkins, which are detailed in his full curriculum vitae. His musical interests have carried him to perform at the New Orleans World's Fair, on many televised shows, appearing with numerous country superstars and ultimately to center stage at the famed Grand Ole Opry Gospel Hour in Nashville, Tennessee. He has composed over 500 songs and his original "Fantasies of You" recording went to the # 1 chart spot on Nashville's Panel Report for nationwide independent air play. He was honored by the Country Music Associations of America with a Lifetime Achievement Award, Inducted into the Tracker Hall of Fame, received the King Eagle Humanitarian Award for "Your Devotion To the Betterment of Mankind", received the 1999 Golden Music Award, Lifetime Achievement Award for Songwriter/Artist/Humanitarian and many other such honors. In 1994, he received Dr. Norman Vincent Peale's America's Awards honoring Unsung Heroes, known as "The Nobel Prize for Goodness," and in 1995, he was awarded an Honorary Doctorate of Humanities Degree by SLU. That same year, he was sworn in by Rudolph W. Giuliani, Mayor of New York City, as the Community Mayor for the State of Louisiana, International Council of Mayors and was an awardee, along with Dr. Stephen Ambrose, for the George Washington Honor Medal.

Told that he could not go directly into solo practice, he boldly returned to New Orleans in 1977 and opened his private practice at the Institute of Cosmetic Plastic Surgery, which became a bona fide success story. He has served as president of the Metropolitan Cosmetic Surgery Society and the Louisiana Cosmetic Surgery Society, and has served the American Academy of Cosmetic Surgeons in numerous national offices and in many capacities. He was awarded a patent certificate for inventing the triple lumen venous catheter in 1977, licensed it to Arrow International, Inc. in 1981, successfully defended it in a multimillion dollar six year patent infringement suit and watched it become recognized as the number one venous catheter in the world. His multilumen catheter has been credited with helping save the lives of over 20 million critically ill patients worldwide and the name of Howes is well-known in the medical field in over 100 countries.

He performed pro bono surgery, since 1982 throughout the Philippines, was honored by the Philippine Ministry of Health in 1985 and since 2004, he holds the Espaldon Professorial Chair in Plastic and Reconstructive Surgery at the University of Santo Tomas in Manila. He was the recipient of the Humanitarian of the Year Award from the Community Mayors of New York, New Jersey and Connecticut in 1996. His philanthropic and humanitarian efforts have been acknowledged by Presidents Ronald Reagan and George H. Bush and he has received a letter of appreciation from former USA President, George W. Bush. He retired from his private practice to pursue his dream of contributing to a better understanding of oxygen biochemistry and of conducting an arduous in depth review of the world's scientific literature on oxygen metabolism. In 2004, he published his first in a series of e-books on oxygen metabolism, which was a 767-page tome entitled, "U.T.O.P.I.A.: Unified Theory of Oxygen Participation In Aerobiosis." Also in 2004, in an unprecedented move, The Johns Hopkins Hospital gave him an appointment as an Adjunct Assistant Professor of Plastic Surgery. In 2005, he published his second e-book, a 931-page tome, entitled, "The Medical and Scientific Significance of Oxygen Free Radical Metabolism." In the last six years, he has written a magnum opus composed of about 15 e-books on electronically modified oxygen derivatives (EMODs) and they are the basis of the Howes Selective World Library Of Oxygen Metabolism, available at www.iwillfindthecure.org. He is offering his library free of charge to all via the world wide web. His mission and his passion is to get the benefits of his innovative theories to the patient's bedside in his lifetime.

THE HOWES SELECTIVE WORLD LIBRARY OF OXYGEN METABOLISM

Dr. R.M. Howes' magnum opus of electronically modified oxygen derivatives (EMODs) in obligate aerobic systems

The thirteenth in a series and a companion to the following books:

#1. U.T.O.P.I.A. © 2004 Unified Theory of Oxygen Participation In Aerobiosis;

767 pages

#2. The Medical and Scientific Significance of Oxygen Free Radical Metabolism © 2005; 934 pages

#3. Hydrogen Peroxide Monograph 1: Scientific, Medical and Biochemical Overview & © 2006; 200 pages

#4. Monograph 2: Antioxidant vitamins A, C & E:E q u i v o c a l Scientific Studies, © 2006; 171 pages

#5. Cardiovascular Disease and Oxygen Free Radical Mythology, © 2006;

308 pages

#6. Diabetes and Oxygen Free Radical Sophistry, © 2006;

366 pages

#7, 8, 9. Reactive Oxygen Species Insufficiency (ROSI)

as the Basis for Disease Allowance and Coexistence:

Extraordinary Support for an Extraordinary Theory

Vol I, II & III. © 2008; 1564 pages

Volume I 501 pages #7 © 2008

Volume II 505 pages #8 © 2008

Volume III 562 pages #9 © 2008

#10. THE HOWES PAPERS

© 2009; 211 pages

#11. Reactive Oxygen Species vs. Antioxidants:

"The Oxypocalypse" or

"The war that never was" © 2010; 550 pages

#12. Death in Small Doses?"

Antioxidant Vitamins: Vitamins A, C & E in the 21st Century

Book One:

A Health Impact Statement For The Layman

© 2010; 93 pages

#13. Antioxidant Vitamins are Making a Killing:

Antioxidant Vitamins: Vitamins A, C & E in the 21st Century

Book Two:

A Health Impact Statement For The Medical Scientist

© 2010; 188 pages

All available at *www.iwillfindthecure.org*

Table of contents:

BOOK ONE:

DEDICATION

To my late Mom and Dad,
Clarence and Magdalena Howes.
Although they had limited wealth,
they had unlimited morality and ethics.
I hope that my quest to eliminate
cancer and heart disease will
always make them proud
to have called me, "son."

RAD!CAL

DOC

R ANDOLPH
x
HOWES

FUNDAMENTAL VALUE OF
CREATIVE IDEAS

In evaluating the fundamental value of an individual's creative ideas, one must not rely solely on the preconceived acceptance of the so called good-old-boy network of experts, how many meetings the author has attended, how many organizations he belongs to, how many degrees he has accumulated, how many articles he has published or his demonstrated skills as a medico/scientific politician and con artist. Instead, I suggest that before accepting or rejecting another's new and creative ideas, there is an absolute requirement for the unbiased evaluation of the intellectual integrity of the ideas themselves as regards their inherent honesty, ascertaining their persuasive strength based on the magnitude of prior established data and the courage to judge for yourself. Anything less is cowardly pandering and appeasement of peers, which is likely to stall scientific progress, just as it has, so many times in the past. Do not stick with a popular but erroneous notion just because it is the convenient and comfortable thing to do. Do not be afraid to open your mind and to step into the future of scientific discovery. (R.M. Howes MD, PhD, 2008)

CHAPTER ONE:

Inform Yourself

If you are taking an antioxidant or an antioxidant vitamin or are thinking of going on antioxidants, this fully referenced book, *Antioxidant Vitamin A, C & E in the 21st Century,* is a "must read" for you. The undeniable legacy of antioxidant vitamin use at today's high doses is an assemblage of confusing and conflicting studies and reports of bad side effects in hordes of unsuspecting **victims**. Only by knowing this information, and in consultation with your healthcare professional, can you make an informed decision about your health care. If you are a user of antioxidant vitamins A, C or E, or multivitamins, you must read this book. Most of the antioxidant side effects I discuss are likely unknown to your busy doctor. Although knowledgeable about routine medical problems, few have heard of increased risks for cancer, heart disease and strokes and fewer still associate increased mortality as being antioxidant-related. As a surgeon, medical research scientist, biochemist and practicing doctor, I was appalled by the lack of information in the medical community on the full range of side effects of the antioxidant vitamins. This book is a selective reference source and summary demonstrating the ineffectiveness and adverse side effects of the antioxidant vitamins A, C and E.

Americans are the biggest pill poppers on the planet. Unrestrained marketing of healthcare supplements permeate all forms of media on a constant and daily basis. The old adage is that "It probably won't hurt me and it might help me. So, why not take it?" Unfortunately, when it comes to the antioxidant vitamins A, C and E, it is becoming manifestly clear that these are agents with unknown or questionable benefits and with known harmful side effects. Thus, the sensible, safe and prudent questions are, "So, why take them at all in the absence of a deficiency state?" "Why waste your money for pills that are only marginally effective, if effective at all or even harmful?" "Is it possible that this entire antioxidant sector of the health industry is driven by market forces and not by medical science?" "Are they just trying to con an unsuspecting public?"

The accumulated evidence on antioxidants
and EMODs can be maddeningly contradictory.
Antioxidant vitamins are no longer about science,
they are about marketing.

Why take pills that are potentially harmful?

Aggressive marketing, testimonials and unrestricted advertising have led to wild claims and to the erroneous belief that antioxidant vitamins, such as A, C and E, are protective from common diseases and that they can effectively help reverse or cure a veritable laundry list of diseases, such as breast cancer, prostate cancer, skin cancer, colon cancer, head and neck cancer (including oral premalignant lesions), bladder cancer, colorectal adenomas, polyps of the colon, cardiovascular disease (including ischemic heart disease, hypertension, atherosclerosis, hyperhomocysteinemia, intimal thickening, lowering of cholesterol and triglycerides), strokes, diabetes (including endothelial dysfunction and insulin resistance), macular degeneration, cataracts, pre-eclampsia, Alzheimer's disease, mild cognitive impairment, Parkinson's disease, tardive dyskinesis, blood platelet disorders, renal insufficiency, and adverse effects of radiation therapy.... and yada, yada, yada.

However, in this far-reaching selective review, I report on **181 scientific reports** (including prospective, cohort and randomized controlled trials, utilizing analysis and/or meta-analysis) that have shown that antioxidant vitamins produce either marginal effects, negligible effects, no effects at all or harmful effects with many of the disease conditions that I just listed in the above paragraph. And, that is not all. I provide alternative possibilities for safe disease prevention and cure, based on prooxidants.

The scale of the antioxidant vitamin use problem is worldwide. In all honesty, I should not be writing a book, which points out the dangers of antioxidant supplements and you should not have to be reading such a book, which describes your increased risk for disease and premature death from these vitamins. Had the investigators, manufacturers and profiteers been honest, these studies would have been stopped long ago and the truth would have been common knowledge. Thus, this book would have been unnecessary.

In a nut shell, **the antioxidant vitamin supplements have failed to live up to their exalted, overstated expectations or to the rosy speculative predictions of the free radical theory.**

Predictions of disease prevention and reversal by common antioxidants, such as vitamins A, C and E, have been based on the free radical theory, which was introduced in the mid 1950s by Dr. Denham Harman. It basically stated that harmful metabolic products of oxygen randomly accumulate over time and serve as the cause for most diseases and aging. It was founded on the following three ideas:

1) **oxygen free radicals are harmful and deleterious, causing disease and aging**

2) **antioxidants will negate or scavenge free radicals and therefore,**

3) **diseases and aging can be prevented, cured and/or reversed by the use of antioxidants, including the common vitamins A, C and E**

ANTIOXIDANT HOGWASH
Today's marketing concepts
with the antioxidant vitamins
have an inadequate scientific basis
and meager biochemical plausibility.

A Global Public Health Issue

However, studies on antioxidant vitamins have been rife with inconsistencies, confusing results and unpredictability. These studies were based on Harman's free radical theory, which is a testable theory. Surprisingly, the free radical theory has repeatedly and blatantly failed many of these tests. But, instead of acknowledging the failure of the antioxidant vitamins, the failed results were said to be merely "disappointing." The inability to reliably repeat studies or to predict their outcomes, for more than fifty years, means that the free radical theory has flat-out failed to meet the requirements of the scientific method and it is thus invalidated, which should be the end of the story. But, marketers of these antioxidant supplements have gone to great lengths to discredit or ignore report after report of these failed studies. Admittedly, study results have to be scrutinized, but eventually a pattern begins to develop, which will reveal underlying truths. Certainly, there are studies extolling the great benefits of the antioxidant vitamins. Yet, proponents of the use of antioxidant vitamins tend to ignore or deny nearly all of the negative studies and continue to push sales of their questionable products.

THE LAMENTABLE FREE RADICAL THEORY
If the free radical theory had been a horse,
it would now be glue.
R. M. Howes, M.D., Ph.D.
1/13/07

For instance, on January 16, 2010, the Orthomolecular News Service issued, in part, the following statement, "Over half of the U.S. population takes daily nutritional supplements. Even if each of those people took only one single tablet daily, that makes 154,000,000 individual doses per day, for a total of over 56 billion doses annually. Since many persons take more than just one vitamin or mineral tablet, actual consumption is considerably higher, and the safety of nutritional supplements is all the more remarkable." Thus, by their own statements, **this is a major public health and safety issue.**

Many people, including doctors, gulp down handfuls of these supplements on a daily basis because of the perception that they promote good health. Such widespread use of antioxidant vitamin supplements and the accumulation of failed studies forces us to evaluate their safety and their impact on overall public health.

In this selective review, I directly address user safety and endeavor to answer the question, "Are antioxidant vitamins making a killing?" Are these agents actually "death in small doses?" There can be no doubt that the number of studies showing adverse effects of the antioxidant vitamins has increased to an impressive body of evidence (60 separate studies).

Of considerable concern is the fact that sixty studies have shown that the antioxidant vitamins can cause serious harmful side effects, including increased risk of cancer, heart disease, strokes and over all mortality. Ironically, these were the very same diseases that they were supposed to cure or prevent. Further, due the prevalent use of the antioxidant vitamins by the general population and especially in those diagnosed with cancer, **this has become a global public healthcare issue.**

Americans are unshakeably mesmerized by the alleged health benefits of nutritional supplements, especially the antioxidant vitamins A, C and E (Blendon et al, 2001).

In fact, **a third of all adults, and half of those older than 55 years of age, reportly take at least 1 supplement daily** (Millen et al, 2004). It seems to be a quick fix but as we all know, **there are no safe quick fixes**.

Let's Get More Specific

Everywhere we turn, someone is hawking the supposed benefits of antioxidants. Rack after rack of supplements flank the aisles of nutrition stores, pharmacies, grocery stores, supermarkets, sporting good stores, discount stores and now, pet stores, feed stores and on and on. Even though studies continually show their lack of effectiveness, the money just keeps rolling in. People seem to feel that they can neglect their health and make up for it by just popping a few pills....magic pills....magical antioxidants.

Even though they are proving to be harmful, many physicians prescribe and use these antioxidant vitamins themselves on a daily basis. Both beta carotene and vitamin E were thought to be free of toxicity but that view is changing rapidly as studies indicate that they can increase mortality rates and risk of common diseases. Tens of millions of Americans and world wide citizens may be hastening their demise, when they do not have to. Yet, many people state that they would continue to take these agents even though scientific evidence points out their harmful potential

(Blendon et al, 2001). That fact alone illustrates the power of unrestrained advertising.

Actually, it appears that the antioxidant vitamins are more popular than ever, even in light of the poorly publicized studies showing their ineffectiveness. And, there are loads of critics of the scientific studies showing the lack of benefits of antioxidants and their harmful potential. They will ferociously defend their territory. They just can not bring themselves to believe the negative data and to toss out the flawed free radical theory from their thinking. Every time a study fails, they state that the results are "disappointing." If antioxidant vitamin users are increasing their risk of disease and an early death, these results are more than disappointing, they are disasterous and an abomination.

As E. Robert Greenberg said in 2005, in referring to many of the included antioxidant vitamin studies, "These research projects have all passed a rigorous peer review, and I do not question the scientific merit of any one of them. But isn't it past the time for the scientific and public health communities to loosen their ties to a theory (i.e., the free radical theory) that lacks predictive ability for human disease?" (Greenberg, 2005).

Deep interest in the relationship that specific foods, supplements, vitamins, antioxidants, or lifestyle factors have to our overall health has resulted in scientific research on the validity of widely publicized claims in disease prevention and cure. No single study provides the last word on any subject and one news report may dramatically overemphasize what appears to be a contradictory or conflicting result, when taken out of proper context. The scientific gold standard, randomized controlled trials (RCTs), are replacing testimonials, observational, epidemiologic or biased reports as being the most reliable source of valid information regarding the effectiveness of antioxidant vitamins A, C and E. Yet, even RCTs can arrive at erroneous conclusions and serve as the center of heated debate.

The Best Advice: Take them only if you have a vitamin deficiency

The best advice about antioxidant vitamins is to take them only if you have a proven vitamin deficiency. Otherwise, the second best advice about antioxidant vitamins is that it is rarely, if ever, advisable to obtain them from synthetic sources, as opposed to a balanced, nutritious diet of fresh fruits and vegetables. Unless one has a known vitamin deficiency, antioxidant vitamin supplements appear to be unnecessary, costly and potentially dangerous.

The overuse of many readily available antioxidant vitamin supplements appears to be a serious breach of human rights, as many of them are only sold to "protect and promote health." They make no claims about "curing" anything. Antioxidant vitamin supplements should be taken with considerable thought and subject to drug regulations and follow-up. People can not continue to ignore antioxidant vitamin supplement warnings. The data has stacked up against them. People, open your eyes and your minds to the preponderance of the data.

Experts are now recommending that, "**Vitamins A, E, D, folic acid, and niacin should be categorized as over-the-counter medications..... Vitamin A should be excluded from multivitamin supplements and food fortificants.**" Further, they state that, "Vitamins have documented adverse effects and toxicities, and most have documented interactions with drugs. Vitamins, such as **fat-soluble vitamins (A, E, D), can cause serious adverse events** (Rogovik, Vohra and Goldman, 2010).

Clinical trials have basically failed to demonstrate a beneficial effect of antioxidant supplements on cancer and cardiovascular disease (CVD) morbidity and mortality. With regard to the meta-analysis, the lack of efficacy has been demonstrated consistently for different doses of various antioxidants in diverse population groups. Still, free radical theory sycophants try to hold their increasingly shaky ground and continue to "peddle for profit" their questionable products.

Over and over, the antioxidant vitamins have produced negative results and over and over, they have been and are being ignored or denied. It is my hope that this selective review will force readers to face the fact that the data showing a lack of effect or a harmful effect is substantial and can no longer be disregarded or passed over. We should also scrutinize the use of multivitamins, since many of these contain antioxidants.

In fact, no consistent data suggests that consuming micronutrients at levels exceeding those provided by a dietary pattern consistent with AHA Dietary Guidelines will confer additional benefits with regard to cancer or CVD risk reduction.

More recently acquired scientific data, i.e., over the last 25-30 years, provides the true picture of the **relative ineffectiveness or null effect of antioxidant vitamin supplementation, their lack of predictive validity and of their untoward effects**. Do not be misled by exaggerations, statistically generated "benefits," half truths or outright lies, regarding these antioxidant vitamin supplements.

On advertising, the 1930s performer, **Will Rogers, famously referred to it as "the art of convincing people to spend money they don't have for something they don't need."**

This current book is primarily a selective systematic overview of **181** interventional initial or follow up studies/reports, published peer reviewed papers and the analysis thereof, showing either marginal effects, negligible effects, no effects or harmful effects of the antioxidant vitamins A (beta carotene), C (ascorbic acid) or E (alpha tocopherol) or combinations thereof. The total number of participants for all of the above studies is well over

8,000,000 subjects or participants, some of which may have been repeats in follow up or parallel studies.

> **You are being radically misled
> by antioxidant vitamin fraudsters.
> Someone is trying to radically mislead you
> concerning antioxidant vitamins and
> antioxidant supplements,
> such that you will make
> "a radical mistake."
> R.M. Howes M.D., Ph.D.
> 3/22/06**

However, I feel that it is not enough to just expose the nullification of the free radical theory and the ineffectiveness and dangers of antioxidant vitamins. I must also offer an improved alternative and I have done so with my UTOPIA (Unified theory of oxygen participation in aerobiosis) (Howes, 2004) theory and my ROSI syndrome (Reactive oxygen species insufficiency) (Howes, 2009) theory for disease allowance and coexistence.

Given the enormous amount of data available on antioxidant vitamin supplementation topic, this overview is not intended to be exhaustive and is selective by design. Yet, it tells an epic story of decades of failed studies, involving millions of participants, and the nullification of the free radical theory.

Even if antioxidant vitamin supplementation is commonly practiced and is increasingly promoted in Western and European countries, supporting evidence is still lacking and equivocal. Data demonstrating predictability is still needed, as are better ways to evaluate any potential benefit from antioxidant vitamin supplementation: 1) an improved understanding of redox mechanisms possibly at the basis of disease causation and the aging process, 2) the determination and establishment of reliable markers of oxidative and reductive damage and overall antioxidant status, 3) the identification of a targeted therapeutic window in which antioxidant vitamin supplementation may be beneficial, 4) a deeper knowledge of prooxidant and antioxidant molecules, which are flip sides of the same redox coin, and 5) an awareness that antioxidants may indiscriminately alter crucial biochemical pathways utilizing EMOD signaling.

Currently, I do not recommend the use of antioxidant vitamins, unless there is a proven vitamin deficiency. **Such caution should be seen as the standard, safe approach for any unproven agent (drug, medicine or therapy) that may be harmful.**

Despite increasing knowledge about the harmful effects of antioxidant vitamins on humans, little has been proven to justify their widespread use.

CHAPTER TWO:

The Facts….Just The Facts

HERE IS WHAT THE STUDIES SHOW: DEAL WITH IT

The following harmful adverse effects are taken directly from the scientific literature and are the results of scientific studies. They are not merely unsupported opinions. These conclusions are distilled from the 181 reviewed studies and the 60 studies indicating an increased risk of adverse side effects of the antioxidant vitamins.

Antioxidant vitamins can lead to increased risk of:
- **lung cancer;**
- **breast cancer;**
- **prostate cancer;**
- **head and neck cancer;**
- **oral pre-malignant lesions;**
- **total mortality;**
- **likelihood of dying by about 5 percent;**
- **esophageal cancer deaths;**

- adenoma recurrence in smokers and drinkers;
- post-trial risk of first-ever non-fatal Myocardial Infarction;
- hemorrhagic stroke deaths;
- increased total and stroke mortality;
- ischemic heart disease deaths;
- deaths from fatal coronary heart disease;
- cardiovascular disease mortality in postmenopausal women with diabetes;
- total fracture;
- hip fracture;
- osteoporotic hip fractures in men and women;
- accelerate the progression of retinitis pigmentosa;
- hospitalization for heart failure;
- heart failure incidence;
- Mother-to-child transmission of HIV;
- rate of low-birth-weight babies;
- rate for gestational hypertension;
- suffered falling more often;
- E supplementation increased tuberculosis and pneumonia risk;
- higher risk of age-related cataract among women;
- vitamin E results in loss of quality-adjusted life years;
- increase in the incidence of cancer among smokers and increased cancer mortality;
- Multivitamin/Minerals associated with doubling in the risk of fatal prostate cancer;
- increase in intima-media thickness over time;
- rate of local recurrence of the head and neck tumor tended to be higher;
- higher rate of second primary head and neck cancers;

- worsening of coronary atherosclerosis in those with two copies of the haptoglobin 2   gene;

- promote the clogging of arteries;

- accelerated thickening of the walls;

- higher mortality rate in men;

- adverse mucocutaneous effects and serum triglyceride elevations;

- cardiac arrhythmias (probucol);

- negated the benefit of cholesterol lowering drugs;

- negatively associated with skeletal health;

- decreased sperm motility;

- induced sperm DNA damage

HERE ARE THE MAJOR MEDICAL AND SCIENTIFIC ORGANIZATIONS (that you were not aware of) WHICH DO NOT RECOMMEND THE USE OF ANTIOXIDANT VITAMINS

The following either do not recommend antioxidant vitamins or have found inconclusive evidence of their benefit:
- The U.S. Food and Drug Administration (FDA)
- The American Heart Association (AHA)
- The American Cancer Society
- The National Cancer Institute (NCI)
- Institute of Medicine of the National Academies
- The American College of Cardiology
- The American College of Chest Physicians (ACCP)
- The American Diabetes Association
- The American Academy of Family Physicians
- Scientific Statement From the American Heart Association and the American Diabetes Association
- The American College of Cardiology/American Heart Association Task Force on Practice Guidelines
- United States Preventive Services Task Force (USPSTF)

- The American Cancer Society Guidelines on Nutrition and Physical Activity for Cancer Prevention
- The Nutrition Committee of the American Heart Association Council on Nutrition, Physical Activity, and Metabolism
- The AHA Scientific Position of the American Heart Association
- The Canadian Task Force on Preventive Health Care (CTFPHC)
- Food and Nutrition Board, Institute of Medicine
- The Food and Nutrition Board of the National Academy of Sciences
- National Academy of Sciences
- The 2006 AHA Diet and Lifestyle Recommendations
- The Medical Letter
- The Oregon Health and Science University
- Food Standards Agency/ the British Nutrition Foundation (BNF)
- Quackwatch
- American College of Cardiology Foundation Task Force on Clinical Expert Consensus Documents
- National Institutes of Health State-of-the-Science Conference
- The American Heart Association Atherosclerosis, Hypertension, and Obesity in Youth Committee, Council of Cardiovascular Disease in the Young, With the Council on Cardiovascular Nursing
- The Physicians Health Study
- The 2008 VITAmins and Lifestyle (VITAL) study
- The Physicians' Health Study II Randomized Controlled Trial
- The Swedish Council of Technology Assessment
- National Heart Foundation of Australia's Nutrition and Metabolism Advisory Committee

This list is a shocking list.

These 32 conclusions or recommendations are apparently some of the best kept secrets in America, since antioxidants are being fortified or added to a wide spectrum of commercial products including foods,

cosmetics, dermatologics, pet products, beverages, energy drinks, energy bars, fruits drinks, fruit juices, chewing gum, shampoos, etc.

Conclusions: Until the effects of antioxidant vitamins are proven in clinical trials, that directly test their impact on major disease end points, tens of millions of Americans may be wasting their money or putting themselves at unnecessary risk. In patients who do not have a vitamin deficiency, consistent beneficial effects of the antioxidant vitamins have not been demonstrated in well designed (randomized, placebo-controlled) clinical trials and their widespread use to the general public is not recommended to prevent disease or to prolong the life span. More caution must be exercised before antioxidants are recommended to ill patients, especially those with immunosuppression, cancer, stroke, bleeding disorders, diabetes or heart disease (Howes, Am J Cos Surg. 2009).

Overall, a considerable number of major health organizations do not recommend the use of antioxidant vitamins and many have issued cautionary notes regarding their casual, injudicious or unnecessary use.

Although their conclusions are not iron clad**, many prestigious scientific organizations have concluded that, "taking antioxidant vitamins - such as vitamins A, C and E - serves no purpose, and in some cases could likely be harmful."**

But, in today's society it is the norm to be taking some sort of drug or pill, ranging from regular antioxidant vitamin supplements to the more dangerous (and potentially lethal) legally prescribed drugs. **So, is anybody listening?**

CHAPTER THREE:

An Epic Chronology Of Antioxidant Vitamin Studies

ANTIOXIDANT VITAMIN FAILURES

I have 181 reports, on over 8 million subjects, showing "disappointing" results with antioxidants in preventing or reversing disease. Thus, prudent questions are, "Why take them in the absence of a deficiency state?" "Why waste money for marginally effective or harmful pills?"

181 Antioxidant Intervention Trial & Analysis Studies:
Antioxidant Failures & Nullification of the Free Radical Theory
R.M. Howes M.D., Ph.D.

This is a selective systematic over view of 181 **interventional initial or follow up studies**, showing either marginal effect, negligible effects, no effects at all. Sixty of these studies/reports showed harmful effects of the antioxidant vitamins A (beta carotene), C (ascorbic acid) or E (alpha tocopherol) or combinations thereof. Total number of participants for all of the above studies is in excess of **8,600,000 subjects**, some of which may have been repeats in follow up or parallel studies. Studies with multivitamins, which contain the antioxidant vitamins, were also included.

The following list will be arranged as: Paper (study) number; Title of Study or Paper; Author reference; and Chronological Year; and Number of participants or trials in the respective study.

1. **Failure of High-dose Vitamin C (ascorbic acid) Therapy to Benefit Patients with Advanced Cancer. A Controlled Trial.** (Creagan et al, 1979) (#159 patients with advanced cancer)

2. **High-dose Vitamin C versus Placebo in the Treatment of Patients with Advanced Cancer Who Have had no Prior Chemotherapy.** (Moertel et al, 1985) (#100 patients with advanced colorectal cancer)

3. **Skin Cancer Prevention Study** (Greenberg et al, 1990) (#1,805 men and women with recent nonmelanoma skin cancer)

4. **Diet in the Epidemiology of Postmenopausal Breast Cancer in the New York State Cohort** (Graham et al, 1992) (#18,586 postmenopausal women)

5. **Women's Health Study (WHS)** (Buring and Hennekens, 1992); (#39,876 healthy women)

6. **Isotretinoin-Basal Cell Carcinoma Study Group** (Tangrea et al, 1992, 1993) (#981 patients with two or more previously treated basal cell carcinomas)

7. **Prospective Study of the Intake of Vitamins C, E, and A and the Risk of Breast Cancer** (Hunter et al, 1993) (#89,494 women)

8. **Serum micronutrients and the subsequent risk of cervical cancer in a population-based nested case-control study.** (Batieha, 1993) (#15,161 women)

9. **A randomized trial of vitamin A and vitamin E supplementation for retinitis pigmentosa.** (Berson, 1993) (#601 patients aged 18 through 49 years with retinitis pigmentosa)

10. **Alpha-tocopherol, Beta-Carotene Cancer Prevention Study (ATBC study)** (Heinonen et al, 1994) (#29,133 men)

11. **Polyp Prevention Study** (Greenberg et al, 1994) (#864)

12. **Effect of vitamin C supplementation on lipoprotein cholesterol, apolipoprotein, and triglyceride concentrations** (Jaques et al, 1995) (#139)

13. **The effect of high-dose ascorbate supplementation on plasma lipoprotein(a) levels in patients with premature coronary heart disease** (Bostom et al, 1995) (#44 patients with premature CHD)

14. **Cholesterol Lowering Atherosclerosis Study (CLAS) (1995)** (Hodis et al, 1995) (#156 men)

15. **Effects of Vitamin E on susceptibility of low-density lipoprotein and low-density lipoprotein subfractions to oxidation and on protein glycation in NIDDM.** (Reaven, 1995) (#21 men with NIDDM)

16. **Excretion of alpha-tocopherol into human seminal plasma after oral administration** (Moilanen and Hovatta, 1995) (#15 unselected male volunteers)

17. **The Beta-Carotene and Retinol Efficacy Trial (CARET)** (Omenn et al, 1996) (#14,254 heavy smokers and 4,060 asbestos workers) (total #18,314)

18. **Cambridge Heart Antioxidant Study (CHAOS)** (Stephens et al., 1996) (#2,002 patients with coronary atherosclerosis)

19. **Physicians' Health Study (PHSI)** (Hennekens et al, 1996) (#22,071 US Physicians and Malignant Neoplasms or CVD)

20. **Dietary Antioxidant Vitamins and Death from Coronary Heart Disease in Postmenopausal Women** (Kushi et al, 1996) (#34,486 postmenopausal women with no cardiovascular disease)

21. **Mortality associated with low plasma concentration of beta carotene and the effect of oral supplementation** (Greenberg et al, 1996) (#1,720 men and women)

22. **The effect of antioxidant treatment on human spermatozoa and fertilization rate in an in vitro fertilization program** (Geva et al, 1996) (#Fifteen fertile normospermic male)

23. **Antioxidant Vitamin Effect on Traditional CVD Risk Factors** (Miller et al, 1997) (#297 retired teachers)

24. **ATBC Sub-Study Shows Increased CVD Deaths** (Rapola et al, 1997) (#1,862 men, with prior myocardial infarction)

25. **Effect of preoperative supplementation with alpha-tocopherol and ascorbic acid on myocardial injury in patients undergoing cardiac operations** (Westhuyzen et al, 1997) (#77 undergoing elective coronary artery bypass grafting)

26. **The influence of antioxidant nutrients on platelet function in healthy volunteers** (Calzada et al, 1997) (#40 healthy volunteers)

27. **The Multivitamins and Probucol Study** (Tardif et al, 1997) (#317 participants)

28. **Vitamin C intake and cardiovascular disease risk factors in persons with non-insulin-dependent diabetes mellitus** (Mayer-Davis et al, 1997) (#Insulin Resistance Atherosclerosis Study (IRAS, n = 520) **and from the San Luis Valley Diabetes Study (SLVDS, n = 422)** (total #942)

29. **Preformed Vitamin A Study Showed No Trend to Reduce Breast Cancer Risk.** (Longnecker, 1997) (#3,543 cases and 9,406 controls)

30. **Effect of Vitamin E and Beta Carotene on the Incidence of Primary Nonfatal Myocardial Infarction and Fatal Coronary Heart Disease** (Virtamo et al, 1998) (#27,271 Finnish male smokers)

31. **SU.VI.MAX** (Vasquez et al., 1998) (#13,017 French adults)

32. **A Sub-Study of SU.VI.MAX** (#1,162 subjects aged older than 50 years)

33. **The Nurses' Health Study and Folic Acid and Colon Cancer** (Giovannucci, 1998) (#88,756 women taking vitamin C and B-carotene, for 8 years)

34. **Effect of B-group vitamins and antioxidant vitamins on hyperhomocysteinemia** (Woodside, et al. 1998) (#101 men)

35. **Relationships of serum carotenoids, retinol, alpha-tocopherol, and selenium with breast cancer risk: results from a prospective study in Columbia, Missouri (United States).** (Dorgan, 1998) (#105 cases of histologically confirmed breast cancer)

36. **Incidence of cataract operations in Finnish male smokers unaffected by alpha tocopherol or beta carotene supplements.** (Teikari, 1998) (#28,934 male smokers)

37. **Effects of alpha-tocopherol and beta-carotene supplements on symptoms, progression, and prognosis of angina pectoris.** (Rapola et al, 1998) (#1,795 male smokers aged 50–69 years who had angina pectoris)

38. **The effects of antioxidant supplementation during Percoll preparation on human sperm DNA integrity** (Hughes et al, 1998) (#150 patients)

39. **GISSI-Prevention Trial** (GISSI-Prevenzione Investigators;1999) (#11,324 patients with recent MI)

40. **Women's Health Study** (Lee et al., 1999) (#39,876 healthy women); 50 mg Beta-carotene (alternate days)

41. **The Health Professionals Follow-Up Study** (Ascherio et al. 1999) (#43,738 men)

42. **Familial hypercholesterolemia, intima-to-media thickness (FH IMT study)** (Raal et al, 1999) (#15 with homozygous familial hypercholesterolemia)

43. **Beta carotene supplementation in prevention of basal-cell and squamous-cell carcinomas of the skin** (Green et al, 1999) (#1,383 participants)

44. **Vitamins A, C and E and the risk of breast cancer: results from a case-control study in Greece,** (Bohlke, 1999) (#830 patients with breast cancer plus 1,548 controls)

45. **Dietary antioxidants and risk of myocardial infarction in the elderly: the Rotterdam Study.** (Klipstein-Grobusch et al, 1999) (#4,802 participants of the Rotterdam Study aged 55–95 y who were free of MI)

46. **A prospective study of vitamin supplement intake and cataract extraction among US women.** (Chasan-Taber et al, 1999) (#47,152 female nurses)

47. **Antioxidant treatment of patients with asthenozoospermia or moderate oligoasthenozoospermia with high-dose vitamin C and vitamin E: a randomized, placebo-controlled, double-blind study** (Rolf et al, 1999) (#31 without genital infection but with asthenozoospermia)

48. **Antioxidant supplementation in vitro does not improve human sperm motility** (Donnelly et al, Fertil Steril. 1999) (#60 patients)

49. **The effect of ascorbate and alpha-tocopherol supplementation in vitro on DNA integrity and hydrogen peroxide-induced DNA damage in human spermatozoa** (Donnelly et al, Mutagenesis. 1999) (#Semen samples with normozoospermic and asthenozoospermic profiles (n = 15 for each control and antioxidant group)

50. **Heart Outcome Prevention Evaluation Study (HOPE)** (Yusuf et al, 2000) (#9,541 patients at high risk for cardiovascular events or diabetes)

51. **Meta-Analysis of Vitamin E in CVD, Ischemic Heart Disease (IHD) and Mortality** (Dagenais et al. 2000) (#51,000 participants)

52. **Vitamin C and the risk of acute myocardial infarction.** (Riemersma et al, 2000) (#180 males with a first AMI and 177 healthy volunteers)

53. **The effects of combined conventional treatment, oral antioxidants and essential fatty acids on sperm biology in subfertile men** (Comhaire et al, 2000) (#27 infertile men)

54. **Dietary antioxidant vitamins, retinol, and breast cancer incidence in a cohort of Swedish women.** (Michels, 2001) (#59,036 women free of cancer)

55. **The secondary prevention HDL Atherosclerosis Treatment study (HATS)** (Brown et al., 2001) (#160 patients with coronary disease)

56. **The Perth Carotid Ultrasound Disease Assessment Study (CUDAS)** (McQuillan et al 2001) (#1,111 subjects)

57. **Randomized Trial of Supplemental ß-Carotene to Prevent Second Head and Neck Cancer** (Mayne et al, 2001) (#264 patients who had been curatively treated for a recent early-stage squamous cell carcinoma of the oral cavity, pharynx, or larynx.)

58. **Age-Related Eye Disease Study Research Group (AREDS)** (AREDS, 2001) (#4,757 participants)

59. **HDL Atherosclerosis Treatment study (HATS)** (Brown et al, 2001) (#160 participants)

60. **Vitamin C and Vitamin E Supplement Use and Colorectal Cancer Mortality in a Large American Cancer Society cohort. (Cancr Prevention Study II cohort - CPS-II)** (Jacobs, 2001) (#711,891 men and women in U.S.A.)

61. **Risk of Ovarian Carcinoma and Consumption of Vitamins A, C and E and Specific Carotenoids: a prospective analysis.** (Fairfield, 2001) (#80,326 women)

62. **Carotenoids, Alpha-tocopherols, and Retinol in Plasma and Breast Cancer Risk in Northern Sweden.** (Hulten, 2001) (#201 cases and 290 referents)

63. **The Vitamin E Atherosclerosis Prevention Study (VEAPS)** (Hodis et al, 2002) (#353 were randomized (176 placebo, 177 vitamin E)

64. **MRC/BHF** (MRC/BHF, 2002) (#20,536); (600 mg vitamin E, 250 mg vitamin C and 20 mg beta-carotene daily)

65. **Antioxidant Vitamins and US Physician CVD Mortality** (Muntwyler et al. 2002) (#83,639 male U.S.A. physicians)

66. **Women's Angiographic Vitamin and Estrogen (WAVE) Trial** (Waters et al, 2002) (#423 postmenopausal women, with at least one 15% to 75% coronary stenosis)

67. **Mega-dose vitamins and minerals in the treatment of non-metastatic breast cancer: an historical cohort study** (Lesperance et al, 2002) (#90 patients with non-metastatic breast cancer who received conventional treatment)

68. **The Roche European American Cataract Trial (REACT)** (Chylack et al. 2002) (#445 patients)

69. **Vitamin E supplementation and macular degeneration** (Taylor et al, 2002) (#1,193 subjects)

70. **Vitamin E on Cardiovascular and Microvascular Outcomes in High-Risk Patients With Diabetes. Results of the HOPE Study and MICRO-HOPE Substudy** (Lonn et al. 2002) (#3,654 with diabetes)

71. **Vitamin C and Vitamin E Supplement Use and Bladder Cancer Mortality in a Large Cohort of US Men and Women (**Cancer Prevention Study II (CPS-II) (Jacobs et al., 2002) (#991,522 US adults in the Cancer Prevention Study II (CPS-II) cohort.)

72. **Supplemental Vitamin C & E and Multivitamin use and Stomach cancer Mortality in U.S.A.** (Jacobs et al. Jan. 2002) (#1,045,923)

73. **Vitamin E and C Supplements and Risk of Dementia** (Laurin et al, 2002) (#3,734 Japanese men)

74. **Retinol intake and bone mineral density in the elderly: the Rancho Bernardo Study.** (Promislow et al, 2002) (#570 women and 388 men)

75. **Vitamin A intake and hip fractures among postmenopausal women.** (Feskanich et al, 2002) (#72,337 postmenopausal women)

76. **A prospective study on supplemental vitamin E intake and risk of colon cancer in women and men.** (Wu et al, 2002) (#87,998 females from the Nurses' Health Study and 47, 344 males from the Health Professionals Follow-up Study) (#135,332 total participants)

77. **The Collaborative Primary Prevention Project (PPP)** (Chiabrando et al., 2002) (#144 participants with CHD risk factors)

78. **Vitamins E & A fail to reduce incidence or mortality of lung cancer: Cochrane Database Syst Rev. 2003.** (Caraballoso et al., 2003) (#109,394 participants)

79. **Use of antioxidant vitamins for the prevention of cardiovascular disease: meta-analysis of randomized trials**. (Vivekananthan et al., 2003) (The vitamin E trials involved a total of #81,788 patients, and the beta-carotene trials involved #138,113)

80. **Antioxidant Vitamins Effect on Alzheimer's Disease: Washington Heights-Inwood Columbia Aging Project** (Luchsinger et al, 2003) (#980 elderly subjects)

81. **Neoplastic and Antineoplastic Effects of Beta Carotene on Colorectal Adenoma Recurrence: Results of a Randomized Trial** (Baron et al, 2003) (#864 subjects who had had an adenoma removed and were polyp-free)

82. **Routine Vitamin Supplementation To Prevent Cardiovascular Disease: A Summary of the Evidence for the U.S. Preventive Services Task Force** (Morris and Carson, 2003)

83. **Midlife Dietary Intake of Antioxidants and Risk of Late-Life Incident Dementia: The Honolulu-Asia Aging Study** (Laurin et al, 2003) (#2,459 men)

84. **Serum retinol levels and the risk of fracture.** (Michealsson, 2003) (#2,322 men)

85. **Impact of simvastatin, niacin, and/or antioxidants on cholesterol metabolism in CAD patients with low HDL.** (Matthan et al, 2003) (#123 HATS participants)

86. **A randomized trial of beta carotene and age-related cataract in US physicians.** (Christen et al, 2003) (#22,071 Male US physicians aged 40 to 84 years)

87. **Supplemental vitamin C increase cardiovascular disease risk in women with diabetes** (Lee et al, 2004) (#1,923 postmenopausal women who reported being diabetic)

88. **Cochrane Database Syst Rev. 2004: Vitamins E & A fail to reduce incidence or mortality of gastrointestinal cancer.** (Cochrane Database Syst Rev. G. Bjelakovic et al, 2004) (#170,525 participants)

89. **ATBC 6-year follow-up study (2004)** (Thornwall et al., 2004) (#29,133 male smokers)

90. **HOPE study of vitamin E on renal insufficiency (2004)** (Mann et al, 2004) (#993 people with a serum creatinine > or =1.4 to 2.3 mg/dL. And renal insufficiency)

91. **Randomized trials of vitamin E in the treatment and prevention of cardiovascular disease (2004)** (Eidelman et al., 2004) (7 large-scale randomized trials)

92. **Effect of supplemental vitamin E for the prevention and treatment of cardiovascular disease** (Shekelle et al, 2004) (#Eighty-four eligible trials)

93. **SU.VI.MAX Study (2004)** (Hercberg et al, 2004) (#A total of 13,017 French adults)

94. **Meta-analysis: high-dosage vitamin E supplementation may increase all-cause mortality** (Miller et al., 2004) (#135,967 subjects)

95. **The role of vitamin E in the prevention of coronary events and stroke. Meta-analysis of randomized controlled trials** (Alkhenizan and Al-Omran, 2004) (#80,645 subjects)

96. **Oats, Antioxidants and Endothelial Function in Overweight, Dyslipidemic Adults** (Katz et al, 2004) (#30) (16 males page 35; 14 postmenopausal females)

97. **Vitamin C Worsens Coronary Atherosclerosis in Those with Two Copies of the Haptoglobin 2 Gene.** (Levy, 2004) (#299 postmenopausal women)

98. **Vitamin C for preventing and treating the common cold. Cochrane Database Syst Rev. 2004;(4):CD000980.** (Douglas, 2004) (#11,350 study participants)

99. **Vitamin E supplementation and cataract: randomized controlled trial.** (McNeil, 2004) (#1,193 eligible subjects with early or no cataract)

100.**Antioxidant vitamins and coronary heart disease risk: a pooled analysis of 9 cohorts.** (Knekt et al, 2004) (#293,172 subjects free of CHD at baseline)

101. **A review of the epidemiological evidence for the 'antioxidant hypothesis' by the British Nutrition Foundation (the Food Standards Agency).** (Stanner et al, 2004) (British Nutrition Foundation independent review)

102.**Impact of antioxidants, zinc, and copper on cognition in the elderly: a randomized, controlled trial.** (Yaffe et al, 2004) (#2,166 elderly persons)

103.**Use of multivitamins and prostate cancer mortality in a large cohort of US men.** (Stevens et al, 2005) (#475,726 men who were cancer-free)

104.**Vitamin A Supplementation for Reducing the Risk of Mother-to-child Transmission of HIV Infection.** (Wiysonge et al, 2005) (#3,033 females)

105.**The Alzheimer's Disease Cooperative Study (ADCS) Group** (Petersen et al, 2005) (#769 subjects)

106.**Vitamin E Supplementation in Alzheimer's Disease, Parkinson's Disease, Tardive Dyskinesia, and Cataract: Part 2** (Pham et al, 2005)

107. **Dementia and Alzheimer's Disease in Community-Dwelling Elders Taking Vitamin C and/or Vitamin E:** (Fillenbaum et al, 2005) (#626 elderly)

108.**HOPE-TOO Extension** (Lonn et al, 2005) (#3,994 original study enrollees)

109.**Women's Health Study (WHS)** (Lee et al, 2005) (#39,876 apparently healthy US women)

110.**A randomized trial of antioxidant vitamins to prevent second primary cancers in head and neck cancer patients** (Bairati et al, 2005 Apr 6) (#540 patients with stage I or II head and neck cancer treated by radiation therapy)

111.**Randomized trial of antioxidant vitamins to prevent acute adverse effects of radiation therapy in head and neck cancer**

patients (Bairati et al, 2005 Aug 20) (#540 patients with stage I or II head and neck cancer treated by radiation therapy)

112. **Effect of intensive lipid lowering, with or without antioxidant vitamins, compared with moderate lipid lowering on myocardial ischemia** (Stone et al, 2005) (#300 patients with stable coronary disease)

113. **Vitamin C and vitamin E for Alzheimer's disease.** (Boothby and Doering, 2005)

114. **Vitamin-mineral supplementation and the progression of atherosclerosis** (Bleys et al, 2006) (searched the MEDLINE, EMBASE, and CENTRAL databases)

115. **Multivitamin/mineral supplements and prevention of chronic disease.** (Huang et al, 2006 May)

116. **The Efficacy and Safety of Multivitamin and Mineral Supplement Use To Prevent Cancer and Chronic Disease in Adults: A Systematic Review for a National Institutes of Health State-of-the-Science Conference.** (Huang et al, 2006 Sept)

117. **Antioxidants Vitamin C and Vitamin E for the Prevention and Treatment of Cancer** (Coulter et al, 2006) (Thirty-eight studies; participant # not available)

118. **Vitamin C levels in Type 2 diabetes and low vitamin C levels does not improve endothelial dysfunction or insulin resistance** (Chen et al, 2006) (#32 type 2 diabetics)

119. **Meta-analysis: antioxidant supplements for primary and secondary prevention of colorectal adenoma (2006)** (Bjelakovic et al., 2006) (#17,620 participants)

120. **Australian Collaborative Trial of Supplements (ACTS)** (Rumbold et al, 2006) (#1,877 subjects)

121. **The Antioxidants in Prevention of Cataracts Study (APC Study): effects of antioxidant supplements on cataract progression in South India.** (Gritz, 2006) (#798)

122. **Vitamins in Pre-eclampsia (VIP) Trial Consortium** (Poston et al., 2006) (#2,410 women at increased risk for preeclampsia, analyzed 2,395)

123. **SU.VI.MAX (2006) Antioxidants do not affect fasting blood glucose** (Czernichow et al, 2006) (#3,146 subjects)

124. **Vitamin E and Risk of Type 2 Diabetes in the Women's Health Study** (Liu et al., 2006) (#38,716 apparently healthy U.S. women)

125. **Vitamin E supplementation and cognitive function in women: The Women's Health Study (2006)** (Kang et al., 2006) (#39,876 healthy US women)

126. **Supplemental and dietary vitamin E, beta-carotene, and vitamin C intakes and prostate cancer risk (PLCO Trial)** (Kirsh et al, 2006) (#29,361 men during up to 8 years of follow-up)

127. **Intakes of Vitamins A, C and E and Folate and Multivitamins and Lung Cancer: a pooled analysis of 8 prospective studies.** (Cho et al, 2006) (#430,281 persons over a maximum of 6-16 years in the studies)

128. **The Melbourne Atherosclerosis Vitamin E Trial (MAVET):a study of high dose vitamin E in smokers.** (Magliano et al, 2006) (#409 male and female smokers)

129. **Mortality in Randomized Trials of Antioxidant Supplements for Primary and Secondary Prevention; Systematic Review and Meta-analysis** (Bjelakovic et al, 2007) (# 232,606 participants)

130. **Multivitamin Use and Risk of Prostate Cancer in the National Institutes of Health–AARP Diet and Health Study** (Lawson et al, 2007) (#295,344 men)

131. **A Randomized Factorial Trial of Vitamins C and E and Beta Carotene in the Secondary Prevention of Cardiovascular Events in Women: Results From the Women's Antioxidant Cardiovascular Study** (Cook et al. 2007) (#8,171 female health professionals at increased risk)

132. **Use of Supplements of Multivitamins, Vitamin C, and Vitamin E in Relation to Mortality** (Pocobelli et al, 2007) (#77,719 subjects aged 50–76 years)

133. **Health Professionals Follow-up Study (2007): Effect of vitamins C, E, A and carotenoids and the occurrence of**

oral pre-malignant lesions (Maserejian et al, 2007) (#42,340 men enrolled in the Health Professionals Follow-up Study) (#207 found with oral premalignant lesions)

134. **Antioxidant meta-analysis for the treatment of macular degeneration (2007)** (Chong et al, 2007) (#149,203 subjects)

135. **Effect of *RRR*-α-tocopherol supplementation on carotid atherosclerosis in patients with stable coronary artery disease (CAD)** (Devaraj et al, 2007) (#90 patients with CAD)

136. **Overview of the Women's Antioxidant Cardiovascular Study (WACS) (2007)** (Zaharris et al, 2007) (#8,171 women)

137. **Serum α-tocopherol, concurrent and past vitamin E intake, and mild cognitive impairment** (Dunn et al, 2007) (#526 subjects)

138. **The role of vitamin E in the prevention of cancer: a meta-analysis of randomized controlled trials.** (Alkhenizan and Hafez, 2007) (#167,025 subjects)

139. **Chemoprevention of Primary Liver Cancer: A Randomized, Double-Blind Trial in Linxian, China.** (Qu et al, 2007) (29,450 subjects)

140. **Risk of Mortality with Vitamin E Supplements: The Cache County Study.** (Hayden et al, 2007)

141. **Multivitamin-multimineral supplements and eye disease: age-related macular degeneration and cataract.** (Seddon, 2007) The Dietary Ancillary Study of the Eye Disease Case-Control Study (EDCCS)

142. **Antioxidant Supplementation Increases the Risk of Skin Cancers in Women but Not in Men.** (Hercberg et al, 2007) (#French adults, 7,876 women and 5,141 men. Total # = 13,017)

143. **Antioxidant Vitamin Supplement Use and Risk of Dementia or Alzheimer's Disease in Older Adults** (Gray et al, 2007) (#2,969)

144. **Antioxidant supplements for prevention of mortality in healthy participants and patients with various diseases.** (Bjelakovic, Nikolova, Gludd, Simonetti and Gludd, 2008 Apr) (#232,550 Cochrane Database Syst Rev.)

145. **Systematic review: primary and secondary prevention of gastrointestinal cancers with antioxidant supplements.** (Bjelakovic, Nikolova, Simonette and Gludd, 2008 Sept) (#211,818 participants)

146. **Vitamins E and C in the prevention of cardiovascular disease in men: the Physicians' Health Study II randomized controlled trial** (Sesso et al, 2008) (#14,641 US male physicians)

147. **Both {alpha}- and beta-Carotene, but Not Tocopherols and Vitamin C, Are Inversely Related to 15-Year Cardiovascular Mortality in Dutch Elderly Men** (Buijsse et al, 2008) (#559 men (mean age ~72 y) free of chronic diseases)

148. **Vitamin E and selenium supplementation and risk of prostate cancer in the Vitamins and lifestyle (VITAL) study cohort** (Peters et al, 2008) (#35,242 men)

149. **VITAL (VITamins And Lifestyle) study 2008** (Slatore et al, 2008) (#77,721 men and women)

150. **Vitamin E for Alzheimers and mild cognitive impairment. Cochrane Database Syst Rev. (2008)** (Isaac et al, 2008) (#769 participants)

151. **Efficacy of Antioxidant Supplementation in Reducing Primary Cancer Incidence and Mortality: Systematic Review and Meta-analysis** (Bardia et al, 2008) (#104,196 participants)

152. **Carotenoids and the risk of developing lung cancer: a systematic review.** (Gallicchio et al, 2008) (Six randomized clinical trials)

153. **Antioxidant enriched enteral nutrition and oxidative stress after major gastrointestinal tract surgery.** (van Stijn et al, 2008) (#21 undergoing major upper gastrointestinal tract surgery)

154. **Vitamin E supplementation may transiently increase tuberculosis risk in males who smoke heavily and have high dietary vitamin C intake.** (Hemila and Kaprio, 2008 Oct) (#29,023 males aged 50-69 years, smoking at baseline, with no tuberculosis)

155. **Vitamin E supplementation and pneumonia risk in males who initiated smoking at an early age: effect modification by body weight and dietary vitamin C.** (Hemila and Kaprio, 2008 Nov) (#21,657 ATBC Study participants who initiated smoking by the age of 20 years)

156. **Oral administration of vitamin C decreases muscle mitochondrial biogenesis and hampers training-induced adaptations in endurance performance.** (Gomez-Cabrera et al, 2008) (#14)

157. **Antioxidant vitamin and mineral supplements for preventing age-related macular degeneration.** (Evans and Henshaw, 2008) (#23,099 participants)

158. **Dietary antioxidants and the long-term incidence of age-related macular degeneration: the Blue Mountains Eye Study.** (Tan et al, 2008) (#2,454 Australian population-based cohort study)

159. **Multivitamin-multimineral supplement use and mammographic breast density.** (Berube et al, 2008) (#Premenopausal (777) and postmenopausal (783) women, total 1,560)

160. **Antioxidant supplements to prevent or slow down the progression of AMD: a systematic review and meta-analysis.** (Evans, 2008) (#23,099 people were randomized in three trials)

161. **Is there a role for supplemented antioxidants in the prevention of atherosclerosis?** (Katsiki and Manes, 2009)

162. **Plasma Carotenoids, Retinol, and Tocopherols and Postmenopausal Breast Cancer Risk in theMultiethnic Cohort Study: a nested case-control study.** (Epplein, 2009) (#286 incident postmenopausal breast cancer cases were matched to 535 controls)

163. **Vitamins E and C in the prevention of prostate and total cancer in men: the Physicians' Health Study II randomized controlled trial (2009)** (Gaziano et al, 2009) (#14,641 male physicians)

164. **Vitamin E, vitamin C, beta carotene, and cognitive function among women with or at risk of cardiovascular disease: The Women's Antioxidant and Cardiovascular Study (2009)** (Kang et al, 2009) (#2,824 participants)

165. **Effects of vitamins C and E and beta-carotene on the risk of type 2 diabetes in women at high risk of cardiovascular disease: Women's Antioxidant Cardiovascular Study (2009)** (Song et al, 2009) (#8,171 female health professionals)

166. **Vitamins C and E and Beta Carotene Supplementation and Cancer Risk: Women's Antioxidant Cardiovascular Study (2009)** (Lin et al, 2009) (#7,627 female health professionals)

167. **Effect of selenium and vitamin E on risk of prostate cancer and other cancers: the Selenium and Vitamin E Cancer Prevention Trial (SELECT) (2009)** (Lippman, 2009) (#35,533 men)

168. **Multivitamin Use and Risk of Cancer and Cardiovascular Disease in the Women's Health Initiative Cohorts** (Neuhouser et al, 2009) (#161,808 participants)

169. **Effects of antioxidant supplements on cancer prevention: meta-analysis of randomized controlled trials** (Myung et al, 2009) (#161,045 total subjects)

170. **Decision Analysis Supports the Paradigm That Indiscriminate Supplementation of Vitamin E Does More Harm than Good** (Dotan et al, 2009) (over 300,000 participants)

171. **Effects of long-term antioxidant supplementation and association of serum antioxidant concentrations with risk of metabolic syndrome in adults (SU.VI.MAX)** (Czernichow et al, 2009) (#5,220 adults)

172. **Total and Cancer Mortality After Supplementation With Vitamins and Minerals: 10 year Follow-up of the Linxian**

General Population Nutrition Intervention Trial. (Qiao et al, 2009) (#29,584 adults)

173. **Vitamin A and retinol intakes and the risk of fractures among participants of the Women's Health Initiative Observational Study.** (Caire-Juvera_et al. 2009) (#75,747 women from the Women's Health Initiative Observational Study)

174. **Modification of the effect of vitamin E supplementation on the mortality of male smokers by age and dietary vitamin C.** (Hemila and Kaprio, 2009 Apr) (#29,023 males aged 50-69 years, smoking at baseline, with no tuberculosis)

175. **Vitamin E supplement use and the incidence of cardiovascular disease and all-cause mortality in the Framingham Heart Study: Does the underlying health status play a role?** (Dietrich et al, 2009) (#4,270 Framingham study participants)

176. **Antioxidants prevent health-promoting effects of physical exercise in humans.** (Ristow et al, 2009) (#39 healthy adults)

177. **Long-term use of beta-carotene, retinol, lycopene, and lutein supplements and lung cancer risk: results from the VITamins And Lifestyle (VITAL) study.** (Satia et al, 2009) (#77,126 (VITAL) cohort Study in Washington State)

178. **Vitamin C supplements and the risk of age-related cataract: a population-based prospective cohort study in women.** (Rautiainen et al, 2010) (#24,593 women)

179. **Micronutrient concentrations and subclinical atherosclerosis in adults with HIV.** (Falcone et al, 2010) (#298 Nutrition for Healthy Living participants)

180. **Multivitamin use and breast cancer incidence in a prospective cohort of Swedish women.** (Larsson et al, 2010) (#35,329 cancer-free women)

181. **Vitamins C and E to prevent complications of pregnancy-associated hypertension** (Roberts et al, 2010) (#10,154)

Total of 181 studies with over 8,600,000 participants

Sixty studies showing harmful effects

HERE ARE THE 60 STUDIES SHOWING HARMFUL
AFFECTS:BRACE YOURSELF

60 FAILED Antioxidant Vitamin
Studies/Reports (SYNOPSIS)

- Adverse mucocutaneous effects and serum triglyceride elevations (Tangrea et al, 1992, 1993)
- Increase the risk of breast cancer (Hunter et al, 1993)
- Supplementation with 400 IU/day of vitamin E has been found to accelerate the progression of retinitis pigmentosa that is not associated with vitamin E deficiency. (Berson,1993)
- Increase in hemorrhagic stroke deaths (Heinonen et al, 1994)
- Increase in ischemic heart disease deaths (Heinonen et al, 1994)
- Increase in lung cancer (Heinonen et al, 1994)
- 8% higher mortality rate in men (Albanes et al, 1996)
- 28% increase in lung cancer; 26% increase in CVD (nonsignificant); 17% increase in total mortality (Omenn et al, 1996)
- Significantly more deaths from fatal coronary heart disease (Rapola et al, 1997)
- Likelihood of cardiac arrhythmias (probucol) (Tardif et al, 1997)
- Vitamin E decreased platelet function (Calzada et al, 1997)
- Acetyl cysteine or ascorbate and alpha tocopherol together induced further DNA damage to human sperm (Hughes et al, 1998)
- Homozygous familial hypercholesterolemia, intima-to-media thickness (FH IMT study) increased with vitamin E supplements (400 mg/day) for 2 years (Raal et al, 1999)

- Progressive motility, average path velocity, curvilinear velocity, straight-line velocity, and linearity were decreased significantly, with the greatest inhibition observed with the highest concentrations of antioxidants. Sperm motility was significantly decreased by antioxidants vitamin C and alpha-tocopherol. (Donnelly et al, Fertil Steril. 1999)

- Both ascorbate and alpha-tocopherol in combination to sperm preparation medium actually induced DNA damage and intensified the damage induced by H_2O_2 (Donnelly et al, Mutagenesis. 1999)

- A possible increase in lung cancer risk (Mayne et al, 2001)

- Negated the benefit of cholesterol lowering drugs on plasma lipid profile and stenosis progression (Brown et al., 2001)

- Increasing retinol became negatively associated with skeletal health at intakes not far beyond the recommended daily allowance (RDA), intakes reached predominately by supplement users (Promislow, 2002)

- A borderline disease-promoting effect of alpha-TOH supplements (Hodis et al, 2002

- Significantly higher all-cause mortality rate and a trend for an increased cardiovascular mortality rate (vitamins E and C) (Waters et al, 2002)

- Breast cancer–specific survival (ie, patients censored only at death from breast cancer) and disease-free survival were shorter in the nutrient-supplemented group than in the non-supplemented group, but the differences were not statistically significant. (Lesperance et al, 2002)

- After controlling for confounding factors, women in the highest quintile of total vitamin A intake ($\geq$3000 µg/d of retinol equivalents [RE]) had a significantly elevated relative risk (RR) of hip fracture compared with women in the lowest quintile of intake. This increased risk was attributable primarily to retinol. Long-term intake of a diet high in retinol may promote the development of osteoporotic hip fractures in women. (Feskanich, 2002)

- **The risk of fracture was highest among men with the highest levels of serum retinol.** Multivariate analysis of the risk of fracture in the highest quintile for serum retinol as compared with the middle quintile showed that the rate ratio was 1.64 for any fracture and 2.47 for hip fracture. **The risk of fracture was further increased within the highest quintile for serum retinol.** Men with retinol levels in the 99th percentile had an overall risk of fracture that exceeded the risk among men with lower levels by a factor of seven. (Michealsson, 2003)

- Increased risk of lung cancer incidence and mortality (Caraballoso et al., 2003)

- Beta carotene led to small but statistically significant increase in all-cause mortality and a slight increase in cardiovascular death (Vivekananthan et al., 2003)

- Beta carotene doubled the risk of adenoma recurrence in smokers and drinkers (Baron et al, 2003)

- Promote the clogging of arteries; accelerated thickening of the walls (Lee et al, 2004)

- 2.3 times the risk of death from stroke and 2 times the risk of dying from coronary artery disease (vitamin C) (Lee et al, 2004)

- A statistically significant increase in mortality, which was particularly strong in patients taking beta carotene and vitamin A (Bjelakovic et al, 2004)

- ß-Carotene seemed to increase the post-trial risk of first-ever non-fatal MI (Thornwall et al., 2004)

- High doses of vitamin E increased mortality (Miller et al., 2004)

- Increased risk of cardiovascular disease mortality in postmenopausal women with diabetes (Lee et al, 2004)

- The relative benefit or harm of vitamin therapy on the progression of coronary artery stenoses in women in the WAVE study was dependent on haptoglobin type. Antioxidant therapy (1,000 mg/day of vitamin C + 800 IU/day of vitamin E) was associated with improvement of coronary atherosclerosis in diabetic women with two copies of the haptoglobin 1 gene but worsening of coronary atherosclerosis in those with two copies of the haptoglobin 2 gene. (Levy, 2004)

- The death rate from prostate cancer was marginally higher among men who took multivitamins regularly (> or =15 times/month) compared to non-users; risk was greatest during the initial four years of follow-up. CONCLUSIONS: Regular multivitamin use was associated with a small increase in prostate cancer death rates. (Stevens et al, 2005)

- Increased risk of heart failure incidence and risk of hospitalization for heart failure (vitamin E) (Lonn et al, 2005)

- Patients receiving alpha-tocopherol supplements had a higher rate of second primary head and neck cancers during the supplementation period; the rate of having a recurrence or second primary cancer was higher during supplementation with alpha-tocopherol (Bairati et al, 2005 Apr 6)

Note: Patients taking an antioxidant were 1.65 times more likely to suffer a return of their original cancer during the three years they were on the supplement. The risk was highest among those taking only vitamin E (1.86 times higher). Five years after they stopped taking the supplement, their recurrence risk had fallen to the same level as those in the placebo group. Although suggestive of harm, these results were not statistically significant.

- The rate of local recurrence of the head and neck tumor tended to be higher in the supplement trial arm (beta carotene and vitamin E) (Bairati et al, 2005 Aug 20)

Note: Researchers were concerned to find that the rate of local recurrence (that is, a return of the original cancer) was 54 percent higher among patients on the combination pill than those on placebo. There was a smaller but still worrisome increase among those on vitamin E only.

- While the trials conducted in South Africa and Malawi did not find evidence that the effect of Vitamin A supplementation was different from that of placebo, the trial in Tanzania found evidence that vitamin A supplementation increased the risk of Mother-to-child transmission of HIV compared with placebo and multivitamins (excluding vitamin A) (Wiysonge et al, 2005)

- Rate of low-birth-weight babies was higher and the rate for gestational hypertension was higher for women in the vitamin C & E group (Poston et al., 2006)

- Vitamin C & E increased risk of being hospitalized antenatally for hypertension and having to take antihypertensive medication (Poston et al., 2006)

- Vitamin C & E increase the rate of babies born with a low birth weight (Poston et al., 2006)

- The mean increase in intima-media thickness over time in the vitamin E group was 0.0041 mm/year faster than placebo in smokers. (Magliano et al, 2006)

- Supplements increase the likelihood of dying by about 5 percent. When looked at separately, they found that Vitamin A increased death risk by 16 per cent, beta carotene by 7 per cent and Vitamin E by 4 per cent (Bjelakovic et al, 2007)

- MVMs associated with a doubling in the risk of fatal prostate cancer (Lawson et al, 2007)

- Increased risk of oral pre-malignant lesions with vitamin E & beta carotene (Maserejian et al, 2007)

- None of these conditions or treatments altered the null main effect with vitamin E, but mortality was increased in vitamin E users who had a history of stroke, coronary bypass graft surgery, or myocardial infarction and, independently, in those taking nitrates, warfarin, or diuretics. (Hayden et al, 2007)

- In women, the incidence of Skin Cancer was higher in the antioxidant group. The incidence of melanoma was also higher in the antioxidant group for women. (Hercberg et al, 2007)

- Antioxidant supplements significantly increased mortality in a fixed-effect model. In the trials with a low risk of bias, the antioxidant supplements significantly increased mortality by vitamin A, beta-carotene, and vitamin E. We found no evidence to support antioxidant supplements for primary or secondary prevention. Vitamin A, beta-carotene, and vitamin

E may increase mortality. Antioxidant supplements need to be considered medicinal products and should undergo sufficient evaluation before marketing. (Bjelakovic, Nikolova, Gludd, Simonetti and Gludd, 2008 Apr) (#232,550 Cochrane Database Syst Rev.)

- Antioxidant supplements had no significant effect on mortality in a random-effects model meta-analysis but significantly increased mortality in a fixed-effect model meta-analysis. CONCLUSIONS: There was no evidence that the studied antioxidant supplements prevented gastrointestinal cancers. On the contrary, they seem to increase overall mortality. (Bjelakovic, Nikolova, Simonette and Gludd, 2008)

- Vitamin E was associated with a small increased risk of lung cancer (Slatore et al, 2008)

- Participants taking Vitamin E suffered a fall more often (Isaac et al, 2008)

- Beta carotene supplementation was associated with an increase in the incidence of cancer among smokers and with a trend toward increased cancer mortality (Bardia et al, 2008)

- Among participants who obtained 90 mg/d or more of vitamin C in foods, vitamin E supplementation increased tuberculosis risk by 72%. This effect was restricted to participants who smoked heavily. Our finding that vitamin E seemed to transiently increase the risk of tuberculosis in those who smoked heavily and had high dietary vitamin C intake should increase caution towards vitamin E supplementation for improving the immune system. (Hemila and Kaprio, 2008 Oct)

- Vitamin E increased the risk of pneumonia in participants with body weight less than 60 kg, and in participants with body weight over 100 kg. The harm of vitamin E supplementation was restricted to participants with dietary vitamin C intake above the median. CONCLUSION: Vitamin E supplementation may cause harmful effects on health in certain groups of male smokers. (Hemila and Kaprio, 2008 Nov)

- The administration of vitamin C significantly (P=0.014) hampered endurance capacity. (Gomez-Cabrera et al, 2008)

- Beta-carotene intake from diet alone predicted neovascular AMD. Higher intakes of total vitamin E predicted late AMD. Higher beta-carotene intake was associated with an increased risk of AMD. (Tan et al, 2008)

- Premenopausal women who were currently using multivitamin-multimineral supplements had higher adjusted mean breast density (45.5%) than past (42.9%) or never (40.2%) users. Regular use of multivitamin-multimineral supplements may be associated with higher mean breast density among premenopausal women. (Berube et al, 2008)

- Vitamin E results in loss of quality-adjusted life years (Dotan et al, 2009)

- Baseline serum zinc concentrations were positively associated with the risk of developing metabolic syndrome (MetS) (Czernichow, S. et al, 2009)

- Treatment with "factor D," a combination of 50 μg selenium, 30 mg vitamin E, and 15 mg beta-carotene, led to esophageal cancer deaths increasing to 14% among those aged 55 years or older. Vitamin A and zinc supplementation was associated with increased total and stroke mortality. (Qiao et al, 2009) (#29,584)

- Women with lower vitamin D intake and retinol had a modest increased risk of total fracture. (Caire-Juvera et al. 2009)

- Among participants with a dietary vitamin C intake above the median of 90 mg/day, vitamin E increased mortality among those aged 50-62 years by 19%. (Hemila and Kaprio, 2009)

- Exercise increased parameters of insulin sensitivity (GIR and plasma adiponectin) only in the absence of antioxidants in both previously untrained and pretrained individuals. (Ristow et al, 2009)

- Longer duration of use of individual beta-carotene, retinol, and lutein supplements (but not total 10-year average dose) was associated with statistically significantly elevated risk of total lung cancer and histologic cell types. Long-term use of individual beta-carotene, retinol, and lutein supplements should not be recommended for lung cancer prevention, particularly among smokers. (Satia et al, 2009)

- Among women aged ≥65 y, vitamin C supplement use increased the risk of cataract by 38%. Vitamin C use among hormone replacement therapy users compared with that among nonusers of supplements or of hormone replacement therapy was associated with a 56% increased risk of cataract. Our results indicate that the use of vitamin C supplements may be associated with higher risk of age-related cataract among women. (Rautiainen et al, 2010)

- Elevated serum vitamin E concentrations are associated with abnormal markers of atherosclerosis and may increase the risk of cardiovascular complications in HIV-infected adults. (Falcone et al, 2010)

- Multivitamin use was associated with a statistically significant increased risk of breast cancer. Use of multivitamins was linked to a statistically significant 19 per cent increased risk of breast cancer. (Larsson et al, 2010)

ANY QUESTIONS?

For all of you radicophobes and pill pushers, do not be upset with me. This is what the literature shows. I am merely the messenger. Actually, I am merely the work horse who put the studies together to help inform you.

If you deny these studies, you are a free radical theory zealot and there is little hope that you will ever view the data objectively.

Still, according to the Orthomolecular Medicine News Service, as of August 4, 2008, some so-called experts ignored or overlooked all of the negative data, as evidenced by Vancouver physician Abram Hoffer, MD. Dr. Hoffer, who also has a PhD in nutritional biochemistry, said, "Vitamin supplements are extraordinarily safe and effective. This is based on fifty years of clinical experience without seeing any life-threatening side effects and no deaths. It is pharmaceutical drugs that are dangerous. Perhaps the drug industry is getting tired of all the bad news about drugs, so instead they are going after nutritional supplements."

And, another British Columbia physician, Erik Paterson, MD, said: "For 33 years I have aggressively prescribed and advocated vitamins in doses vastly higher than the usual government recommendations for my family and my patients. I have never seen any adverse reactions, even though I have been on the alert for them all this time."

Folks, what is wrong with this picture?

CHAPTER FOUR:

The Gigantic Antioxidant Vitamin Experiment

Follow the Money

A gigantic human experiment is underway. Individuals, without known vitamin deficiencies, are consuming ever increasing quantities of antioxidant vitamins on both a voluntary and an involuntary basis. Voluntarily, many people take antioxidants on a daily basis because they have been led to believe that they are good for their over all health and that they are protective of common diseases, such as cancer, heart disease, Alzheimer's disease and diabetes.

Involuntarily, people are ingesting larger quantities of antioxidant vitamins which have been incorporated into everyday foods and are being genetically engineered into farm crops, such as tomatoes and berries, which contain very high antioxidant levels. If a little is harmful, then a lot is even more harmful. So, why are they doing this?

Yes, you got it. "Follow the money!"

Unfortunately, reliable scientific studies are increasingly showing that antioxidant vitamins are producing negligible effects or having no effects at all. Even worse, many studies are demonstrating the harmful potential of these same antioxidant vitamins. Amazingly, unscrupulous profiteers are going full steam ahead with unrestricted marketing of these potentially dangerous products, as though they are truly "miracle pills." And, more and more antioxidants are entering the marketplace everyday. Yet, oxidation remains one of the most important processes protecting us from pathogens and disease.

Violating The Scientific Method

Predictability and repeatability are the hallmark of the scientific method. If studies can not be repeated and if predictions of a theory are inconsistent, then the theory upon which they are based is nullified. Such is the case with the free radical theory. Yet, amazingly, this invalidated theory continues to be one of the most widely accepted in providing a possible explanation for disease causation and aging. This theory has more holes in it than a Swiss cheese factory.

The available scientific literature shows that the effects of antioxidant vitamins A, C and E are highly inconsistent, non-repeatable and totally unpredictable, as evidenced by a host of cohort studies and randomized controlled trials (RTCs) in humans. Laboratory and in vitro studies are much more predictable but this has not translated over to human in vivo studies. Free radicals may be bad for rats but people are not rats.... well, most of us are not. This outdated and outmoded theory must be discarded and replaced with a creative, more accurate, scientifically based theory. My UTOPIA theory (Unified theory of oxygen participation in

aerobiosis) (Howes, 2004) and my ROSI theory (Reactive oxygen species insufficiency) serve such a purpose and represent a major step forward (Howes, 2009).

Extrapolation of data obtained from in vitro studies to the living/breathing human cell has been fraught with errors. The complexities in the "living/breathing" cell are light years removed from the simplicity of "dead" test tube studies, which are clearly laden with countless metabolic artifacts. Perhaps the most important aspect of these artifacts is due to the fact that in vitro studies take place outside of the living totality of a respiring aerobic organism and are conducted in the "glass-casket" test tube, housed inside the sterile confines of the laboratory-morgue. This is, indeed, a far cry from the beautifully integrated biochemical engine room of a living cell, which is incorporated into a living and fully functional organism.

Analysis of The Meta-analysis

It appears that we are trying to analyze the data to death. Seemingly, everyone has an agenda to prove. **Some want to write more papers, obtain more grants, sell more products or make more profits.** However, some actually seek the scientific truth regarding the antioxidant vitamins. Relative to evaluating the data on antioxidant vitamins, we have witnessed the analysis of the raw data, the analysis of the collective data, the meta-analysis of the overall data and the analysis of the meta-analysis. Yet, supporters of the free radical theory still believe in the miraculous abilities of antioxidants, even after repeated studies have shown their marginal effects or total lack of effect. Even worse, some studies have shown their dangerous and harmful potential.

Everyday some new "antioxidant concoction" is aggressively marketed with an exotic sounding name or with outlandish and overstated claims that encourage individuals to take nigh toxic levels of these vitamins, antioxidants and potentially dangerous supplements. The theory they project is that these agents are good for you, therefore, the more of them you ingest, the healthier you will be, but, **this is blatantly wrong**. Please remember the wisdom of Paracelsus, "only the dosage makes the poison," in regards to everything you ingest. Scientific studies have determined that a well balanced diet is preferentially the best choice. **Do not be misled by exaggerations, fuzzy math, statistically generated "benefits," or outright lies, regarding many vitamins and antioxidant supplements.**

Various epidemiological and observational studies have produced conflicting results on the protective effect of antioxidants. Most studies of primary or secondary disease prevention have frequently failed to show a protective effect. These conflicting and confusing results may be the result of numerous confounding factors.

Also, please do not confuse the poor results of antioxidant vitamins with the beneficial effects of prooxidant vitamins, such as vitamin D3. Vitamin D3 is currently developing into an upcoming superstar.

CHAPTER FIVE:

Science Is Getting A Little Crazy

Ignore the negative studies

In all fairness, one can find selective data to support almost any position on almost any subject, e.g., there are studies showing support, studies which are neutral and studies which are negative. Take global warming, for instance. So-called experts have diametrically opposed views on the subject and the presumed scientific data to back up their respective position. Well then, who is right? Can both be right? Or, is neither right? Yes, science is getting a little crazy. Could "science" be bad for your health?

Actually, one must look for truth in the overall data, if you can find it, and follow its lead. I have done that, but in this book, I readily admit that I have intentionally sought out studies which have demonstrated the failures or ineffectiveness of the antioxidant vitamins. The total data on the subject of antioxidant vitamins would be too large for any one book or even a series of books. Also, I literally found so many so-called "disappointing antioxidant studies" that I have stopped looking for more. They have been there all along but most authors have chosen not to discuss them and those selling such products have intentionally ignored or avoided them. It appears that they believe that if they hide them that they will just go away. But, I will not let that happen. It is time to bring them to the "cleansing" light of day and let people know the truth about these potentially harmful products.

All of life is dependent upon the interactions of millions of proteins, carbohydrates and lipids. Additionally, it is dependent upon the actions of billions and trillions of electronically modified oxygen derivatives (EMODs). These are the modulating agents for cellular energy production and they form the molecular basis of life itself. Many of these EMODs have been referred to and demonized as free radicals. More specifically, oxygen radicals have been called reactive oxygen species, reactive oxygen metabolites, active oxygen reactants and a whole host of less accurate and perplexing terms. The old terminology needs to be discarded and replaced with the more accurate term, EMODs.

The term "EMODs" merely indicates that the electron structure of ground state oxygen has been altered or changed. It makes no determination of charge or radicality.

Even though hydrogen peroxide, singlet oxygen and hypochlorous acid are not free radicals, they have been erroneously lumped or categorized under the nefarious free radical umbrella. Inaccuracies are common place in oxidation/reduction (redox) studies and this lends itself to even more confusion.

All of us seek answers to our health problems, which makes us willing to believe many of the exaggerated claims that we hear regarding antioxidant vitamins but it is far from being that simple. Plus, we all like an easy way out, i.e., just pop a pill and all will be fine. WRONG! As a result, rumors, lies and errors spread, statistics get misinterpreted and relatively small or irrelevant connections become headline news. There are a lot of half truths and outright lies out there. So, be cautious. Be very cautious.

In actuality, we do not know specifically the causes of cancer, heart disease, diabetes, arthritis, etc. nor do we know how to prevent them. We do know some important so-called risk factors. But, that is about it. If we knew the cause of these diseases, then we could prevent them now. But, we can't. The cancer and heart disease advocacy movements have done a terrific job in increasing awareness of these diseases, but an unfortunate side effect has been the acceptance of erroneous theories and flat out lies. The free radical theory tops this reprehensible list.

Many studies have resulted in improved treatments but we also need much more research to figure out prevention and causes of most common diseases. Demand new hypotheses. Demand truth in the reporting of data. Demand protection from fraudsters. Demand and encourage creative ideas to eradicate these diseases once and for all.

Today, antioxidant vitamins are primarily about marketing and not about biochemistry or boosting health. If they can sell it, they will and therefore, it must be O.K. Study after study has exposed the half truths and broken promises of the supplement manufacturers. Yet, pharmaceutical companies and supplement manufacturers continue to push sales of these potentially dangerous chemicals and to influence and control of governmental regulation of such products. Actually, they have managed to keep the government out of it. Basically, these antioxidant vitamins are unregulated.

These products are sold as dietary supplements in the United States. Unlike drugs (which must be tested before being allowed to be sold), the companies that make supplements are not required to prove to the Food and Drug Administration (FDA) that their supplements are safe or effective, as long as they don't claim the supplements can prevent, treat, or cure any specific disease.

Some such products may not contain the amount of the herb or substance that is written on the label, and some may include other substances (contaminants). Actual amounts per dose may vary between brands or even between different batches of the same brand. Regulation standards are scant.

Most such supplements have not been tested to find out if they interact with medicines, foods, or other herbs and supplements. Even though some reports of interactions and harmful effects may be published, full studies of interactions and effects are not often available. Because of these limitations, any information on ill effects and interactions should be considered incomplete.

Thus, millions of citizens globally continue to ingest these questionable agents on a daily basis and are totally unaware of their harmful potential. **Even more shocking is the fact that most regular vitamin and supplement users said they would continue to use these products even if scientific evidence showed they were not useful.** This demonstrates the remarkable power of unrestrained marketing and the current danger to public health in general.

The Vitamin Cartel

Overall, the vitamin and supplement industry, which garners sales of over $23 billion annually, has been found to be manipulated by a few dozen chemical and pharmaceutical corporations in an illegal cartel-like manner. On May 20, 1999, Assistant U.S Attorney General, Joel Klein, announced nearly $1 billion in criminal fines against a cartel of vitamin manufacturers, which was allegedly headed by pharmaceutical heavy weight Hoffman-LaRoche. Klein made the following statement regarding the vitamin and supplement industry:

"The vitamin cartel is the most pervasive and harmful criminal antitrust conspiracy ever uncovered. The criminal conduct of these companies hurt the pocketbook of virtually every American consumer—anyone who took a vitamin, drank a glass of milk, or had a bowl of cereal: this cartel was truly extraordinary. It lasted almost a decade and involved a highly sophisticated and elaborate conspiracy to control everything about the sale of these products. These companies fixed the price; they allocated sales volumes; they allocated customers; and in the United States they even rigged bids to make absolutely sure that their cartel would work. The conspirators actually held annual meetings to fix prices and to carve up world markets, as well as frequent follow-up meetings to ensure compliance with their illegal scheme. The enormous effort that went into maintaining this conspiracy reflects the magnitude of the illegal revenues it generated as well as the harm it inflicted on the American economy."

In fact, there is currently a proposed settlement of a class action lawsuit regarding the indirect purchase of certain Vitamin Products. The law suit is called *Richardson, et al. v. Akzo Nobel Inc, et al.* No. 99-197, pending in the U.S. District court for the District of Columbia. The settling defendants have agreed to pay $25.03 million and the court will hold a final fairness hearing on June 18, 2010.

The vitamin industry used spin to go from the word **"supplementation"** to a more acceptable and appealing word, **"fortification."** In 2007, nutrition expert, Dr. Jeff Blumberg stated that, "we have more than 20,000 different antioxidants in our diet. There aren't 20,000 pills we can take. One of the reasons that dietary supplements can't replace a healthful diet is because we don't know what's important to put in every pill." We also do not know the synergistic effect of nutrient combinations.

Author, Michael Pollan, said in a 2007 New York Times article, "People don't eat nutrients, they eat foods, and foods can behave very differently than the nutrients they contain…as soon as you remove these useful molecules from the context of the whole foods they're found in, as we've done in creating antioxidant supplements, they don't work at all." In other words, it is believed by some that there is a synergism amongst the complex of nutrients in most foods.

Each and every one of us is basically serving as a lab rat for global experiments involving the fortification of our foods with antioxidant supplements. This is equivalent to an unauthorized, world wide, clinical experiment. This experiment could be tantamount to a gradual poisoning of mankind globally and the results of which will only be seen over decades and generations. Vitamin pushers try to convince us that just because we do not immediately keel over dead, after ingesting antioxidant vitamins, that they must be safe. However, their effects are going to be long term and found only with long term studies or in examples of deaths from accidental mega-dose ingestion. Also, deaths which are caused by increased risk of cancer, heart disease and stroke will not be attributed to the ingestion of these products. Based on current studies, they may well have been responsible for many of these deaths. This type of data is now emerging, as is evidenced by the results of RCTs. These same RCTs show that for agents such as vitamin A, it may only take small quantities above the daily requirement to push it into an area of potential harm and hypervitaminosis.

Because of the widespread use of antioxidant supplements by 10% to 30% of the adult population (80-160 million people) in North America and Europe, **there exists a serious public health issue and the potential for harm or increased mortality is highly significant and relevant.** (Bjelakovic et al, 2007).

T.J. Wheeler reported that a 2001 survey of American adults found that **59% used dietary supplements. The main reasons for use were to feel better (72%), prevention of illness (67%), treatment during illness (51%), longer life (50%), strength (37%), weight management (12%). Thirty three percent (33%) of adults took supplements on the advice of their physician** (Wheeler, 2001).

Regulations of dietary supplements state that "Structure and function claims" must have scientific support, but need not be approved by FDA (can even be kept secret!). Consumers do not generally understand this provision and tend to think that claims

49

have been approved. In an editorial, Fontanarosa wrote, "...these products nearly always include at least one 'structure/function' claim...Yet the only way such claims can be valid is if the dietary supplement actually promotes or has inherent biological activity...**If dietary supplements have or promote such biological activity, they should be considered to be active drugs**. They make drug-sounding claims. On the other hand, if dietary supplements are claimed to be safe because they lack or have minimal biological activity, then their ability to cause physiologic changes to support 'structure/function' claims should be challenged, and their sale and distribution as products to improve health should be curtailed (Fantanarosa et al, 2003). Amen, brother.

In other words, if they have drug activity, they should be regulated like drugs. But, they are not. In fact, they are hardly regulated at all. One regulation is, that if they are in a pill form, they have to be able to dissolve in your stomach. That is about it.

Antioxidant Vitamins Should be Considered Drugs

A February 2010 paper entitled, "Safety considerations and Potential Interactions of Vitamins: Should Vitamins Be Considered Drugs?" by Alexander L. Rogovik, Sunita Vohra, and Ran D. Goldman in the Annals of Pharmacotherapy, recommends that, "**Vitamins A, E, D, folic acid, and niacin should be categorized as over-the-counter medications..... Vitamin A should be excluded from multivitamin supplements and food fortificants.**" Further, Rogovik et al state that, "Vitamins have documented adverse effects and toxicities, and most have documented interactions with drugs. While some vitamins (biotin, pantothenic acid, riboflavin, thiamine, vitamin B_{12}, vitamin K) have minor and reversible adverse effects, others, such as **fat-soluble vitamins (A, E, D), can cause serious adverse events**. Two water-soluble vitamins, folic acid and niacin, can also have significant toxicities and adverse events." (Rogovik, Vohra and Goldman, 2010).

Manufacturers of dietary supplements **claim that their products are powerfully beneficial, on the one hand, but harmless on the other.** To claim both, does not make sense and to claim either without trials demonstrating efficacy and safety is deceptive, misleading and dangerous.

Products do not need to be shown to be safe; they just have to give "reasonable assurance" that there is not a significant risk of harm. Burden is on the FDA to show that a product is unsafe. "To police an industry with **1,000 manufacturers offering 20,000 products**, the FDA has a core staff of **eight people**." (Boston *Globe*, Aug. 22, 1999). It is now estimated that there are **30,000 supplement products, with 1000 new ones entering the market place each year.**

It is reported that, the American diet provides 120% of the recommended dietary allowances for β-carotene, vitamin A, and vitamin C, and dietary vitamin E deficiency has rarely been reported in the United States (Maxwell, 1999) (Herbert et al, 1990) (Herbert, 1994) (Herbert, 1997) (Seifried et al, 2003).

Basically, the data shows that vitamin deficiencies are rare in the USA. So, what is the problem? Why are so many people gulping down handfuls of vitamins every day? Is someone trying to sell you something?

CHAPTER SIX:

False Profits....er, Prophets

The field of antioxidant research is controversial and confusing to many clinicians and scientists because the results of many studies conflict with others, making simple conclusions as to efficacy and safety difficult. Antioxidant vitamins fall under regulatory guidelines similar to those for foods and supplements but cannot be marketed for disease treatment or disease prevention. Health promotion is the primary mode of marketing for dietary supplements, although such use transcends some of the regulatory barriers.

The Food and Drug Administration's oversight of vitamins and other dietary supplements was side stepped in 1994. Unlike most medications, most supplements sold today never had to be proven safe, much less proven to bring any health benefit.

Mae West said, "Too much of a good thing is wonderful"....but , she was wrong

There is an additional growing concern that some people may get a risky or harmful vitamin overload. Yet, in health oriented individuals, use of vitamin supplements and foods fortified with vitamins has recently skyrocketed as erroneous speculative reports suggested that high doses of certain nutrients would help prevent cancer and many other serious diseases. That's where safety questions arise, because it has been known that too much of certain nutrients or **hypervitaminosis can be bad**.

Many of the nonrandomized and uncontrolled studies, that suggested a beneficial effect of antioxidant vitamins, also showed that people who take vitamins tend to take better care of their health in other ways, such as eating plenty of fruits and vegetables, exercising and not smoking and it therefore was difficult to determine whether the vitamins were responsible for any health benefits.

According to Patsy Brannon, a Cornell University nutritionist, concern especially arises with super doses that exceed the government's "recommended daily amount," or RDA. **Between 1 percent and 11 percent of supplement users may be exceeding the upper limits set for certain nutrients, if they add together their doses from vitamin pills and their vitamin fortified diets**. Too much vitamin A can cause birth defects, and too much vitamin E can cause bleeding problems. Too much vitamin C causes diarrhea and increases oxalate excretion, which may cause kidney stones.

In discussing the history of the free radical theory and the use of antioxidant vitamins, such as vitamins A, C and E, free radical research pioneer, Barry Halliwell, said that, "In the beginning, it was simple: we said free radicals are bad, antioxidants are good." However, much has changed and over the past half a century and these unfounded charges have steadfastly remained unproven. Further, the free radial theory, upon which these notions were based, has failed to be verified by the scientific method because of a glaring lack of predictability. In fact, recent findings from some randomized controlled trials (RCTs) have necessitated that they were shut down early, due to increases in disease risk. Antioxidant vitamin adverse side effects were so obvious that it would have been medically unethical to continue with such trials (ATBC, CARET and SELECT studies) and knowingly endanger participants.

Some trials resulted in increased morbidity and increased risk of mortality from antioxidant use. This was a real shocker to the oxymorons.

Following the 1992 U.S. National Cancer Institute research for testing of beta carotene, Halliwell, from the National University of Singapore, said, "It was a shock. It (beta carotene) not only did no good but had the potential to do harm." Subsequently, an expert panel convened by the National Institutes of Health has concluded that there is no evidence to recommend beta carotene supplements for the general population, and strong evidence to recommend that smokers avoid it.

The same surprising story was repeated with vitamin E, in which recent studies have been almost universally "disappointing." Further, in 2005, Dr. Edgar Miller of the Johns Hopkins Medical Institutions, published a meta-analysis review of 19 studies in Annals of Internal Medicine showing that vitamin E increased overall mortality. Yes, he did catch hell from the manufacturers of these dubious products but his reputation and qualifications have made it difficult for them to discredit him, even though they have tried.

Even though vitamin E appeared to be a good antioxidant in vitro, there has been accumulating serious scepticism that it acts in the same manner in vivo (Howes, Philica, April 5, 2007).

Following a large RCT on vitamin C, Halliwell said, "Vitamin C is another disappointment. People are still trying to defend it, but you don't get an effect on free radical damage unless you start with people with a vitamin C deficiency. I think it is a lost cause."

Yet, the prevailing prejudice against EMODs was manifestly illustrated in the November 2003 issue of Readers Digest. In quoting Dr. Bruce Ames, a biochemist at the University of California at Berkley, he stated that, "free radical oxidation doesn't just rise with aging--it causes it. The more that mitochondria 'leak' free radicals (i.e., oxygen radicals, EMODs), the more those radicals end up damaging the mitochondria, which in turn leak even more free radicals." In bold print, the article states, "The ultimate irony: The thing we need most to live--oxygen--is what's killing us." Statements such as this, which appear in both the lay press and in scientific publications, point out the currently accepted non-sense/non-science dogma which states that oxygen and its radicals are highly toxic, even lethal. To the contrary, the overall data shows that these conclusions are, at best, dubious.

The glowing predictions for vitamin E alone or in combination with vitamin C and beta carotene have been stifled by a compelling body of clinical trial evidence and by the association of certain adverse effects with antioxidant vitamin usage.

Antioxidants, which had been wildly touted as the savior from the alleged damaging effects of electronically modified oxygen derivatives (EMODs), were quickly being shown to be of marginal help or no help at all. Antioxidants, which were believed to nullify, scavenge or eliminate free radicals, were failing their expectations and were losing the role as the answer to so-called "free radical induced diseases" in man. Scientists had erroneously assumed three things: 1) that the free radical theory was correct, 2) that oxygen free radicals were always deleterious and 3) that antioxidants would successfully counteract the alleged damaging effects of oxygen free radicals. They have been proven wrong on all three points.

Harman had planted the seed of "oxidant confusion," which led to the growth of a sprawling tree of dead ends and half truths, which were rooted in the shadow of the free radical hypotheses. Its run away growth smothered most of the real truth in regards to the essentiality of oxygen free radicals and human disease causation. It has stymied creative thinking concerning prooxidants for over half a century.

Other Scientists Chime In

Despite the widely held enthusiasm for the free radical theory, I can hardly find a single proven medical application or clinical breakthrough, which has been based on the free radical theory (see "The Howes Selective World Library of Oxygen Metabolism, available at www.thepundit.com or www. iwillfindthecure.org).

When confronted with non-supportive evidence, the medico-scientific establishment and supplement manufacturers did what any purveyor of profitable misinformation would do, i.e., they either ignored it, denied it or called it a paradox. Interestingly, they simultaneously sought out supportive evidence, no matter how flimsy, and then embarked on an aggressive propaganda campaign to 'indoctrinate' or persuade as many people as possible to accept this allegedly supportive evidence. Television ads were hawking antioxidants everywhere. Printed media was filled with ads proclaiming the wonders of antioxidants. All the while, studies were taking the wind out of the billowing sails of the antioxidant fleet. Yet, the end result was that the supplement industry grew to a $23 billion industry and that the general public received a highly distorted interpretation of the data that had little resemblance to the truth. This has been the biased situation with the free radical theory for the last fifty years.

Antioxidant vitamins as food supplements cannot be recommended in the primary or secondary prevention against cardiovascular disease or cancer. That is a fact. Any way you look at it, antioxidants have failed to protect, reverse or stop the major diseases facing mankind.

Marketing has placed antioxidants in products ranging from pizza dough to cake mix, from water to energy drinks, from doughnuts to dog food and from bread to bubble gum.

In 2005, Johns Hopkins expert, Simeon Margolis, M.D., Ph.D, posted the following cautions: "I urge you not to be taken in by unproven claims that a dietary supplement can treat diabetes -- or any other disorder, for that matter."

The Mayo Clinic website states that, "Many ads sound too good to be true: All you have to do is take a pill, and you'll suddenly find yourself muscle-bound and full of youthful energy. What those ads don't tell you is you'll also empty out your wallet and possibly harm your body using an unproven therapy. Proponents believe that antioxidants can prevent chronic diseases, such as heart disease and diabetes but experimental data has failed to confirm this. There's no proof that antioxidants in pill form can improve your general health or extend your life. In fact, they can have the opposite effect."

The National Cancer Institute states that, "Considerable laboratory evidence from chemical, cell culture, and animal studies indicates that antioxidants may slow or possibly prevent the development of cancer. However, information from recent clinical trials is less clear. In recent years, large-scale, randomized clinical trials reached inconsistent conclusions."

The Heart and Vascular Institute of the Cleveland Clinic joined in and stated the following: "*Natural products, herbal supplements, alternative dietary therapies, antioxidants, micronutrients or plain old vitamin pills...* No matter what you call them, if you take these products prior to a heart operation, they can cause real problems during or after your surgery. Previous studies of these and other natural or alternative therapies such as ginger, coenzyme Q-10, and vitamin E, have found that side effects from natural agents can be as serious as a heart attack, stroke or excess internal bleeding."

Writer, Lisa Melton said that, "If it is an **antioxidant,** such as cranberry capsules, green tea extract, effervescent vitamin C, pomegranate concentrate, beta carotene, selenium, grape seed extract, high-dose vitamin

E, pine bark extract or bee spit, we will swallow it by the bucket-load." Well said, Lisa.

The Antioxidant Craze

In 2002, C. T. Ryan presented a brief summary on antioxidants and cancer prevention. She stated, "Antioxidants were once confined to the vocabulary of scientists and nutritionists. The word "antioxidant" is now plastered on everything from magazine headlines to grocery ads. Basically, antioxidant means "against oxygen." Even though diets rich in fruits and vegetables (and thus naturally high in antioxidants) are thought to protect against cancer, **there is no convincing evidence** that the same benefits can be achieved by taking antioxidants as supplements. Keep in mind that fresh fruits and vegetables can also be high in oxidants, such as hydrogen peroxide and that antioxidants usually become free radicals themselves.

Since EMODs have been linked to all major diseases and degenerative conditions, including dandruff and hangovers, antioxidant consumption has been successfully promoted upon the general population.

Everyday some new "potion" is aggressively marketed with an exotic sounding name or with outlandish claims that encourage individuals to take almost toxic levels of vitamins, antioxidants and dietary supplements. The theory they project is that these agents are good for you, therefore, the more of them you ingest, the healthier you will be, but, this is wrong. Again, please remember the wisdom of Paracelsus, "only the dosage makes the poison," in regards to everything that you ingest.

CHAPTER SEVEN:
Where Are The bodies?

Here Are The Dead Bodies

**Adverse consequences of antioxidant
vitamins and increased risk of death:
Any agent which causes an increased risk of
the following can contribute to the number
of dead bodies. They need repeating.**

Antioxidant vitamins can lead to increased risk of:
- lung cancer, 18%, 28%;
- lung cancer incidence and mortality;
- breast cancer;
- prostate cancer;
- multivitamins doubled risk of fatal prostate cancer
- head and neck cancer;
- skin cancer;
- melanoma;
- oral pre-malignant lesions, especially in smokers;
- total mortality, 17%;

- likelihood of dying by about 5%;
- esophageal cancer deaths 14%;
- doubled adenoma (polyp) recurrence in smokers and drinkers;
- had a higher rate of second primary cancers during the supplementation period
- hemorrhagic stroke deaths, 50%;
- increased total and stroke mortality;
- supplements increase the likelihood of dying by about 5%
- vitamin A increased death risk by 16%,

beta carotene by 7%,

vitamin E by 4 %;

- significant increase in all-cause mortality and a slight increase in cardiovascular death;
- mortality was increased in vitamin E users who had a history of stroke, coronary bypass graft surgery, or myocardial infarction and, independently, in those taking nitrates, warfarin, or diuretics;
- participants with a dietary vitamin C intake above the median of 90 mg/day, vitamin E increased mortality among those aged 50-62 years by 19%
- increased post-trial risk of first-ever non-fatal Myocardial Infarction (heart attack);
- ischemic heart disease deaths, 11%;
- significantly more deaths from fatal coronary heart disease;
- 2.3 times risk of death from stroke and 2 times risk of dying from coronary artery disease in diabetic postmenopausal women;
- higher rates of heart failure and hospitalizations for heart failure
- total fracture;
- hip fracture;
- osteoporotic hip fractures in men and women;

- accelerate the progression of retinitis pigmentosa (eye disease);
- increased risk of age-related macular degeneration;
- higher risk of age-related cataract among women;
- among women aged ≥65 y, vitamin C supplement use increased the risk of cataract by 38%;
- vitamin C use among hormone replacement therapy users was associated with a 56% increased risk of cataract
- increased risk of Mother-to-child transmission of HIV;
- increased rate of low-birth-weight babies;
- increased rate for gestational hypertension;
- increased in having to take antihypertensive medication antenatally (after birth)
- suffered falling more often;
- E supplementation increased tuberculosis 72% and pneumonia risk 14%;
- vitamin E results in loss of quality-adjusted life years
- increase in the incidence of cancer among smokers and increased cancer mortality
- Multivitamin/Minerals associated with doubling in the risk of fatal prostate cancer
- increase in intima-media thickness over time in smokers
- rate of local recurrence of the head and neck tumor tended to be higher
- higher rate of second primary head and neck cancers
- worsening of coronary atherosclerosis in those with two copies of the haptoglobin 2   gene
- promote the clogging of arteries;
- accelerated thickening of the walls
- higher mortality rate in men
- adverse mucocutaneous effects and serum triglyceride elevations

- cardiac arrhythmias (probucol)
- negated the benefit of cholesterol lowering drugs (statin plus niacin)
- negatively associated with skeletal health
- 2 studies suggested poorer survival with concurrent administration of antioxidants and cytotoxic therapy in non-metastatic breast cancer
- C hampered endurance capacity
- multivitamins associated with higher mean breast density in premenopausal women
- multivitamins statistically significant increased risk 19 % of breast cancer
- supplementing the general public with vitamin E results in loss of quality-adjusted life years (loss of about four months)
- decreased sperm motility
- induced sperm DNA damage

I believe that just as there can be a dangerous build up of natural antioxidants, such as urate or bilirubin, this same condition could possibly occur with synthetic antioxidants (even those contained in multivitamins), such as vitamins A, beta carotene, ascorbate and vitamin E (tocopherol). Their effects may be augmented by the build up of common synthetic food antioxidants, such as BHT and BHA.

Since supplement manufacturers have not provided the public with adequate safety information, I believe that it is time for a class action law suit to control and regulate the supplement industry, as it relates to antioxidants. Adequate scienfitic data is in, the conclusions are becoming clear and it is time to act on behalf of the people. **Marketing has placed antioxidants in products ranging from pizza dough to cake mix, from water to energy drinks, from doughnuts to dog food and from bread to bubble gum.**

Genetic engineers are mutating foods to create fruits and vegetables which contain mega-loads of antioxidants, effectively bringing us into the age of "fortified Franken-foods." These antioxidants have been and will be incorportated into the general food supply, even though individuals may not want to ingest higher levels of these questionable and potentially dangerous antioxidants.

It would also appear that the insidious influence of antioxidant vitamins would be difficult to verify on autopsy, because it is so widespread and at the heart of energy production. However, certain cases of antioxidant doses have clearly resulted in "dead bodies."

The Antioxidant Killer, Uric Acid (urate)

First, consider the lethal potential of common natural antioxidants, such as uric acid, bilirubin and estrogen.

Hyperuricemia has been associated with increased morbidity in patients with hypertension and is associated with increased mortality in women and elderly persons. Hyperuricemia is clearly a powerful predictive factor for ischemic cardiovascular disease (CVD; and poor outcomes in these conditions), as recently reviewed. **The recently published National Health and Nutrition Examination Survey I (NHANES I) study of 5926 subjects concluded that increased uric acid is independently and significantly associated with cardiovascular mortality. In univariate Cox proportional hazard analyses, serum urate concentration was associated with CVD mortality. Uric acid levels also tended to be associated with death from any cause during follow-up.** (Niskanen et al, 2004).

Hyperuricemia has a strong association with the relative risks of death in all causes, coronary heart disease, stroke, hepatic disease and renal failure, and indicated that serum uric acid seems to be a considerable risk factor for reduced life expectancy (Tomita et al, 2000).

Men with hyperuricemic gout have a higher risk of death from all causes. Among men without preexisting CHD, the increased mortality risk is primarily a result of an elevated risk of CVD death, particularly from CHD (Choi and Curhan, 2007).

The Antioxidant Killer, Bilirubin

Free bilirubin is the most toxic substance produced by the human body. In normal adults, however, the bilirubin is conjugated in the liver, i.e. converted to a nontoxic form known as bilirubin-glucuronide.

Several reports have emphasized the antioxidant role **of bilirubin, which in human neonatal plasma seems to have a greater antioxidant capacity than urates, α-tocopherol, or ascorbates** (Miller et al, 1993).

Hyperbilirubinemia frequently occurs in the first five days of life of a newborn baby and may clear up within seven to fourteen days. This condition known as "physiological jaundice of newborns" or "neonatal jaundice" is due to incomplete development of certain mechanisms of the body resulting in a decreased ability to conjugate bilirubin with glucronic acid. Specifically, the key enzyme, UDP-glucuronyl transferase, is not present in the newborn, requiring several weeks to be fully induced. As a result, the bilirubin cannot be conjugated and is retained in the body for some time. The hyperbilirubinemia may be severe, lasting longer, and resulting in kernicterus.

Kernicterus can result in severe neurological deficits, mental retardation, loss of IQ and death. **The most popular treatment for neonatal juandice is phototherapy, which ironically generates large amounts of EMODs, especially excited singlet oxygen.** The light penetrates the skin, generates singlet oxygen and converts bilirubin to a less toxic substance, which is eliminated through the urine. In short, the lethal antioxidant hyperbilirubinemia death sentence is revoked and given a pardon by an EMOD, singlet oxygen.

In adults, hyperbilirubinemia, commonly referred to as "Gilbert's Disease", frequently results in death and the study appeared in the Oct. 30, 2008 *New England Journal of Medicine* (Morris et al, 2008). It is indeed ironic that the highly maligned EMODs must come to the rescue in the treatment of antioxidant induced lethal kernicterus.

The Antioxidant Killer, Estrogen

Long-term estrogen administration to post-menopausal women appears to have deleterious effects on rates of cardiovascular events such as myocardial infarction, strokes or venous thromboembolism (HERS) (Hulley et al, 1998) and Women's Health Initiative, **WHI** (WHI, 2002). **I believe that it must be kept in mind that estrogen is considered to be an antioxidant. Thus, I am not surprised by the fact that it actually increases the risk of developing EMOD insufficiency syndrome diseases.**

Older women who take hormone pills that combine estrogen and testosterone more than double their risk of breast cancer, according to a study of more than **70,000 nurses.** "This type of hormone therapy may help with mood, libido and bone mineral density, but the possible risk of breast cancer may outweigh these benefits," said study co-author Rulla Tamimi of Harvard Medical School. The findings, published in 7/24/06 issue of Archives of Internal Medicine, add to the evidence that **certain types of hormone supplements, such as estrogen-progestin pills, increase women's risk of breast cancer, strokes and heart attacks.** Earlier research **also found a greater breast cancer risk in women with higher natural levels of testosterone.**

Tragic deaths of 38 infants by lethal IV antioxidant vitamin E

A fatal syndrome characterized by progressive clinical deterioration with unexplained thrombocytopenia, renal dysfunction, cholestasis, and ascites developed in certain infants throughout the United States who had received E-Ferol, an intravenous vitamin E supplement. (THE TRAGIC CASE HISTORY OF INTRAVENOUS VITAMIN E (The New York Times) May 27, 1984
By PHILIP M. BOFFEY)

Prolonged exposure to E-Ferol was associated with progressive intralobular cholestasis, inflammation of hepatic venules, and extensive sinusoidal veno-occlusion by fibrosis. E-Ferol, contained 25 units per milliliter of dl-alpha-tocopheryl acetate solubilized with 9% polysorbate 80 and 1% polysorbate 20. They proposed that vasculocentric hepatotoxicity is the basis for the observed clinical syndrome that represents the cumulative effect of one or more of the constituents of E-Ferol (Bove et al, 1985).

All affected infants received E-Ferol; some affected infants received up to 1 ml or more daily. **Both outbreaks ceased shortly after use of E-Ferol was discontinued. Three were jailed for selling drug (vitamin E) that killed 38 babies.**

E-Ferol Aqueous Solution was the brainchild of James B. Madison, executive vice president of operations at O'Neal, Jones and Feldman (OJF), a drug distribution firm in St. Louis. Madison, with the permission of his boss, Larry K. Hiland, president of OJF, asked Ronald Carter of Carter-Glogau Laboratories, a drug manufacturer in Glendale, Ariz., to develop the formula. They believed their product was a nutritional supplement, not a drug. But because the product was labeled for treating a disease--retrolental fibroplasia--the solution was legally a drug.

By April 23, 1984, FDA had completed recall audits of all the wholesale distributors and the 159 hospitals that had received E-Ferol, ensuring that all of the product was off the market, as it remains today. **But by that time, the infant death toll attributable to E-Ferol had reached 38.**

On Sept. 30, 1988, after a seven-week trial, a jury returned guilty verdicts against Carter-Glogau, Ronald M. Carter, Sr., and Larry K. Hiland for distributing an unapproved and misbranded drug with the intent to defraud and mislead, and for participating in a conspiracy to market the drug without testing and without FDA approval. Hiland, the former president of OJF, was also found guilty of mail fraud in connection with the promotion of E-Ferol and was sentenced to a federal prison.

The **Center for Drug Evaluation and Research, Food and Drug Administration, Rockville, Maryland, concluded that the use of E-Ferol in these neonatal intensive care units was associated with increased morbidity and mortality among exposed infants** (Arrowsmith et al, 1989).

Research has shown infants who received E-Ferol injections are at an increased lifetime risk for reproductive problems, cervical and vaginal cancer, and other health problems. The drug was never FDA approved, but the companies sold E-Ferol to hospitals anyway, allegedly saying that it didn't need approval because it was a supplement.

"The E-Ferol scandal is one of the most shocking examples of corporate crime in American history."

There are the bodies! **The studies (RCTs) on vitamin E and beta carotene also argue for their toxicity and increased mortality.** Please refer to the section on "Antioxidant intervention trials."

Vitamin E deficiency is rare, and may occur in people with intestinal absorption problems, malnutrition, very low-fat diets, several genetic conditions, very low birth weight premature infants, or infants taking unfortified formulas. Supplementation with vitamin E may be necessary in these conditions and should be under strict medical attention. Prolonged vitamin E deficiency may cause severe medical complications.

Possible Vitamin A Deaths

1-28-2002 http://www.nutraingredients-usa.com/Research/Vitamin-A-deaths-blamed-on-Indian-government accessed 10-4-09

The Indian government has been accused of causing the deaths of more than 20 children last year (2001) by wrongly administering doses of vitamin A in a UNICEF-backed anti-blindness campaign.

In a report, the Assam Human Rights Commission said there was evidence that some of the deaths were the fault of the government workers who did not examine whether the children could take the medication.

"If one looks at the cause of death from the medico-legal aspect, there is every possibility that some of the children died due to Vitamin A poisoning or allergy to Vitamin A," said the commission Assam's leading human rights group.

The group placed the blame for the deaths on "agencies or instrumentalities or the public functionaries of the state government."

The report added that few supervisors at the anti-blindness campaign's booths noticed if the children were in ill health before administering the vitamin dose. "Vitamin A might have precipitated their deaths," the 12 page report said.

The investigation conducted by the State Department of Health and UNICEF revealed that, in most of the cases, deaths were due to causes unrelated to vitamin A (UNICEF, 2001). Controversially, this can be viewed as a possible cover up due to associated medico-legal liabilities.

Nutrient Intoxication

Fortification of foods has been associated with overdoses. Nutrient intoxication has been reported after consumption of fortified foods, primarily in instances when mistakes were made in over-fortifying the food product (e.g., **superabundant amounts of niacin improperly added to pumpernickel bagels** and **over fortification of milk with vitamin D**) (Niacin intox, 1983) (Blank et al, 1995) (Jacobus et al, 1992). Thus, it is possible that nutrient intoxication could occur with the antioxidant vitamins, due to it frequent and common place use with fortified foods and due to genetic engineering to produce fruits and vegetables with higher natural content of these same antioxidants.

CHAPTER EIGHT:

A, C & E and Multivitamin Summaries

16 Vitamin A (beta carotene) studies - summary

Vitamin A, beta carotene, has been found to have no effect or benefit: on occurrence of new nonmelanoma skin cancers (basal or squamous cell cancers); no reduction in relative mortality rates from all causes or from cardiovascular disease; no effect on incidence of cancer, heart disease (CVD), or total mortality; no significant effect on second head and neck cancer or lung cancer; no overall benefit or harm of 12 years of beta carotene supplementation on cataract or cataract extraction.

 Vitamin A, beta carotene, has shown adverse effects such as: adverse mucocutaneous effects and serum triglyceride elevations; 28% increase in lung cancer; 26% increase in heart disease (CVD) (nonsignificant); 17% increase in total mortality; point estimates suggested a decrease in second head and neck cancer risk but a possible increase in lung cancer risk; negatively associated with skeletal health; significantly elevated relative risk of hip fracture; may promote the development of osteoporotic hip fractures in women; risk of fracture was highest among men with the highest levels of serum retinol; modest increase in total fracture risk; beta carotene doubled the risk of adenoma (polyp) recurrence; increased the risk of Mother-To-Child-Transfer of HIV;

The incidence of lung cancer and deaths from all causes decreased but did not disappear completely after the supplementation ceased.

Thus, vitamin A could increase risk of lung cancer, heart disease, increased total mortality, osteoporosis and fractures, polyp recurrence and transfer of HIV.

35 Vitamin E studies - summary

Studies have vitamin E to have no effect or benefit such as: reduce risk of developing breast cancer, prostate cancer or colon cancer; has no benefit in reducing risk of stroke, cardiovascular diseases, ischemic heart disease, non-fatal myocardial infarction, cancer or total mortality; does not delay progression from amnestic mild cognitive impairment to Alzheimer's disease; does not prevent the development or progression of early or later stages of age related macular degeneration; does not reduce the incidence of or progression of nuclear, cortical, or posterior subcapsular cataracts; and provides no significant benefit for type 2 diabetes in initially healthy women.

Not only is it ineffective in preventing diseases, it can cause serious adverse effects. Unfortunately, vitamin E has been shown in some scientific studies to increase the overall mortality rate by 4%; increase the incidence of heart failure and hospitalization for heart failure; increase the rate of vessel blockages; decreased platelet function; increase the rate of falling in Alzheimer's patients; increase the risk of tuberculosis and pneumonia; and supplementing the general public with vitamin E results in loss of quality-adjusted life years (loss of about four months).

Thus, vitamin E could increase the risk of mortality, increase hospitalizations and heart failure, decrease platelet function, increase blood vessel blockages, increase tuberculosis and pneumonia in smokers and falls in Alzheimer's patients.

12 Vitamin C (ascorbic acid) studies - summary

Vitamin C, ascorbic acid, studies have shown no effect or benefit such as: no benefit to patients with advanced cancer; no effect against advanced malignant disease regardless of whether the patient has had any prior chemotherapy; no effect on lipoprotein cholesterol, apolipoprotein, and triglyceride concentrations; no important lowering effect of high-dose ascorbate on plasma Lp(a) in patients with premature CHD; not associated with improved CVD risk factor status among persons with diabetes; did not decrease the incidence of colds; does not improve endothelial dysfunction or insulin resistance in type 2 diabetics; low plasma vitamin C was not associated with an increased risk of acute myocardial infarction (AMI), irrespective of smoking status.

Vitamin C, ascorbic acid, studies have shown adverse effects such as: associated with an increased risk of cardiovascular disease mortality in postmenopausal women with diabetes; worsening of coronary atherosclerosis in those with two copies of the haptoglobin 2 gene; decreases muscle mitochondrial biogenesis and hampers training-induced adaptations in endurance performance; associated with higher risk of age-related cataracts among women.

Thus, vitamin C could increase the risk of cardiovascular disease in female diabetics, block the good effects of exercise and increase cataracts in women.

105 Combinations of Vitamin A, C & E studies - summary Vitamins A, C and E

Combinations of these vitamins may have no effect or benefit such as: retinol, lutein, alpha- and gamma-tocopherol, and selenium were not related to **cervical cancer** risk; neither beta carotene or vitamins C and E reduced the incidence of **adenomas**; no benefit was found in the **Cholesterol Lowering** Atherosclerosis Study (CLAS) with vitamins E, C or multivitamins; no decreased risk of death from **coronary heart disease** with vitamins A and C; vitamin C, E and beta carotene had no significant effect on the **systolic and diastolic blood pressures, fasting serum lipids** (total cholesterol, high-density lipoprotein cholesterol, and LDL cholesterol) and **fasting glucose**; no significant differences in **major coronary events** with vitamins A & E; preoperative supplementation with alpha-tocopherol and ascorbic acid on myocardial injury in patients undergoing cardiac operations provided no measurable reduction in myocardial injury after the operation; vitamin C or beta-carotene had no effect on **platelet function**; combination of vitamins C and E and beta carotene had no effect in reducing **the rate of restenosis** in patients after angioplasty; vitamin E had no influence on **nonfatal myocardial**

infarction; beta carotene has no primary preventive effect on **major coronary events**; vitamins C & E, beta carotene, selenium, and zinc made no differences in terms of **cancer incidence**, or in **cardiovascular disease incidence**, or **all-cause death** and no beneficial effects of long-term daily low-dose supplementation of antioxidant vitamins and minerals on **carotid atherosclerosis** and **arterial stiffness**; no benefit with respect to **colon cancer** with vitamin C and beta carotene; no protective effects of alpha- and beta-carotene, alpha-tocopherol, retinol, or selenium for **breast cancer**; neither alpha tocopherol nor beta carotene supplementation affected the incidence of **cataract surgery**; no evidence of beneficial effects for alpha tocopherol or beta carotene supplements in male smokers with **angina pectoris**; Vitamin E and vitamin C supplements and specific carotenoids did not substantially reduce risk for **stroke**; Vitamin E supplementation fails to slow (or inhibit) the progression of **intima-to-media thickness** in healthy men and women at low risk for cardiovascular disease; Vitamins A, C and E and the Risk of Breast Cancer, among post-menopausal women, found no association between any of the micronutrients evaluated and risk of **breast cancer**; vitamin C or vitamin E had no effect on **myocardial infarction**; vitamin C, E, or A did not have decreased risks of **cataract**; no overall association between intake of ascorbic acid, beta-carotene, retinol or vitamin E and **breast cancer** incidence; antioxidant supplementation alone had no significant effect on **plasma lipid profile** and **stenosis progression**; vitamins A, C and E, lycopene and alpha- and beta-carotene had no benefit against **atherosclerosis**; vitamin C, vitamin E, and beta carotene had no apparent effect on risk of development or progression of age-related **lens opacities or visual acuity loss**; no effect of vitamin C or E supplement use on overall **colorectal cancer** mortality; Vitamins A, C and E and specific carotenoids showed no evidence of an association between dose or duration of any specific vitamin and **ovarian carcinoma** risk; no significant associations between **breast cancer** risk and plasma levels of alpha -tocopherol or retinol were found; vitamin E, vitamin C and beta-carotene did not produce any significant reductions in the 5-year mortality from, or incidence of, any type of **vascular disease, cancer, or other major outcome**; vitamin E, vitamin C, and multivitamin supplements were not associated with a significant decrease in **total CVD or CHD mortality**; no benefit was seen from vitamin C supplements for **bladder cancer**; no association between **stomach cancer mortality** and regular use of vitamin E or multivitamins, regardless of duration of use; Supplemental intake of both vitamins E and C does not alter the risk for

dementia or Alzheimer's disease (AD); Neither dietary, supplemental, nor total intake of carotenes and vitamins C and E was associated with a decreased risk of AD; beta-carotene, flavonoids, and vitamins E and C were not associated with the risk of **dementia or its subtypes**; vitamin E supplements should not be recommended for primary or secondary prevention of AD; Vitamins E & A failed to reduce incidence or **mortality of gastrointestinal cancer**; beneficial or harmful effect of antioxidants or zinc and copper on **cognition in older adults**; Neither use of any vitamins C and/or E nor high-dose use reduced the time to dementia or AD; no incremental effect of supplemental vitamins C and E on any **myocardial ischemia outcome**; no evidence of a protective effect of antioxidants (vitamins E and C, ß-carotene, or selenium) or B vitamin supplements on the **progression of atherosclerosis**; effects of supplementation with beta-carotene, vitamins A, C, E and selenium alone or in combination on progression of primary or **secondary colorectal adenomas**; vitamin C and vitamin E during pregnancy did not reduce the risk of **pre-eclampsia in nulliparous women**, the risk of intrauterine growth restriction, or the risk of death or other serious outcomes in their infants; beta carotene, vitamins C and E did not affect **cataract progression** in a population with a high prevalence of cataract whose diet is generally deficient in antioxidants; Vitamins E, C and beta-carotene showed no statistically significant benefit of treatment in the U.K. **cataract** group; vitamin C, vitamin E, ß-carotene, Se, and Zn do not affect **fasting blood glucose**; no association between **prostate cancer** risk and dietary or supplemental intake of vitamin E, beta-carotene, or vitamin C; vitamins A, C and E and folate do not reduce **lung cancer** risk; no overall effect of ascorbic acid, vitamin E, or beta carotene on the individual **secondary outcomes of myocardial infarction, stroke, coronary revascularization, or CVD d**eath; no overall effects of ascorbic acid, vitamin E, or beta carotene on cardiovascular events among women at high risk for CVD; Multivitamin use was not related to **total mortality**; vitamins A and E, zinc, lutein, zeaxanthin, alpha-carotene, beta-carotene, beta-cryptoxanthin and lycopene have either a very slight or no effect on primary prevention of early age-related macular degeneration; no indication of an important role for carotenoids, tocopherols, or vitamin C in **lowering the risk of CVD death**; multivitamins, vitamin C, vitamin E, and folate were not associated with a decreased risk of **lung cancer**; no evidence that alpha-tocopherol and beta-carotene supplementation prevented or delayed the onset of **age-related macular degeneration (AMD)**; Neither vitamin E nor vitamin C had a significant effect on **prostate, colorectal, lung, or**

other site-specific cancers; vitamin E, C and beta carotene did not slow cognitive change among women with preexisting cardiovascular disease or cardiovascular disease risk factors; no significant overall effects of vitamin C, vitamin E, and beta-carotene on risk of developing type 2 diabetes in women at high risk of CVD; vitamin C, vitamin E, or beta carotene offers no overall benefits in the **primary prevention of total cancer incidence or cancer mortality**; vitamins C and E, beta-carotene, zinc, and selenium did not affect the risk of **metabolic syndrome** (MetS);

Combinations of these vitamins have shown adverse effects such as:

-   **Combinations of A & E showed 50% increase in hemorrhagic stroke deaths among vitamin E group; 11% increase in ischemic heart disease deaths among beta-carotene group; 18% increase in lung cancer among beta-carotene group and eight percent more men in this group died, as compared to those receiving placebo;**

-   **vitamin C or E did not protect women from breast cancer and a low intake of vitamin A may increase the risk of breast cancer;**

-   **beta-carotene and combined alpha-tocopherol and beta-carotene groups significantly increased deaths from fatal coronary heart disease;**

-   **vitamin E decreased platelet function;**

-   **antioxidants alone produced a nonsignificant increase of homocysteine;**

-   **homozygous familial hypercholesterolemia, intima-to-media thickness (FH IMT study) increased with vitamin E;**

-   **when used in combination with simvastatin/niacin, antioxidants negated the benefit of the latter on plasma lipid profile and stenosis progression;**

-   **vitamin E plus vitamin C had an unexpected significantly higher all-cause mortality rate and a trend for an increased cardiovascular mortality rate;**

-   **combination with high doses of beta-carotene, vitamin C, niacin, selenium, coenzyme Q10, and/or zinc showed death** from breast cancer and disease-free survival were shorter in the nutrient-supplemented group, but the differences were not statistically significant;

- results suggest poorer survival with concurrent administration of antioxidants and cytotoxic therapy;

- Vitamins E & A fail to reduce incidence or mortality of lung cancer but there was a statistically significant, increased risk of lung cancer incidence and mortality in people with risk factors for lung cancer who took both vitamins;

- Beta-carotene and vitamin A and beta-carotene and vitamin E significantly increased mortality in gastrointestinal cancer patients;

- ß-Carotene seemed to increase the post-trial risk of first-ever non-fatal MI;

- alpha-Tocopherol supplementation produced unexpected adverse effects on the occurrence of second primary cancers and on cancer-free survival in head and neck cancer patients and quality of life was not improved by the supplementation;

- vitamin C and vitamin E does not prevent pre-eclampsia in women at risk, but does increase the rate of babies born with a low birth weight;

- beta carotene, vitamin A, and vitamin E, singly or combined, significantly increased mortality (Vitamin A increased death risk by 16%, beta carotene by 7% and Vitamin E by 4%);

- beta carotene, vitamin A, and vitamin E, singly or combined, significantly increased mortality;

- increased risk of oral pre-malignant lesions was observed with vitamin E, especially among current smokers and with vitamin E supplements. Beta-carotene also increased the risk among current smokers;

- vitamin C, vitamin E, ß-carotene, selenium, and zinc found the incidence of skin cancer (SC) was higher in women in the antioxidant group and the incidence of melanoma was also higher in the antioxidant group for women;

- vitamin E was associated with a small increased risk of lung cancer;

- Among participants who obtained 90 mg/d or more of vitamin C in foods, vitamin E supplementation increased tuberculosis risk by 72%;

- Vitamin E increased pneumonia risk in males who initiated smoking at an early age and with body weight less than 60 kg, and in participants with body weight over 100 kg;

- Higher beta-carotene intake was associated with an increased risk of age-related macular degeneration (AMD);

- combinations of A and E showed E to accelerate the progression of retinitis pigmentosa;

- Baseline serum antioxidant concentrations of beta-carotene and vitamin C were negatively associated with the risk of metabolic syndrome (MetS);

- Vitamin A and zinc supplementation was associated with increased total and stroke mortality;

- Among smoker participants with a dietary vitamin C intake above the median of 90 mg/day, vitamin E increased mortality among those aged 50-62 years by 19%;

- vitamins C & E prevent health-promoting effects of physical exercise (insulin sensitivity);

- Longer duration of beta-carotene, retinol, and lutein supplements was associated with statistically significantly elevated risk of total lung cancer and histologic cell types;

- elevated serum vitamin E concentrations are associated with abnormal markers of atherosclerosis and may increase the risk of cardiovascular complications in HIV-infected adults;

- sperm motility was significantly decreased by antioxidants vitamin C and alpha-tocopherol

- both ascorbate and alpha-tocopherol in combination to sperm preparation medium actually induced DNA damage and intensified the damage induced by H_2O_2

8 Multivitamin studies - summary

Multivitamins may have no effect such as: no benefit in preventing **cardiovascular disease or cataract**; insufficient evidence to prove the presence or absence of benefits from use of multivitamin and mineral supplements to **prevent cancer and chronic disease**; multivitamin-multimineral supplement with a combination of vitamin C, vitamin E, beta-carotene, and zinc (with cupric oxide) is recommended for age-related macular degeneration (AMD) but **not cataract**; multivitamin use has little or **no influence on the risk of common cancers, CVD, or total mortality** in postmenopausal women;

Multivitamins may have adverse effects such as: a small increase in **prostate cancer** death rates; use of multivitamins more than seven times per week, when compared with never use, was associated with a doubling in the risk of **fatal prostate cancer**; multivitamin-multimineral supplements may be associated **with higher mean breast density** among premenopausal women; multivitamins was linked to a statistically significant **19% increased risk of breast cancer.**

Thus, multivitamins could increase fatal prostate cancer in men and breast cancer in women.

CHAPTER NINE:

Free Radical Theory
Fails The Scientific Method

Human antioxidant clinical trials have failed to demonstrate consistency or predictability

For the most part, **human antioxidant clinical trials have failed to demonstrate consistency or predictability** in the prevention, reversal or cure of the following: cardiovascular disease, atherosclerosis, cancer of all types, diabetes, macular degeneration, pre-eclampsia, hypertension, strokes, or any of the other diseases that have been tested for with reliable scientific studies.

Fortunately, the free radical theory is testable.

Unfortunately, it has repeatedly failed the tests.

It lacks predictability.

It does not allow for repeatable results.

Antioxidant vitamin study results are an inconsistent and confusing mess.

Many vitamins and supplements classified as antioxidants are actually *redox agents*, meaning they act as antioxidants in some instances and prooxidants in others.

VITAMIN E (Alpha-tocopherol) OVERVIEW

The following was excerpted and summarized from the AOL website. The content was provided by some of the **Faculty of the Harvard Medical School**. http://www.aolhealth.com/complementary/vitamin-e-alpha-tocopherol

Vitamin E deficiency is rare, and may occur in people with intestinal absorption problems, malnutrition, very low-fat diets, several genetic conditions, very low birth weight premature infants, or infants taking unfortified formulas. Supplementation with vitamin E may be necessary in these conditions and should be under strict medical attention.

Vitamin E possesses antioxidant activity, but it is **not clear if there is any benefit of this property in humans.**

Vitamin E: Unclear results; Inconsistent evidence

(content was provided by some of the Faculty of the Harvard Medical School Members)

Treatment with vitamin E for the following health problems has yielded these results:

- **Anemia: unclear mixed results**

- **Angina: unclear results**

- **Asthma: Initial research suggests no benefits of vitamin E**

- **Atherosclerosis: unclear mixed results**

- **Bladder cancer: promising preliminary evidence but unclear conclusions**

- **Cancer prevention (general): controversy, with mixed results of studies. At this time, based on the best available scientific evidence, and recent concerns about the safety of vitamin E supplementation, vitamin E cannot be recommended for this use**

- **Cancer treatment: There is no reliable scientific evidence that vitamin E is effective as a treatment for any specific type of cancer. Caution is warranted in people being treated with some types of chemotherapy or radiation, because it has been proposed that the use of high-dose antioxidants** may actually reduce the anti-cancer effects of these treatments.

- Heart Disease in dialysis: evidence is inconclusive
- Cataract prevention: conflicting evidence
- Chemotherapy nerve damage protection: inconclusive evidence
- Colon cancer protection: inconclusive evidence
- Dementia/Alzheimer's disease: inconclusive evidence
- Diabetes mellitus: inconclusive evidence
- G6PD deficiency: conflicting evidence
- Glomerulosclerosis (kidney disease): inconclusive evidence
- Heart disease prevention: Numerous studies of vitamin E oral supplementation have suggested no benefits in the prevention of cardiovascular disease, and there is recent evidence to suggest that regular use of high-dose vitamin E (400 IU/day or greater) increases the risk of death (from "all causes") by a small amount. In 2005, the Women's Health Study reported a 24% reduction in cardiovascular deaths in women taking 600 IU of vitamin E daily (with 10 year follow-up), but no change in total death rate or number of heart attacks or strokes. Based on the balance of available scientific evidence, and in light of recent safety concerns, chronic use of vitamin E cannot be recommended for this purpose, and high-dose vitamin E should be avoided
- High cholesterol: inconclusive evidence
- Immune system function: mixed results, unclear conclusions
- Intermittent claudications: inconclusive evidence
- Macular degeneration: inconclusive evidence
- Parkinson's disease: inconclusive evidence
- Pre-menstrual syndrome: inconclusive evidence
- Pneumonia prevention: inconclusive evidence, although initial research suggests that vitamin E is not beneficial.

- Retinitis pigmentosa: vitamin E does not appear to slow visual decline in people with retinitis pigmentosa and may be associated with more rapid loss of visual acuity.

- Scar prevention: vitamin E on the skin does not appear to reduce surgical wound scarring. Because of a risk of rash, some authors have recommended against the use of this therapy.

- Stroke: Evidence from the Women's Health Study published in 2005 suggests that regular vitamin E supplementation with 600 IU daily does not reduce the risk of stroke. Prior evidence was indeterminate for stroke prevention or stroke recovery. At this time, based on the best available scientific evidence and recent safety concerns, vitamin E cannot be recommended for this use.

- Supplementation in preterm and very low birth weight infants: There are numerous studies of vitamin E given to premature infants to try to prevent potentially serious complications such as intraventricular hemorrhage (bleeding into the brain), retinopathy (eye damage), or death. The quality of published research is variable, and is not clearly conclusive. With intravenous dosing of vitamin E, the risk of sepsis (life-threatening blood infection) and bleeding into the brain may actually be worse (particularly with high-dose vitamin E). With dosing by mouth, the risk of bleeding into the brain appears to be decreased. Some research suggests that blood levels of tocopherol greater than 3.5 mg/dl are associated with a reduced risk of severe retinopathy, but an increased risk of sepsis. Therefore, the current scientific evidence does not support the routine use of intravenous vitamin E at high doses, or supplementation with a goal of serum tocopherol levels greater than 3.5 mg/dl.

- Tardive dyskinesis: inconclusive evidence

Unproven uses of vitamin E:

Abortifacient Acne, Aging skin, Air pollution protection, Allergies, Amiodarone pulmonary toxicity prevention, Bee stings, Benign prostatic hypertrophy,y Beta-thalassemia, Bronchopulmonary dysplasia in premature infants, Bursitis, Cardiomyopathy, Chemotherapy extravasation, Chronic cystic mastitis, Chronic hepatitis B, Chronic progressive hereditary chorea, Congestive heart failure, Crohn's disease, Cystic fibrosis, Dermatitis, Diaper rash, Doxorubicin hair loss prevention, Duchenne muscular dystrophy, Dyspraxia, Energy enhancement, Frostbite, Gastric ulcer, Gastroesophageal cancer prevention, Granuloma annulare, (used on the skin) Hair loss, Heart attack, Heart transplant rejection prevention, Hereditary spherocytosis, Huntington's disease, Hypertension, Impotence, Inflammatory skin disorders, Labor pain, Leg cramps, Liver spots, Lung cancer prevention, Male fertility, Menopausal symptoms, Menstrual disorders, Miscarriage, Mucositis, Muscle strength, Myotonic dystrophy, Neuromuscular disorders, Nitrate tolerance, Oral leukoplakia, Osteoarthritis, Pancreatic cancer prevention, Peptic ulcers, Peyronie's disease, Physical endurance, Poor posture, Porphyria, Post-angioplasty restenosis prevention, Pre-eclampsia prevention, Preventing aging, Radiation-induced fibrosis, Reperfusion injury protection during heart surgery, Restless leg syndrome, Rheumatoid arthritis, Sickle cell disease, Skeletal muscle damage, Skin disorders, Sperm motility, Sunburn, Thrombophlebitis, Uveitis.

Dangers of vitamin E: Skin reactions/rashes such as contact dermatitis and eczema have been reported with the use of vitamin E on the skin, for example ointments or vitamin E containing-deodorants.

Research suggests that regular use of high-dose vitamin E supplements (400 IU/day or greater) may increase the risk of death (from "all causes") by a small amount.

High doses of vitamin E (greater than 400 IU/day) might increase the risk of bleeding (particularly in patients with vitamin K deficiency), including hemorrhagic stroke (bleeding into the brain). Caution is advised in patients with bleeding disorders or taking drugs that may increase the risk of bleeding.

In rare cases, vitamin E supplementation has been associated with dizziness, fatigue, headache, weakness, or blurred vision (particularly when used in high doses). In rare cases, vitamin E supplementation has also been associated with abdominal pain, diarrhea, nausea, diarrhea or flu-like symptoms (particularly when taken at high doses, such as greater than 2000 IU/day). The risk of necrotizing enterocolitis may be increased with large doses of vitamin E.

In rare cases, vitamin E supplementation has been associated with gonadal (sex organ) dysfunction and diminished kidney function.

Oral vitamin E should be avoided in patients with retinitis pigmentosa, as is does not appear to slow visual decline, and may be associated with more rapid loss of visual acuity.

Interactions with vitamin E and drugs

Interactions with vitamin E and drugs, herbs and other supplements have not been thoroughly studied. The interactions listed below have been reported in scientific publications. The amount of bleeding risk associated with vitamin E remains an area of controversy, and caution is warranted in patients with a history of bleeding disorders or taking blood-thinning drugs such as aspirin, anticoagulants such as warfarin (Coumadin) or heparin, anti-platelet drugs such as clopidogrel (Plavix), and non-steroidal anti-inflammatory drugs such as ibuprofen (Motrin, Advil) or naproxen (Naprosyn, Aleve).

Concern has been raised that antioxidants may interfere with some chemotherapy agents (such as alkylating agents, anthracyclines, or platinums), which themselves can depend on oxidative damage to tumor cells for their anti-cancer effects. Studies in this area are mixed, with some reporting interference, others noting benefits, and most suggesting no significant interaction.

Cholesterol lowering drugs, Cholestyramine (Questran) and Colestipol (Colestid) can reduce dietary vitamin E absorption and blood levels of vitamin E. Vitamin E may increase absorption and blood levels of cyclosporine. Gemfibrozil (Lopid) may decrease blood levels of vitamin E.

Dietary vitamin E absorption may be reduced by isoniazid (INH, Lanizid, Nydrazid), Olestra ("Olean" fat substitute), Orlistat (Xenical), and Sucralfate (Carafate). Anti-seizure drugs such as Phenobarbital, phenytoin, or carbamazepine may decrease blood levels of vitamin E.

Large doses of vitamin E may deplete vitamin A stores in the body. Mineral oil may reduce dietary vitamin E absorption. Increased intake of omega-6 fatty acids may increase vitamin E requirements, particularly at high doses. High doses of vitamin E appear to increase the body's vitamin K requirement and may cause blood clotting abnormalities in patients with vitamin K deficiency. Blood levels of vitamin E may be decreased with zinc deficiency.

Summary of vitamin E evaluation

Vitamin E has been suggested as a treatment for many conditions. Research supports use in individuals with vitamin E deficiency, although this condition is rare. There is not enough scientific evidence to support the use of vitamin E for any other medical condition. Recent research suggests that regular use of high-dose vitamin E supplements (400 IU/ day or greater) may increase the risk of death (from "all causes") by a small amount. Chronic use of vitamin E should be approached cautiously, and high-dose vitamin E should be avoided. Caution is warranted in patients with a history of bleeding disorders or taking blood-thinning drugs. Like other antioxidants, use during chemotherapy and radiation therapy may interfere with cancer treatment, and should be discussed with the treating physician.

This vitamin E information was prepared by the professional staff at Natural Standard (www.naturalstandard.com), based on thorough systematic review of scientific evidence. The material was reviewed By some members of the **Faculty of the Harvard Medical School** with final editing approved by Natural Standard.

CHAPTER TEN:

The most obvious reason for the failure of the Free Radical Theory is that the theory is wrong. Prooxidants are not normally deleterious, in living systems. They are crucial, low toxicity agents that sustain all aerobic life forms, provide pathogen defense and neoplasia protection. It is possibly that simple.

If you do not breathe or ingest oxygen, you die rather immediately.

Reasons For The Free Radical Theory Failure

A group of researchers at the University of New South Wales in Australia, led by Roland Stocker, studied a cholesterol-lowering drug called Probucol (Lorelco) in laboratory rodents with vascular disease. Probucol reduces the risk of heart disease in humans, but is no longer prescribed in the US and Australia because of adverse side effects: a tendency to lower good cholesterol along with the bad and the potential to induce an irregular heartbeat. Probucol is still available in Canada and Europe.

In their new study, Stocker and his colleagues show that the protective effect of probucol has nothing to do with its ability to scavenge oxygen free radicals, as the free radical-scavenging part of the drug alone was ineffective in protecting animals against heart disease. Instead, a different part of the probucol molecule was doing the beneficial work.

In fact, **contrary to widely accepted opinion, the group found no relationship between the levels of oxidized cholesterol in blood vessels and the severity of heart disease**. This might help explain the "disappointing results" of clinical trials with other free radical-scavenging antioxidants, such as vitamin E, which have shown no protective effect against heart disease in humans.

Stocker and Keaney stated that the causative relationship between oxidative events and atherosclerosis in general and the pathophysiological importance of LDL oxidation in particular have been challenged by **the overall poor performance of antioxidant strategies in limiting atherosclerosis and its cardiovascular events**, the overall lack of clear disease stage dependency in the vessel wall contents of oxidized molecules and antioxidants, and by the reported dissociation of atherosclerosis and lipoprotein oxidation in the vessel wall of animals.

That about sums it up for antioxidant failures in the prevention or cure of atherosclerotic or cardiovascular heart disease.

The story is essentially the same for cancer prevention or cure. That is, the underlying principles of the free radical theory have been wrong. Thus, the predicted outcomes of clinical trials have not worked as predicted.

In fact, because the free radical theory was flawed, none of the clinical trials could show consistent positive results. Such is the case with unsound theories. Still, many in the medical and scientific community just can't give it up or come up with a creative theory of their own.

The Long And Short Of It

We are witnessing the largest global human experiment in the history of the planet with injudicious antioxidant vitamin use.

With the antioxidant vitamins, you get proven risks with unproven health benefits.

In the past decade, randomized, controlled clinical trials have shown that ß-carotene and vitamin E supplements, which were widely believed to be safe, increase mortality and morbidity (Miller et al, 2005) (Bjelakovic et al, 2007).

No dietary supplement, including selenium, has proven useful so far for the prevention of cardiovascular disease or cancer in the general U.S. population.

CHAPTER ELEVEN:

Improved, New Alternate Theories:

1) UTOPIA AND
2) ROSI SYNDROME

I have developed and presented in my e-books the ROSI syndrome, whereby reactive oxygen species insufficiency "allows" for disease manifestation, including atherosclerotic plaque formation and cancer growth. (available at www.iwillfindthecure.org)

Here is what I now believe relative to my ROSI syndrome:
- we require a continuously operative prooxidative defensive system
- this system is based on a sufficiency of EMOD generation
- an immune competent system is also based on a sufficiency of EMOD production
- conditions such as HIV/AIDS has an EMOD insufficiency, which results in higher risk of infections, cancer and other diseases

- Chronic granulomatous disease (CGD) has an EMOD insufficiency and results in higher risks of infections, cancer, other diseases and early death
- Pregnancy can be an immunodeficiency condition, to allow the development of the "foreign body fetus" and has an insufficient EMOD production and results in higher risk for gestational diabetes, arthritis and other diseases
- Atherosclerosis develops at sites of intimal injury or at sites with insufficient EMOD production. This allows for the formation of a pimple-like lesion, just as it would on the external epidermis, which ultimately breaks open and causes clot formation. Adequate EMOD levels would not allow for the seeding of this lesion or of xenografts with viable pathogens and would oxidize microaggregates for excretion. Plaques have relatively high levels of antioxidants
- All of the major diseases such as cancer, atherosclerosis, diabetes, strokes and arthritis require a prooxidant system to constantly prevent the development or progression of these conditions

The most important and most basic reason for the failure of the free radical theory is that the theory is an erroneous theory. It has repeatedly been invalidated.

Prooxidants are not deleterious by nature, in living systems.

Instead, they are of low toxicity and are crucial agents for sustaining all aerobic life.

They are crucial agents for pathogen and neoplasia protection and they promote electron and proton flow.

It may be that simple.

The biggest EMOD source of all is EXERCISE, which medical science has repeatedly validated is good for us. Antioxidants can block the good effects of exercise.

If antioxidant therapies are to ever be successful, **antioxidant therapies must become: more specific for site of action,**

not have deleterious effects on other signaling pathways, be targeted to a specific reactive oxygen species or cellular compartment, and be "time sensitive" so they deliver the correct therapy at precisely the correct time.

First, we must remember that EMODs are ubiquitous and omnipresent.

EMOD SOURCES

Exponential numbers of oxygen molecules are hurriedly scurrying throughout my body and brain, shuttling down my electron transport chain and transferred by NOX and cytochrome P_{450} enzymes, carrying on instantaneous corporeal and cellular cross talk, protecting me and generating energy-rich ATP, thus, allowing me to utilize the combined prooxidant je ne sais quoi to present this material to you.

EMODs are formed via important biological systems, including the electron transport chain, NADPH oxidase, xanthine oxidase, prostaglandin synthesis, reduced riboflavin, nitric oxide synthetase, reperfusion injury, the cytochrome P450s, activated neutrophils and phagocytic cells. Outside sources of EMODs include drugs, antibiotics that depend on quinoid groups or bound metals for their action such as nitrofurantoin, and anti-cancer drugs such as doxorubicin, cisplatin, bleomycin and methotrexate, and pesticides, transition metals, tobacco smoke, alcohol, environmental radiation and high temperature, radiation treatment, inhalation of inorganic particles such as asbestos and silica, and ozone inhalation and even fever. NOX enzymes are even involved in the respiratory burst that occurs during fertilization.

One must use extreme care when altering antioxidant defenses. The redox balance is a critical aspect of all aerobic life. EMODs are signaling mechanisms for a vast range of vital metabolic pathways and biochemical networks.

Allowance of disease

During the course of my research over the past decade, I have been struck by the significance of oxygen's electronic modification derivative levels on "allowance" of diseases, such as cancer, atherosclerosis, diabetes, arthritis, strokes, and cataracts. I have tried to reduce my analysis of the causation to the simplest explanation, which ties together the clustering of these diseases. Homeostatic levels of electronically modified oxygen derivatives (EMODs) are crucial to maintaining health, protecting against pathogens and holding neoplastic cells in abeyance.

Oxygen consumption and cellular oxygen levels decrease with aging and these decreases are directly related to the onset of disease, irrespective of other considerations such as genetics, inheritance, smoking, diet, exercise, etc. Let me present the following interesting facts:

- **Skin has one of the lowest levels of oxygen and has one of the highest rates of cancer**

- **The thyroid synthesizes lots of hydrogen peroxide, as a substrate for thyroxin (tetraiodothyronine) synthesis, and has a very low incidence of carcinoma**

- **Muscle has a very high rate of oxygen consumption and has a very low incidence of rhabdomyosarcoma cancer**

- **Fat has one of the lowest oxygen levels and lipomas are one of the most common tumors**

- **The retina has the highest oxygen utilization rate of all tissues and cancers therein are an extremely rare occurrence**

- **The heart has a very high oxygen utilization rate and has a very low rate of tumor or cancer formation**

- **Areas of chronic inflammation predispose to cancer formation and inflammation is pathognomonic of hypoxia**

- **The brain has a very high oxygen utilization rate and has a relatively low rate of tumor and cancer formation. Also, the brain has high lipid and iron content and low antioxidant levels, yet, free radical chain reactions of lipid peroxidation do not spontaneously or continuously occur.**

The brain is particularly vulnerable to oxidative stress. Factors include the brain's:

- High energy requirement
- High oxygen consumption
- Richness in polyunsaturated fatty acids (over 70% fat in brain tissue)

- High levels of transition metals (e.g., iron, copper)
- Relatively low antioxidant defenses

It is also notable that **dopamine can generate quinones (which many consider as a main free radical), hydrogen peroxide and free radicals** and that treatment with Levodopa may increase oxidative stress in the brain.

- **Areas of inflammation on the vascular wall are sites for plaque formation and plaques have high levels of antioxidants. Further, vascular xenografts, which produce no EMODs, are sites for bacterial vegetation formation.**

- **High glucose levels can suppress EMOD levels and are associated with diabetes, cancer, atherosclerosis, obesity and cataract formation**

- **Physical activity, which increases EMODs 10-15 fold, offers protection against CVD, type 2 diabetes, colorectal cancer, breast cancer, age-related cognitive decline, and all-cause mortality**

- **Hypoxia is a component of most neoplastic growths**

- **Hypoxia is present in the aging prostate and BPH**

- **Hypoxia is associated with metastasis, recurrence and resistance to radiation and chemotherapy**

- **EMOD generating methods, such as irradiation, chemotherapy, PDT, hyperbaric oxygen, the Howes singlet oxygen tumoricidal system, etc. kill cancer cells via prooxidant mechanisms**

- **Antioxidants, such as vitamin E, NAC, and beta carotene, block the killing of neoplastic cells in vitro**

- **Tumor size decreased two-   and threefold in sildenafil-treated (Viagra) animals**

- **The prevalent antioxidant uric acid is directly associated with cardiovascular disease, gout and high levels suppress cognitive function**

- **The antioxidant bilirubin is directly associated with kernicterus and brain damage. In its free state it is one of the most toxic agents known**

Cancer, Apoptosis and Reactive Oxygen Species: A New Paradigm

Showing that a theory has failed is important but it is more important to replace it with an improved alternative. That is what I have done.

Apoptosis or cellular suicide is an important means of eliminating precancerous and cancerous cells from the body. Cellular apoptotic execution is frequently modulated by levels of EMODs serving as the effector stimulus initiating subsequent cellular death. Studies have shown that antioxidants can modify or block apoptosis in many tumorous or neoplastic cell types. Caution should be exercised to prevent creating insufficient EMOD levels and to avoid the injudicious use of antioxidants, especially in subjects with compromised immunity or with cancerous or precancerous conditions. Allowance of cellular proliferation could represent an EMOD insufficiency state and an EMOD insufficiency syndrome may explain clustering or coexistence of common diseases, such as cancer, atherosclerosis, diabetes and obesity. In reality, sufficient prooxidant levels can induce cancer cell apoptosis, which can be blocked or nullified by certain antioxidants (Howes, Philica. Feb 26, 2007) (Manda et al, 2009) (Lopez-Lazaro, 2010).

Total inhibition of oxidant production (free radical production) is predictably going to be detrimental because of the important physiologic roles of reactive oxygen species in regulating the redox state, which is **critical** for cell growth/differentiation (Pani et al, 2000).

Radiation treatments and many chemotherapeutic agents kill cancer by relying on oxidation reactions. This is also true for photodynamic therapy (PDT). The antioxidants can interfere with the apoptotic process causing the cells to live (not to commit suicide) and allowing the cancer to spread by using the resources of the cell.

Dangers of Antioxidants in Cancer Patients: A Review

Many chemotherapeutic agents, radiation therapy and photodynamic therapy kill cancer cells oxidatively, via the production of reactive oxygen species. These EMODs, formerly called oxygen free radicals, play a prominent, if not crucial, role in the induction of apoptotic killing of tumorous cells and pathogens. A long-standing concern with antioxidants is that they could theoretically interfere with the effectiveness of chemotherapy and radiation treatment of cancer. In spite of claims to the contrary, antioxidants can counter the effects of oxygen free radicals and as such, they can protect cells exhibiting metaplasia, dysplasia or neoplasia, allowing them to grow and metastasize.

Significant in vitro data exists showing that antioxidants can block EMOD-induced apoptosis for a wide variety of cancerous cell types, such as leukemia, lymphoma, retinoblastoma, myeloma, pheochromocytoma and human cancers of the breast, lung, pancreas, liver, colon, rectum and endometrium. This data can not be ignored. Commonly used antioxidant vitamins, such as vitamins A, C and E, possess antioxidant qualities. It is concluded that extreme caution should be exercised before recommending antioxidant administration to patients with pre-malignant lesions or in patients with known cancerous growths until this issue is definitively scientifically clarified (Howes, Philica. Feb 7, 2009).

Unlike some critics, I do not believe that the antioxidant vitamins are just "a way to make expensive urine." I believe that they can be inherently harmful but that they can also function usefully as prooxidant precursors. They are "pre-oxidants or co-oxidants." The main problem occurs when antioxidants reduce EMODs to an insufficiency level.

Studies have repeatedly demonstrated the ability of antioxidants to block electronically modified oxygen derivative (EMOD)-activated apoptosis of neoplastic cells. This is especially concerning for individuals predisposed to malignancies, those exposed to carcinogenic agents, those with established cancer or those who may be undergoing chemical or radiation treatment for cancer. Before recommending that individuals take antioxidants for chemoprevention, a better understanding of free radical-mediated biochemistry must be considered. Over supplementation with antioxidants may actually produce an environment that is beneficial to the tumor and allow it to survive.

It has now been proven that EMODs act as secondary cellular messengers and regulate the activity of over 200 transducing proteins and genes necessary to the normal functioning of the human body. Injudicious use of nonspecific antioxidants could modify or harmfully alter any one of these sensitive and essential systems. These EMOD dependent controlling systems range from sperm and ova activities to growth and suicidal cellular death. It is becoming increasingly clear that EMODs are central to the maintenance of a healthful condition.

Antioxidants can block crucial EMOD functions, including sperm and ova function, apoptosis, the respiratory burst, protein translation, phagocytosis and detoxification.

(Salganik, 2001) (Simon et al, 2000) (Kimura et al, 2005).

Excessive antioxidants could dangerously interfere with these protective functions, while temporary depletion of antioxidants can enhance anti-cancer effects of apoptosis. Investigators have recently shown that efficient apoptotic signaling, which is primarily prooxidant induced, tells a cancer cell to kill itself.

Further, the EMOD, hydrogen peroxide (H_2O_2) has a ubiquitous presence in cells and is continuously being generated by the plasma membrane, cytosol and several different sub-cellular organelles including peroxisomes, endoplasmic reticulum, nucleus and by almost 100 enzyme systems (Chance et al, 1979) (Thannical and Fanburg, 2000).

A Great Biochemical Wonder, EMODs

It ranks amongst the greatest biochemical wonders of evolution that the most crucial and widespread small molecular EMODs, which are purportedly the alleged "enemies within" are ever present and essential occupants of the most sensitive intracellular organelle control systems for obligate aerobes. In fact, EMODs, such as hydrogen peroxide, can not be excluded from cells or their intracellular compartments.

The naïve notion that the EMODs are inherently deleterious is counterintuitive to the very basis of the concept of the Darwinian process itself and to sound evolutionary biochemical principles.

Because of public health concerns and the widespread use of antioxidant vitamins, we can no longer ignore these warnings or attempt to explain them away as so-called "paradoxes."

There are no magical antioxidant cures.

We must ask, "How could the magnanimous wisdom of evolution produce a ubiquitous, omnipresent, allegedly highly damaging, powerful, toxic molecule such as hydrogen peroxide, which, by design, is freely mobile and highly permeable through biological membranes enabling its unfettered diffusion out of and within the cell from any intracellular production site?" The logical answer to this query is that peroxide is an essentiality for normal aerobic cellular functioning. By design, it is of low toxicity and allowed access to highly sensitive control areas wherever and whenever it is needed. (Howes, 2010).

In fact, many of the peroxidases and oxidase enzymes can not function without hydrogen peroxide serving as a substrate or co-factor.

Consumer confidence with the antioxidant vitamins is being rapidly eroded as additional randomized controlled trials (RCTs) show their lack of effectiveness or their harmful potential, including their associated risk to increasing mortality. Their effect is a slow, prolonged harmful influence, as opposed to the drop-dead effect of cyanide. (Howes, Philica, April 5, 2007).

Because of public health concerns and the widespread use of antioxidant vitamins, we can no longer ignore these warnings or attempt to explain them away as so-called "paradoxes."

Actually, it is my belief that the oxygen paradox....is resolved!

Antioxidant vitamin recommendations as of 2004

This abstract by Chertow sums up the general over view for the use of antioxidant vitamins as of 2004. These guidelines are still useful in 2010. Basically, if you have a known vitamin deficiency, correct it. If not, be careful.

In general, evidence does not support the use of supplements, and supplements are not recommended unless patients are deficient. Use of vitamins in excess may have adverse effects. Vitamin supplements are indicated in patients deficient in vitamins due to inadequate dietary intake or intestinal disease. Treatment with proper amounts of vitamins and antioxidants is best accomplished with a balanced diet including 3 servings of vegetables and 2 servings of fruits. Regarding supplementation of specific vitamins: carotene cannot be recommended in view of the possible harm and lack of benefit in clinical studies. Vitamin A (retinol) and Vitamin D should be repleted if deficient by laboratory assay. Excesses should be avoided. Vitamin A supplements, particularly in pregnancy, should not exceed 10,000 IU daily or a supplement should not exceed 25,000 units weekly. Vitamin E (alpha-tocopherol) alone in doses of 400 units is of questionable value, and larger doses may cause intracranial hemorrhage or interact negatively with lipid-lowering drugs. Vitamin E should not be used in patients who have bleeding disorders or patients on anticoagulants or acetylsalicylic acid (ASA). Vitamin C (ascorbic acid) losses in urine may be excessive in diabetic patients and may require repletion to 200 mg in nonsmokers and 250 mg in smokers (Chertow, 2004).

As was stated in 2002 by Hasanain and Mooradian, "Given the lack of data to substantiate the benefit and safety of ingestion of antioxidant vitamins in excess of the recommended dietary allowance, physicians should avoid the recommendation of vitamin supplementation to their patients." (Hasanain and Mooradian, 2002).

CHAPTER TWELVE:

Now You Have The Facts, You Decide

I have shown you **181** studies that demonstrate the lack of efficacy for the antioxidant vitamins in treating a wide array of disease conditions. I have also shown you the studies showing the harmful potential of the antioxidant vitamins.

I presented data from **181** scientific, peer reviewed published articles. These studies contained over eight million (8,600,000) participants or subjects. Certainly, there are studies showing miraculous results in disease prevention or reversal with antioxidants but this becomes meaningless when it is deciphered through the filter of the overall data.

There is no consistency of action or results for the antioxidants, whether it be vitamin A, α-carotene, beta-carotene, beta-cryptoxanthin, lycopene, and lutein+zeaxanthin, alpha tocopherol, gamma tocopherol or ascorbic acid.

We do not know the contribution of metal-mediated formation of free radicals (e.g. Fenton chemistry) with iron, copper, chromium, cobalt, vanadium, cadmium, arsenic or nickel. Nor do we know the precise role of antioxidants such as enzymatic antioxidants (superoxide dismutase (Cu, Zn-SOD, Mn-SOD), catalase, glutathione peroxidase, peroxidoreductase) and non-enzymatic antioxidants (Vitamin C, Vitamin E, carotenoids, thiol antioxidants (glutathione, thioredoxin and lipoic acid), flavonoids, selenium and others). Certainly, many of these have multiple biochemical functions other than serving only as an EMOD antagonist. Again, I believe that they may be in many cases serving as "pre-oxidants or co-oxidants" and as assistants in maintaining adequate electron and proton flow. Yet, my basic conclusion is that antioxidant restriction is of more importance for health than is antioxidant supplementation.

Studies utilizing singular biomarkers of oxidative activity yield inconsistent results. I have looked at the results with about 20 different oxidation biomarkers (such as 8-hydroxy-2'-deoxyguanosine (8-OhdG) and 8-iso-prostaglandin-F2alpha (8-iso-PGF2alpha), malonyldialdehyde, etc.) and results do not match between the differing biomarkers. This makes the interpretation of data extremely difficult, especially on articles concerning so-called oxidative stress or antioxidant capacity. If the various markers do not match or yield comparable results, how can they be useful? What are they measuring? Does any body really know?

Even though oral supplementation of vitamin C (ascorbic acid) and vitamin E (D-alfa-tocopherol acetate) alone and in combination have been shown to decrease oxidative DNA damage in animal studies in vivo, in vitro, and in situ, this has not been supported in human clinical trials or RCTs. The studies in humans are the most important of all. So what if they reduce cancer or heart disease in a rodent? We need to know how they affect human health and their potential for disease prevention. Thus far, they have been an uber-disappointment (failure).

In theory, the antioxidants are supposed to donate an electron to oxygen. In doing so, the antioxidant becomes itself a weaker oxidizing free radical and it awaits being recharged by another antioxidant (e.g., vitamin C can be recharged by alpha lipoic acid and glutathione and vitamin C can recharge vitamin E). Thus, I believe that antioxidants may serve a useful purpose as "pre-oxidants or co-oxidants" and aid in maintaining homeostatic electron and proton flow. Electron and proton flow creates and supports the electromagnetic forces essential for life survival. Further, I believe that the primary purpose of antioxidants is not to wipe out EMODs, for to do so, would kill all aerobic cells and organisms. Such a scenario would be counter to evolutionary principles and biochemical mechanisms.

In conclusion, careful attention should be given to the nearly 40 year time period covered by the studies I have presented. The overall data demonstrates the confusion and inconsistencies associated with antioxidant studies. However, conclusive statements can now be made about the unnecessary use of dietary antioxidants, their potential to do harm and the fact that synthetic vitamin supplements can not replace natural vitamins from fresh fruit and vegetables. Yet, they may have a role in establishing a redox balance in the body or serving as pre-oxidants and in maintaining electron and proton flow, while serving as co-oxidants. We must remember that the small molecular weight antioxidants are non-specific in their reactivity and that this feature likely means that they can interfere with vital oxidative metabolic events. In that regard, they would best be viewed in a new light as "pre-oxidants or co-oxidants" and in need of regulation.

There are no magical antioxidant cures.

The take-home message is that the antioxidant vitamins have unsubstantiated benefits and known potential to do harm!

Even fruit and vegetable benefits have come under fire

It has been said that, "Dietary fruits and vegetables provide a reasonable amount of compounds that act as physiological antioxidants." (Herrera et al, 2009).

Yet, even this bit of assumed sage advise is coming under scrutiny. In 2010, a study of over 500,000 Europeans in the Journal of the National Cancer Institute has found that **eating more fruit and vegetables has only a modest effect on protecting against cancer. The studies failed to substantiate the suggestion that as many as 50% of cancers could be prevented by boosting the public's consumption of fruit and vegetables and the researchers estimated that only around 2.5% of cancers could be averted by increasing their fruit and vegetable intake.**

In a companion editorial, **Harvard Professor Walter Willet said that this research strongly confirmed the findings of other studies, showing "that any association of intake and fruits and vegetables with risk of cancer is weak at best".**

What more do you need to know?
STUDY RESULTS IN 21st CENTURY
Supplements and synthetic vitamins
do not substitute for a healthy diet
and 60 scientific reports have shown that
they increase the risk of diseases,
including cancer, heart disease, diabetes, stroke, etc.
and overall mortality.

Should we just wait for the body count to climb? Please remember that the effects of antioxidants will be incremental and ever so gradual and not instantaneous, as seen with cyanide. You are not going to immediately keel over graveyard dead if you take one but life-shortening events may be gradually occurring. We could be witnessing a slow poisoning of the population, accompanied by a weakening of their immune systems and the creation of EMOD insufficiencies, both of which make individuals more susceptible to disease and neoplasia. We must acknowledge the current data, indicating their harmful potential and ignore the extravagant claims of pushers of antioxidants and supplement profiteers.

In David Michaels' book, *Doubt is Their Product: How Industry's Assault on Science Threatens Your Health*, he makes a quote that is applicable to those who defend the antioxidant vitamin supplement industry. His approach is somewhat applicable to the antioxidant vitamin issue. Michaels states, "They profit by helping corporations minimize public health and environmental protection and fight claims of injury and illness. In field after field, year after year, this same handful of individuals and companies comes up again and again... They have on their payrolls (or can bring in on a moment's notice) toxicologists, epidemiologists, biostatisticians, risk assessors, and any other professionally trained, media-savvy experts deemed necessary. They and the larger, wealthier industries for which they work go through the motions we expect of the scientific enterprise, salting the literature with their questionable reports and studies. Nevertheless, it is all a charade. The work has one overriding motivation: advocacy for the sponsor's position in civil court, the court of public opinion, and the regulatory arena [where these studies benefit their sponsors] not because they are good work that the regulatory agencies have to take seriously but because they clog the machinery and slow down the process. Public health interests are beside the point. Follow the science wherever it leads? Not quite. This is science for hire, period, and it is extremely lucrative."

The food industry and the vitamin supplement industry are now being influenced by the pharmaceutical industry. The injudicious use of antioxidant vitamins by such a large portion of the population is, indeed, a significant public health issue. Antioxidant vitamin pushers can deny the truth but they can not change the truth. Fortification of foods with antioxidants, which have harmful potential, constitutes an unprecedented, global, human experiment.

If these antioxidant vitamins have the claimed potent pharmacologic activity ascribed to them, some body had better be watching their long term effects with extreme care.

Foods reportedly contain over 20,000 different antioxidants, which can not be safely replaced by a handful of synthetic antioxidant vitamins. The antioxidant vitamins should be reserved for those with a specific and proven vitamin deficiency. Otherwise, save your money and perhaps save your health and your life.

Antioxidant vitamins have lacked predictive validity and have failed to demonstrate consistently beneficial results but have shown untoward or null effects on health promotion and disease prevention. Their therapeutic value in disease treatment is, at best, dubious.

In fact, relative to cancer, current investigators say that, "The prospects for cancer prevention through micronutrient supplementation have never looked worse, micronutrient supplementation may be harmful and that the likelihood that micronutrient supplementation will be included in any public health policy for cancer control has become vanishingly small."

Others have cautioned that, "The recent announcement of early termination of the Selenium and Vitamin E Cancer Prevention Trial's (SELECT) interventions because of lack of efficacy and observation of possible adverse events (i.e., small and not statistically significant increases in type 2 diabetes in those receiving selenium alone and in prostate cancer incidence in the vitamin E (alone) group) should serve as a reminder that the unexpected can happen in these well-designed trials." (Lippman et al, 2009)

The ATBC study, the CARET study and the SELECT studies were all shut down early, due to the obvious fact that the antioxidant agents being tested were causing alarming and unexpected harmful adverse effects.

Now that you have the facts, you decide!

ANTIOXIDANT VITAMINS ARE MAKING A KILLING

These findings need repeating one final time and were taken directly from the data and are the results of scientific studies and not from unsupported opinions.

Antioxidant vitamins can lead to increased risk of:

- lung cancer;
- breast cancer;
- prostate cancer;
- head and neck cancer;
- oral pre-malignant lesions;
- total mortality;
- likelihood of dying by about 5 percent;
- esophageal cancer deaths;
- adenoma recurrence in smokers and drinkers;
- post-trial risk of first-ever non-fatal Myocardial Infarction;
- hemorrhagic stroke deaths;
- increased total and stroke mortality;
- ischemic heart disease deaths;
- deaths from fatal coronary heart disease;
- cardiovascular disease mortality in postmenopausal women with diabetes;
- total fracture;
- hip fracture;
- osteoporotic hip fractures in men and women;
- accelerate the progression of retinitis pigmentosa;
- hospitalization for heart failure;
- heart failure incidence;
- Mother-to-child transmission of HIV;
- rate of low-birth-weight babies;
- rate for gestational hypertension;
- suffered falling more often;
- E supplementation increased tuberculosis and pneumonia risk;
- higher risk of age-related cataract among women;

- vitamin E results in loss of quality-adjusted life years
- increase in the incidence of cancer among smokers and increased cancer mortality
- Multivitamin/Minerals associated with doubling in the risk of fatal prostate cancer
- increase in intima-media thickness over time
- rate of local recurrence of the head and neck tumor tended to be higher
- higher rate of second primary head and neck cancers
- worsening of coronary atherosclerosis in those with two copies of the haptoglobin 2   gene
- promote the clogging of arteries;
- accelerated thickening of the walls
- higher mortality rate in men
- adverse mucocutaneous effects and serum triglyceride elevations
- cardiac arrhythmias (probucol)
- negated the benefit of cholesterol lowering drugs
- negatively associated with skeletal health
- decreased sperm motility
- induced sperm DNA damage

An insidious threat to their overall well being

There is good scientific reasoning to believe that the antioxidant vitamins A and E and to a lesser degree, C, (and even selenium) are capable of causing adverse effects, that they can cause serious diseases, which will shorten one's life and that they may directly, albeit slowly, hasten one's demise. I cite 60 such studies showing harmful outcomes to support this view. To deny the crucial role of prooxidant EMODs in normal metabolic processes and disease protection is to deny scientific truth and its related teachings.

Please remember my previously quoted caveat concerning long time follow up on subjects in the CARET study: "A 6-year follow-up of a large, randomized trial in people with a history of smoking has found that the overall harm associated with beta-carotene supplementation on cardiovascular disease mortality disappeared quickly after participants stopped taking the supplements. However, **the risk of lung cancer may persist**, especially in females and former smokers, according to the study in the December 1, 2004 issue of the Journal of the National Cancer Institute. Gary E. Goodman, M.D., of the Fred Hutchinson Cancer Research Center in Seattle, and colleagues followed the more than 18,000 participants in CARET for 6 years after the trial was stopped, until the end of 2001. The increased risk of cardiovascular disease mortality quickly disappeared after participants stopped taking the supplements. However, women had a higher risk of death from cardiovascular disease or from any cause than men. In addition, the incidence of lung cancer and deaths from all causes decreased but **did not disappear completely after the supplementation ceased.** The excess risk of lung cancer was restricted primarily to females and former smokers. The results of CARET and ATBC emphasize that chemoprevention trials require careful monitoring of all disease endpoints ... even after the study intervention is discontinued." (Goodman et al, 2004)

When considered in its totality, my review presents a compelling argument that antioxidant vitamins have considerable proven potential to do harm. In the absence of vitamin deficiency states, one should consider refraining from the injudicious use of antioxidant vitamins, especially if you are undergoing cancer therapy. Even considering the glowing profiteer testimonials regarding the antioxidant vitamins, there is an obligation to bring these possible antioxidant dangers to the attention of the general public and to create an awareness of the increased potential risk of developing cardiovascular disease, cancer, strokes and overall mortality by the unsupervised and imprudent use of antioxidant vitamins.

I believe that the sheer volume of the scientific studies, to date, is such that it constitutes a growing legal liability for those pushing these potentially dangerous products on the general public and **an insidious threat to their overall well being**. Before purchasing antioxidant vitamins, remember the old admonition, "Caveat emptor (buyer beware)." Be very aware of what you are doing to your body!

Antioxidant Vitamins Are Making A Killing:

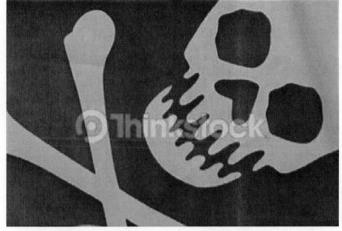

Invalidation and Nullification of the Free Radical Theory

**Vitamins A, C and E
Negligible Results, Half Truths and Potential Harm
As Demonstrated by Failed Intervention Trials**

BOOK TWO:
ANTIOXIDANT VITAMIN STUDIES
FOR THE MEDICAL SCIENTIST

BY

PROF. HON. RANDOLPH M. HOWES, M.D., Ph.D.
Orthomolecular Surgical Scientist and Biochemist
R.M. Howes © 2010

Antioxidant Vitamins Are Making A Killing:

Antioxidant Vitamins A, C & E in the 21st Century

**Vitamins A, C and E
Negligible Results, Half Truths and Potential Harm
As Demonstrated by Failed Intervention Trials**

**Invalidation & Nullification of the Free Radical Theory
A Selective Review**

A HEALTH IMPACT STATEMENT

BY

PROF. HON. RANDOLPH M. HOWES, M.D., Ph.D.

Orthomolecular Surgical Scientist and Biochemist

Adjunct Assistant Professor of Plastic Surgery, The Johns Hopkins Hospital, Baltimore, Md., U.S.A., Espaldon Professor of Plastic and Reconstructive Surgery, University of Santo Tomas, Manila, Philippines. Adjunct Professor of Biological Sciences, Southeastern Louisiana University, Hammond, La., U.S.A.

Founder, Director and Chairman of the Scientific Advisory Board;

U.S. Medical and Scientific Research Foundation, Inc.

Table of contents:

BOOK TWO:

CHAPTER ONE:

The Flawed Free Radical Theory

Many authors have stated that, "In the past several years, unprecedented progress has been made in the recognition and understanding of roles of reactive oxygen species in many diseases. These include atherosclerosis, vasospasms, cancers, trauma, stroke, asthma, hyperoxia, arthritis, heart attack, age pigments, dermatitis, cataractogenesis, retinal damage, hepatitis, liver injury, and periodontitis, which are age related." (Lee, Koo and Min, 2004).

Unfortunately, **they have implied a cause and effect relationship between reactive oxygen species (ROS) and over 100 diseases. Now, some authors say over 200 diseases are caused by ROS, actually it is as many diseases as they can think of, including aging.** I do not agree with their assessment and a review of the literature will clearly reveal that the evidence linking these conditions to reactive oxygen species is **merely circumstantial**. Proof is lacking. Misinterpretation of the data is common place. Data is confusing and contradictory, such that arriving at scientific proof is impossible, and following the faint truth-trail, in search for the scientific Holy Grail of cellular biochemical reality, is rife with difficulty. **Separating "fact from factitious" has become increasingly challenging.**

Large scale clinical trials in the 20th and early 21st century reached differing conclusions concerning many diseases and about the effects of antioxidants on a host of these diseases, including cancer and cardiovascular disease. **Conclusions were spread all over the scientific smorgasbord. Predictability of results was no where to be found.**

It is not necessary to prove things which are obvious, such as "everything ages." Whether one is a learned scientist, doctor, Croesus, soothsayer, president, farmer or housewife, we basically live to about the same age. It is not necessary to "prove" this, because all one has to do is simply look around. This is substantiated by actuarial tables.

In spite of vitamin and dietary supplement ingestion by some estimates of almost 60% of the USA population, **we are still experiencing an epidemic in cancer and heart disease**. We have had 50 years to apply the teachings of the free radical theory of oxidative stress and aging and they have failed to ward off or cure the diseases of present day man. Books with flamboyant titles, such as "Stop Aging Now" by Jean Carper and "Live Now, Age Later" by Isadore Rosenfeld, M.D, have misled the general population into believing that vitamins, antioxidants and dietary supplements can stop the aging process and prevent or reverse the diseases which commonly affect mankind. To this I say, **"Stop Jean Carper Now."** This ole' gal is making a fortune off of these vitamin supplements and grinning all the way to the bank. Just check out her website.

Enter The Lamentable Free Radical theory

Free radicals have been vilified and oxygen radicals have especially been belittled.

Harman called the products of oxygen metabolism "toxic." Here is the definition of toxic:

TOXIC tox·ic 1. **involving something poisonous** 2. **deadly: causing serious harm or death** Encarta ® World English Dictionary 2005.

ANGELINA JOLIE AND BRUCE AMES

Harman is saying that oxygen and its metabolic products (free radicals) are deadly and/or even lethal. In fact, not only is oxygen a radical, it is a diradical. Many authors horrifyingly emphasize oxygen's radical character and state that it is the very substance which is killing us, by causing a multitude of diseases and aging. This has been especially promoted by biochemist Dr. Bruce Ames, who has turned this concept into a **cash cow** by selling a product called Juvenon.

Angelina Jolie's suprapubic tattoo states, *"Quod me nutrit me destruit"* - "That which nourishes me, destroys me".

Antioxidant biochemist, Bruce Ames' quote states, "The ultimate irony: The thing we need most to live, oxygen, is what's killing us."

Great minds run in the same path! Ames pushes the product, Juvenon.

Juvenon advertisements have large headlines which state, "POSTPONE CELLULAR AGING. JUVENON: The Supplement That Can Slow Down the Clock On Aging Cells." A disclaimer in micro-script at the bottom of the page states," The statements made here have not been evaluated by the FDA. **The product is not intended to diagnose, treat, cure or prevent any disease.**" Ames considers aging a disease. I vehemently oppose this type of hype and speculation. These theories do not even hold up to Gumpian (as in Forest) analysis.

The Free Radical Fairy Tale

**Extraordinary theories necessitate
extraordinary proof.
The free radical theory is falsified by a glut of
non-supportive, paradoxical, conflicting, confusing,
inconclusive evidence and a modicum of
supportive documentation.
It exhibits
extreme vulnerability as regards
its logicality.
R. M. Howes, M.D., Ph.D.
11/15/06**

Denham Harman and his sycophants (or what I call sick-o-phants) believe that oxygen and its EMODs are inherently toxic and responsible for the myriad of human diseases and aging. However, logically neither oxygen free radicals nor EMODs can be highly toxic. First, we are bathed in and continually breathe in and transport ground state triplet diradical oxygen from the air (21% or one in five molecules in the air is a diradical oxygen molecule) across the alveolar membrane and into waiting oxygen-hungry red blood cell. This occurs from the time of fetal development until our last breath.

EMODs Are Crucial Cellular Controlling Agents

EMOD (redox) CONTROL (signaling, regulation)
EMODs regulate vital pathways i.e., energy metabolism, survival/ stress responses, apoptosis, inflammatory response, oxygen sensing, redox homeostasis, fertilization, survival kinase activation, ion channel regulation, apoptosis signaling, preconditioning, necrosis, inflammatory system, regulation of vascular tone, the activity of HIF (hypoxia inducible factor) etc.

Let me give you a basic axiom: if you do not breathe, you are going to die. Without oxygen, you are going to die. It is that simple.

Ground state triplet oxygen is not only a free radical, but it is a diradical and is essential for sustaining the life of all aerobic organisms, inclusive of humans. That, alone, invalidates the free radical theory. If you care to test the essentiality of diradical oxygen, simply stop breathing for about 5 minutes and we will continue our discussion. Any takers?

O_2 is present in the human body in quantities exceeding that of all other elements combined. Any compound present in such high concentrations and continuously being taken into and carried throughout the entirety of the body can hardly be considered "toxic." Dictionary definition of "toxic" reads, "Involving something poisonous; deadly." Thus, if oxygen were truly toxic, we would all be dead but we are not and many people live to be centenarians, all the while consuming huge quantities of oxygen.

Basically, we breathe in and cycle about a pint of air with each breath and we repeat this about 21,600 times in a day, 7,884,000 times a year and 551,880,000 times in the lifetime for a 70 year old.... **at rest!** This calculates out to almost 70 million gallons of ground state oxygen. This observation begs the question, "How toxic can oxygen really be?" Clearly, if there is any oxygen toxicity, it must be extremely low, if at all, or no aerobes would survive. The whole oxygen free radical story is truly a fairy tale, with even less credibility than Peter Pan.

It is readily conceivable that a person who exercises a lot, could inhale 100 million gallons of diradical oxygen in a life time, because exercise increases oxygen consumption 10-15X that of a resting state.

Sure, there are free radicals and true, I can make them wreak havoc in the chemistry lab. But, the living/breathing human cell compartmentalizes, controls and exquisitely regulates their biochemical activity. Thus, the proposed widespread cellular destruction does not occur in the living/breathing cell.

CHAPTER TWO:

Exercise Should Kill Us

NO WANTON EMOD DESTRUCTION

In 2000, expert Barry Halliwell said, "As opposed to earlier concepts, ROS (EMODs) interaction with proteins does not invariably lead to irreversible oxidative damage. H_2O_2 is poorly reactive: it can act as a mild oxidizing or as a mild reducing agent, but it does not oxidize most biological molecules readily, including lipids, DNA and proteins, especially in the absence of transition metal ions."

During metabolism for energy production, EMODs are copiously generated in steady state levels and are markedly increased with health-rendering exercise. Ergo, EMODs must be of extremely low toxicity, if at all toxic, in the living/breathing organism or **exercise would kill us**. In fact, lactic acid builds up when an athlete competes at a pace that exceeds the body's capacity to bring in enough oxygen to burn fuel aerobically. If a runner stops all movement, circulation slows and the body retains lactic acid and an acidic environ even further increases EMOD production. Additionally, antioxidant vitamins have been shown to negate the health benefits of exercise.

Dr Michael Ristow, from the University of Jena in Germany, and colleagues wrote in the 2009 journal Proceedings of the National Academy of Sciences: "We find that antioxidant supplements prevent the induction of molecular regulators of insulin sensitivity and endogenous antioxidant defense by physical exercise." In other words, the **antioxidant vitamins C and E can "undo" the benefits of exercise, weaken the body's own exercise-induced free radical defense system** and increase the risk of diabetes by decreasing insulin sensitivity (Ristow et al, 2009).

In 2007, Ivor Benjamin of the University of Utah, found the first bona fide example of the role that reductive stress can play in disease. Mice with one of the mutant genes, áB-crystallin, specifically in the heart develop the same symptoms seen in human patients, including heart enlargement, progressive heart failure, and an early death. They further show that the animals' hearts are under reductive stress. They found the mice had "markedly reduced" oxidative stress levels due to an abundance of a natural antioxidant known as glutathione, producing excess levels of the reduced glutathione and a condition of **reductive stress**. This supports my ROSI syndrome (Reactive Oxygen Species Insufficiency) (Howes, 2009) and my Unified Theory (Howes, 2004).

In short, EMODs have pervasive distribution and steady state levels in all aerobic cells, tissues and organs. Basically, EMODs are everywhere. Ergo, they must be of low toxicity and crucial for normal homeostatic cellular functioning. Again, in April of 2008, I spoke with Dr. Denham Harman and re-emphasized my belief that his free radical theory was and is invalid. He suggests that his work has led investigators, like me, to look for the real answers for disease and aging causation. He applauded my diligence and efforts in trying to further clarify the role of EMODs in health and disease. We remain good friends and I visited him on April 5th of 2010, but…..

Dr. Harman, "How could so many have been so wrong for so long?" R. M. Howes, M.D., Ph.D. 6/6/06

Perpetually repeated false impressions (i.e., regurgitated lies) have led to the acceptance of flawed theories and disproved hypotheses. Yet, the inaccuracies and the theories, relative to oxygen free radicals, appear to live on and they are now, more than ever, erroneously referred to in the scientific literature as proven facts. Sadly, the free radical theory of oxidative stress and aging seems to be indelibly tattooed into the frontal lobes of the minds of current medical scientists, who have accepted and embellished this fairy tale rumor with the zeal of a child embracing the perceived reality of Snow White, Mickey Mouse and Jolly Old St. Nick.

The unrestricted promotion and unrestrained advertising of antioxidants as therapeutic agents are inappropriate and misleading because their efficacy is unproven, their toxicology is uncertain and their potential for harm is mounting. Today's antioxidant marketing promotes unsubstantiated benefits and tries to equate the effectiveness of synthetic antioxidant vitamins with those obtained from fresh fruits and vegetables in the maintenance of overall health. There are currently no known "magical cures" as regards antioxidant vitamins, unless one has a known and specific vitamin deficiency.

The current rage is to combat "harmful oxygen free radicals" but there is little in the lay press to document the many crucial areas of activity of the electronically modified oxygen derivatives (EMODs). In fact, I believe that the family of prooxidant EMODs act synergistically to sustain health and to protect us from pathogens and neoplasia. The scientific data backs up my position (www.iwillfindthecure.org).

INEXTRICABLE EMODs

The two most critical energy-generating processes of life, photosynthesis and oxygen respiration, inextricably involve EMOD participation and interactions. You can go without food for a few weeks, without water for a few days but you can only go for a few minutes without oxygen. There is nothing with a greater evolutionary effect or influence on human survival than oxygen.

Likewise, I believe that antioxidants can work synergistically with EMODs to maintain electron and proton flow. It would make no sense to completely wipe out either group. They are flip sides of the same oxidation/reduction (redox) coin.

Actually, I believe that many of the antioxidants serve as "pre-oxidants or co-oxidants." This is a new concept which I am introducing. Once they give up an electron, they go in search of another electron because they have now turned into an oxidant themselves.

Yes, I have been quoted saying that, **"If the free radical theory had been a horse, it would now be glue."** Additionally, I have pointed out numerous times that the free radical theory has been invalidated because, for over half a century, it has lacked predictability and therefore fails to meet the criteria of the scientific method. It is invalid. Get it? Invalid! Please, can we move on? This is not a matter of opinion, it is a matter of scientific fact.

In a JAMA 2007 study, it was shown that, "Health claims from observational data can persist long after being debunked in randomized controlled trials (RCTs). Observational studies may take on a life of their own in the literature, hanging on even after they have been discredited by randomized controlled trials (Tatsioni et al, 2007).

Epidemiological and observational erroneous conclusions may continue to inexplicably be supported in certain so-called scientific circles as a means of securing grants or supporting specialties or reputations. For example, favorable observational citations to beta-carotene and vitamin E persisted long after RCT evidence contradicted their effectiveness and it was as though the authors did not consider the contradicting evidence. Tatsioni et al. concluded that, **"Claims from highly cited observational studies persist and continue to be supported in the medical literature despite strong contradictory evidence from randomized trials."**

This "persistence of contradicted claims in the literature" has helped perpetuate the nullified free radical theory. Unproven theories must be abandoned and replaced by better theories, which more precisely fit the data. My theory of "Reactive oxygen species insufficiency as the basis of disease allowance and coexistence" fulfills that goal (Howes, 2009). It is hard to correct or stop the momentum of a good lie.

Denham Harman: The First (well, nearly the first) Oxy-moron

In *Science* in 1954, Rebeca Gerschman and her colleagues first introduced the notion that free radicals are toxic agents. Gerschman published a paper entitled, "Oxygen poisoning and X-irradiation: a mechanism in common." This paper led to some supposed link between oxygen free radicals, products of radiation and cellular damage. Later this was used as the mud bed upon which the free radical theory of aging and oxidative stress would be built. In 1956, along came Dr. Denham Harman, who proposed the free radical theory and a little later, he whipped up the free radical theory of aging. For oxygen, things have not been the same since. The free radical theory of aging simply argues that aging results from the accumulated damage generated over time by EMODs (oxygen free radicals) (Harman, 1956).

Harman's theory stated that diseases and the aging process resulted from the "stochastic" or randomly accumulated damage caused by EMODs (reactive oxygen species, ROS), most of which are crucial components of normal cellular metabolism (Harman, 1981) (Beckman and Ames, 1998) (Finkel and Holbrook, 2000) (Balaban et al, 2005).

EMODs were defined as being deleterious and harmful. The investigators' approach was as simple as one, two and three:

1. Electronically modified oxygen derivatives (EMODs) were believed to be harmful and they were accused of causing over 100 pathophysiologies.
2. Antioxidants would therefore nullify or negate the effects of these deleterious EMODs.
3. Based on Harman's free radical theory, diseases, such as cancer, atherosclerosis and diabetes (including aging), would be reversed, prevented or cured by the judicious use of antioxidants.

It now appears that, contrary to most doom and gloom formulations of the free radical theory of aging, which argue EMODs are flying all over the place and uncontrolled and thus cause wanton damage that accumulates with age, EMODs are under strict metabolic control. In fact, a compartmentalization of oxidative events appears to exist in terms of physiological stimuli, signaling mechanisms, and functional consequences, clearly demonstrating that EMODs are crucial and constructively functional in all aerobic cells.

In the studies testing the validity of the free radical theory, paradoxes are pervasive in the free radical literature. If something does not fit the free radical theory, call it a "paradox," ignore it and move on. Oh, if life were so simple.

Authors have been reluctant to accept experimental results which were contrary to the dogma of the free radical theory. However, assuming the invalidity of the free radical theory eliminates many so-called paradoxes and offers a level of understanding that was hitherto unavailable.

Radicophobes can ignore the truth or
they can reject the truth but
they can not change the magnificent truths
regarding the crucial role
of EMODs in the life process
of all aerobes
or the inherent splendor of oxygen.
R. M. Howes M.D., Ph.D.
1/26/09

The notion that antioxidants could theoretically reduce disease occurrence or be curative, have been pushed by zealots and was based on the flawed free radical theory. Denham Harman believed that oxygen free radicals produced harmful oxidation products, which randomly accumulated with aging, and they were allegedly responsible for over 100 diseases and aging (Harman, 2000).

Previously, this theory had been extended to particularly apply to redox damage occurring within the mitochondrion (Harman, 1972).

The free radical theory had predicted that the DNA of the mitochondrion (mtDNA) is especially vulnerable to oxidative damage because it is one of the primary sites for the production of oxygen free radicals within the cell and it has low antioxidative defenses. The mitochondrion lacks catalase and does not have histones to protect its DNA, as does nuclear DNA (nDNA). Since 1988 several research groups (including Barry Halliwell's group) had reported greater levels of oxidative damage in mitochondrial DNA than in nuclear DNA, while others had suggested that the greater damage in mtDNA might be due to artifactual oxidation.

However, the popular theory that mtDNA is more heavily damaged *in vivo* than nDNA **does not stand on firm ground**. Using an improved GC-MS method and pure mtDNA, Halliwell's analyses revealed that **the**

damage level in mtDNA is not higher, and may be somewhat lower, than that in nDNA (Lim et al, 2005). If so, the mitochondrial theory of aging is wrong.

Inherent in the free radical theory was the concept that the harmful effects of oxidation and accumulated oxidized products could be diminished or alleviated by the sensible use of antioxidants. Although there was initially widespread enthusiasm for the antioxidant studies, it has become apparent, that **the overall analysis of the data had failed to conclusively validate or confirm the free radical theory.** In fact, more than fifty years of investigations has revealed the invalidity of the free radical theory, due to its failure to predict repeatable scientific outcomes attributable to the use of antioxidants.

The dream of stopping the aging process or of wiping out hordes of diseases, with the use of antioxidants, has turned into a meta-analysis nightmare for the sycophants of the free radical theory. Even worse for believers in the free radical theory, RCTs have been revealing the potential dangers associated with antioxidant use.

Even a cursory review of the overall literature shows that **the free radical theory lacks predictability** and is basically a meaningless and confusing approach. **Observations and predictions are neither logical nor predictable.**

Patients treated with antioxidants should have predictably decreased the incidence and increased protection against cancer, arteriosclerosis and cataracts. This did not happen and there are strong indicators that **harm** may be done by ingestion of these same antioxidants, including an increased risk of these same diseases that they were supposed to cure. From now on, **investigators are going to have to deal with the fact that the free radical theory has been proven to be wrong and they need to stop trying to force the data to fit a flawed theory.**

Established rules dictate that scientific studies be used to determine if a theory is valid or invalid. The free radical theory does not fulfill the criteria of the scientific method and has been invalidated, over and over again.

Unless the free radical theory can explain the inconsistencies and failures of antioxidant supplements, in the prevention or cure of aging and diseases attributable to oxygen free radicals, the theory is passé. Enough said.

Electronically modified oxygen derivatives, (EMODs, aka, ROS) and antioxidants are conceivably potentially double-edged swords in disease prevention, allowance and promotion. Whereas generation of EMODs once was considered as damaging to overall health, continued research has shown that EMODs play critical and essential roles in normal physiological processes including response to growth factors, the immune response, and apoptotic elimination of damaged cells (cancer kill).

Actually, nearly all compounds of the body can be either detrimental or beneficial, dependent upon whether or not they are in the right amounts, in the right places and at the right times. For decades, extreme and unjustified scrutiny has focused on EMODs. Now it is time to take an equally critical look at the common antioxidants, vitamins A, C & E.

On an April 2010 trip to lecture at Creighton Medical School, Dr. Robert C. Allen and I visited with Dr. Denham Harman. Upon entering his office, he was seen reading my book, UTOPIA, he looked up and said, "I was looking for the place where you called me the first oxy-moron." I replied, "Yes sir, that was me. It's in there." We had a good laugh and a great visit. He further stated that, "Your book is loaded with information."

Actually, we have been friends for many years, irrespective of our conflicting personal beliefs on oxygen metabolism. Further, I would never personally disrespect this fine 93 year old scholar.

CHAPTER THREE:

Early Support For The Antioxidant Vitamins

"Old Data" Lauds Antioxidants

Newspaper headlines at the New York Times, in 1979 read as follows: "Cancer-Blocking Agents Found in Foods; Origin of New Techniques." Antioxidants were touted as newly discovered cancer cures.

"Old data" from epidemiologic and prospective cohort studies of **antioxidants and heart disease rates amply appeared to support the preventive role of antioxidants** in heart disease. Some of these studies were as follows:

"Vitamin E consumption and the risk of coronary heart disease in men." (Male health professionals study) (Rimm et al, 1993)

"Antioxidant vitamin intake and coronary mortality in a longitudinal population study."(National Health and Nutrition Examination Survey-I) (Knekt et al, 1994)

"Vitamin E consumption and the risk of coronary disease in women."(Nurses' Health Study) (Stampfer et al, 1993)

"The Scottish Heart Health Study. Dietary intake by food frequency questionnaire and odds ratios for coronary heart disease risk. II. The antioxidant vitamins and fibre."(Scottish Heart Health Study) (Bolton-Smith et al, 1992)

"Inverse correlation between plasma vitamin E and mortality from ischemic heart disease in cross-cultural epidemiology."(World Health Organization cross-cultural study) (Gey et al, 1991)

However, these types of studies can show only an associative, not a causative, relationship between antioxidant consumption and reduced rates of heart disease.

As of 1997, everything looked rosy, regarding supplements and cancer. Patterson et al's report reviewed published epidemiologic research on the associations of vitamin and mineral supplementation with cancer risk and stated the following: "Although the literature on nutrition and cancer is vast, few reports to date have addressed supplemental nutrients directly (seven clinical trials, 16 cohort, and 36 case-control studies). These studies offer insight into effects of nutrients that are distinguishable from effects of other biologically active compounds in foods. Randomized clinical trials have not shown significant protective effects of beta-carotene, but have found protective effects of: alpha-tocopherol against prostate cancer; mixtures of retinol/zinc and beta-carotene/alpha-tocopherol/selenium against stomach cancer; and selenium against total, lung, and prostate cancers. Cohort studies provide little evidence that vitamin supplements are associated with cancer. Case-control studies have reported an inverse association between bladder cancer and vitamin C; oral/pharyngeal cancer and several supplemental vitamins; and several cancers and vitamin E. A randomized clinical trial, a cohort study, and a case-control study have all found inverse associations between colon cancer and vitamin E. Overall, there is modest evidence for protective effects of nutrients from supplements against several cancers. Future studies of supplement use and cancer appear warranted; however, methodologic problems that impair ability to assess supplement use and statistical modeling of the relation between cancer risk and supplement use need attention." (Patterson et al, 2007)

Initial Antioxidant Optimistic Studies

Linxian (Chinese) Cancer Prevention Study Country:China;   Study Type: Primary prevention; randomized, double-blind, placebo-controlled intervention; The results showed that a combination of beta-carotene, vitamin E and selenium **significantly reduced** incidence of both gastric and cancer and cancer overall. A randomized study of **29,584 residents in rural China over a 5-year period reported no significant benefit of vitamin C supplements in reducing cardiovascular mortality.** [9%

lower total mortality; 13% reduction in cancer mortality; 21% decrease in stomach cancer mortality; no significant reduction in total or CV mortality] (Blot et al, 1993).

These impressive results have not been duplicated in later studies and raise serious doubt about their validity.

A World Health Organization cross-cultural study, which surveyed 12 different populations in Europe, showed a significantly lower rate of cardiac death in groups with high dietary intake of vitamin C or vitamin E.

Independent studies from Finland and the United States also demonstrated similar beneficial effects of a diet rich in antioxidants, including vitamins C and E, beta carotene, and selenium (Luoma et al, 1995) (Verlangieri et al, 1985).

Supplemental vitamin C claimed to prevent disease and saves lives. Unbelievably, just 500 mg daily resulted in a 42 percent lower risk of death from heart disease and a 35 percent lower risk of death from any cause (Enstrom et al, 1992).

More **confusion** was added with the **Scottish Heart Health Study**, which reported **significant benefits from vitamins C and E and beta carotene but only in men**; no benefit was observed in women (Bolton-Smith et al, 1992).

Yet, even more confusion soon set in. Outcomes of prospective cohort studies were inconsistent. **The Nurses' Health Study,** which surveyed more than **88,000 women over an 8-year period**, showed that women who consumed the highest amount of vitamin E for more than 2 years, in both diet and supplements, had a much lower risk of heart disease compared with those who took the lowest amount. However, **use of vitamin C and beta carotene supplements did not lead to any reduction in heart disease risk**. A similar study involving nearly **40,000 male** health professionals showed risk reductions of up to 40% in men with the highest vitamin E intakes. Use of beta carotene supplements led to smaller reductions in risk but only in smokers. **No benefit was shown for vitamin C supplements** (Rimm et al, 1993).

On the other hand, **the first National Health and Nutrition Examination Survey (NHANES)** reported a **significantly lower risk of cardiovascular death in persons with high intakes of vitamin C.** This study, however, did not take into consideration other antioxidants that the study participants might have consumed in addition to vitamin C (Knekt et al, 1994).

A number of observational studies reported that certain dietary patterns are associated with positive health outcomes. For example, **diets high in fruits and vegetables, low-fat dairy products, or whole grains had been associated with decreased risk of heart disease, blood pressure, and cancer** (Ness and Powles, 1997) (Law and Morris, 1998) (Appel et al, 1997) (Sacks et al, 2001) (Bazzano et al, 2002) (Hu et al, 2000) (Strandhgen et al, 2000) (Steinmetz and Potter, 1996).

Yet, as already discussed, **single nutrients or a combination of nutrients such as beta carotene, vitamins C and E, folate, and fiber, which are contained in the foods associated with beneficial effects in both observation and intervention studies, had shown disappointing results** (Alberts et al, 2000) (Schatzkin et al, 2000) (Gibbons et al, 2003) (Kris-Etherton et al, 2004) (Morris and Carson, 2003).

Hyped as a miracle cure, vitamin C had been claimed to be helpful in fighting over thirty major diseases, including pneumonia, herpes zoster (shingles), pancreatitis, hepatitis, arthritis, some forms of cancer, leukemia, atherosclerosis, high cholesterol, diabetes, multiple sclerosis, and chronic fatigue. (Levy, 2002)

The retinue or "oxy-morons" of the free radical theory had lined up as much support as possible.

The early nineties brought some more good news with the **Women's Health Study** (Buring and Hennekens, 1992) (#39,876). A study of women in Iowa provided evidence that **an increased dietary intake of vitamin E may decrease the risk of colon cancer, especially in women under 65 years of age** (Bostick et al, 1993).

On the other hand, a 2002 study of 87,998 females from the Nurses' Health Study and 47,344 males from the Health Professionals Follow-up Study failed to support the theory that an increased dietary intake of vitamin E may decrease the risk of colon cancer (Wu et al, 2002).

Also in 2002, the American Cancer society released the results of a long-term study that evaluated the effect of regular use of vitamin C and vitamin E supplements on bladder cancer mortality in almost **1,000,000 adults** in the U.S. The study, conducted between the years 1982 to 1998, found that **subjects who regularly consumed a vitamin E supplement for longer than 10 years had a reduced risk of death from bladder cancer. No benefit was seen from vitamin C supplements** (Jacobs et al., 2002).

In 1997, observational studies found that **lens clarity,** which is used to diagnose cataracts, **was better in regular users of vitamin E supplements** and in persons with higher blood levels of vitamin E. A study of middle-aged male smokers, however, did not demonstrate any effect from vitamin E supplements on the incidence of cataract formation (Teikari et al, 1997).

The antioxidant hypothesis spawned a number of large clinical trials whose results were reported between 1994 and 2000. The **conclusions of these studies were as follows:**

(1) There was little or no cardiovascular benefit from vitamin E in the dose ranges studied.

(2) There was no cardiovascular benefit from ß-carotene.

(3) There was no cancer benefit from vitamin E, and at least in smokers over the short term, new cancer risk may be increased with ß-carotene. (Brown et al, 2002).

Overall, in the past, there was seemingly little dispute that the more dietary antioxidants people within a population consumed, the lower the rate of their heart disease and death. But, things were about to change.

Clouds of Doubt Gather and Turn to Antioxidant Doom and Gloom

A series of large, negative intervention studies on vitamin E and/ or beta carotene supplements and cardiovascular disease started to accumulate (Hennekens et al, 1996) (Greenberg et al, 1996) (Virtamo et al, 1998) (GISSI-Prevenzione Investigators;1999) (Yusuf et al. 2000) (de Gaetano et al, 2001) (Lonn et al. 2002) (Hodis et al, 2002) (MRC/BHF, 2002) (Katz et al, 2004) (Lonn et al, 2005).

In 2003, after reviewing the data, a joint committee of **the American College of Cardiology** (Gibbons et al, 2003) **and American Heart Association (AHA)** (Kris-Etherton et al, 2004) **concluded that "... there is currently no basis for recommending that patients take vitamin C or E supplements or other antioxidants for the express purpose of preventing or treating coronary artery disease."**

In 2004, **the AHA Nutrition Committee** similarly concluded that **"At this time, the scientific data do not justify the use of antioxidant vitamin supplements for cardiovascular disease risk reduction."** (Kris-Etherton et al, 2004).

Also, at about that same time, an evidence-based review conducted for **the US Preventive Services Task Force** concluded that " ... **randomized,** controlled trials of specific supplements [to prevent cardiovascular disease] have failed to demonstrate a consistent or significant effect of any single vitamin or combination of vitamins on incidence of or death from cardiovascular disease," (Morris and Carson, 2003) as did another comprehensive review ((Eidelman et al., 2004) and an evidence-based review (Shekelle et al, 2004).

The available scientific studies offer little evidence that supplementation with vitamin E has any benefit on cardiovascular disease prevention or treatment. Indeed, supplementation with vitamin E at the doses tested appears to provide no benefit: large placebo-controlled, randomized trials have reported no benefit in terms of all-cause mortality, cardiovascular mortality, myocardial infarction, or blood lipids (e.g., the MRC/BHF trial, GISSI, HOPE, PPP, ATBC). (Shekelle et al, 2004).

Lack of consistency in the evidence casts doubt on any of the reported associations having a cause-and-effect relationship. There is good evidence that vitamin E supplementation has no clinically important effect on lipid levels. (Shekelle et al, 2004).

Please remember that for a cause and effect relationship to be genuine, there must be the same effect each time the cause is initiated.

Taken together, these reviews, conducted independently, using somewhat different inclusion criteria and methods for synthesis, provide strong convergent validity that supplementary use of vitamin E has no effect on cardiovascular outcomes.

In short, these findings make it unlikely that a particular antioxidant intervention will be found that proves to be markedly effective or beneficial.

In 2005, researchers were examining vitamin A as a potentially new risk factor for osteoporosis. Animal, human, and laboratory research suggested an association between greater vitamin A intake and weaker bones. According to Binkley, animal, human, and in vitro data all indicate that excess vitamin A stimulates bone resorption and inhibits bone formation and that this combination would be expected to produce bone loss and to contribute to osteoporosis development and may occur with relatively low vitamin A intake. It is possible that unappreciated hypervitaminosis A contributes to osteoporosis pathogenesis (Binkley and Krueger, 2000) (Forsyth et al, 1989).

The **Nurses Health Study** looked at the association between vitamin A (retinol) intake and hip fractures in over **72,000 postmenopausal women**. **Women who consumed the most vitamin A in foods and supplements (3,000 mcg or more per day as retinol equivalents, which is over three times the recommended intake) had a significantly increased risk of experiencing a hip fracture as compared to those consuming the least amount** (less than 1,250 mcg/day). The effect was lessened by use of estrogens. These observations raised questions about the effect of retinol because retinol intakes greater than 2,000 mcg/day were associated with an increased risk of hip fracture as compared to intakes less than 500 mcg (Feskanich et al, 2002).

A longitudinal study in more than **2,000 Swedish men** compared blood levels of retinol to the incidence of fractures in men. The investigators found **that the risk of fractures was greatest in men with the highest blood levels of retinol** (more than 75 mcg per deciliter [dL]). Men with blood retinol levels in the 99th percentile (greater than 103 mcg per dL) had an overall risk of fracture that exceeded the risk among men with lower levels of retinol by a factor of seven. (Michaelsson et al, 2003).

"Are the antioxidant companies driven by market forces and not by medical science and are profiteers duping an unsuspecting public?"

In chapter four, I present a large collection of selective data showing marginal effect or lack of effectiveness of the antioxidant vitamins.

CHEMOPREVENTION

**First, there was a chemoprevention "wave of hope."
Then, there were the "disappointing antioxidant results" of failed studies.
Chemoprevention has run its course
and led us to a antioxidant dead end.**

CHAPTER FOUR:

An Epic Chronology Of Antioxidant Vitamin Studies

ANTIOXIDANT VITAMIN FAILURES

I have 181 reports, on over 8 million subjects, showing "disappointing" results with antioxidants in preventing or reversing disease. Thus, prudent questions are, "Why take them in the absence of a deficiency state?" "Why waste money for marginally effective or harmful pills?"

181 Antioxidant Intervention Trial & Analysis Studies:
Failures & Nullification of the Free Radical Theory
R.M. Howes M.D., Ph.D.

This is a selective systematic over view of 181 **interventional initial or follow up studies,** showing either marginal effect, negligible effects, no effects at all. Fifty seven of these studies/reports showed harmful effects of the antioxidant vitamins A (beta carotene), C (ascorbic acid) or E (alpha tocopherol) or combinations thereof. Total number of participants for all of the above studies is in excess of **8,600,000 subjects**, some of which may have been repeats in follow up or parallel studies. Studies with multivitamins, which contain the antioxidant vitamins, were also included.

The following list will be arranged as: Paper (study) number; Title of Study or Paper; Author reference; and Chronological Year; and Number of participants or trials in the respective study.

1. **Failure of High-dose Vitamin C (ascorbic acid) Therapy to Benefit Patients with Advanced Cancer. A Controlled Trial.** (Creagan et al, 1979) (#159 patients with advanced cancer)
2. **High-dose Vitamin C versus Placebo in the Treatment of Patients with Advanced Cancer Who Have had no Prior Chemotherapy.** (Moertel et al, 1985) (#100 patients with advanced colorectal cancer)
3. **Skin Cancer Prevention Study** (Greenberg et al, 1990) (#1,805 men and women with recent nonmelanoma skin cancer)
4. **Diet in the Epidemiology of Postmenopausal Breast Cancer in the New York State Cohort** (Graham et al, 1992) (#18,586 postmenopausal women)
5. **Women's Health Study (WHS)** (Buring and Hennekens, 1992); (#39,876 healthy women)
6. **Isotretinoin-Basal Cell Carcinoma Study Group** (Tangrea et al, 1992, 1993) (#981 patients with two or more previously treated basal cell carcinomas)
7. **Prospective Study of the Intake of Vitamins C, E, and A and the Risk of Breast Cancer** (Hunter et al, 1993) (#89,494 women)
8. **Serum micronutrients and the subsequent risk of cervical cancer in a population-based nested case-control study.** (Batieha, 1993) (#15,161 women)

9. **A randomized trial of vitamin A and vitamin E supplementation for retinitis pigmentosa.** (Berson, 1993) (#601 patients aged 18 through 49 years with retinitis pigmentosa)

10. **Alpha-tocopherol, Beta-Carotene Cancer Prevention Study (ATBC study)** (Heinonen et al, 1994) (#29,133 men)

11. **Polyp Prevention Study** (Greenberg et al, 1994) (#864)

12. **Effect of vitamin C supplementation on lipoprotein cholesterol, apolipoprotein, and triglyceride concentrations** (Jaques et al, 1995) (#139)

13. **The effect of high-dose ascorbate supplementation on plasma lipoprotein(a) levels in patients with premature coronary heart disease** (Bostom et al, 1995) (#44 patients with premature CHD)

14. **Cholesterol Lowering Atherosclerosis Study (CLAS) (1995)** (Hodis et al, 1995) (#156 men)

15. **Effects of Vitamin E on susceptibility of low-density lipoprotein and low-density lipoprotein subfractions to oxidation and on protein glycation in NIDDM.** (Reaven, 1995) (#21 men with NIDDM)

16. **Excretion of alpha-tocopherol into human seminal plasma after oral administration** (Moilanen and Hovatta, 1995) (#15 unselected male volunteers)

17. **The Beta-Carotene and Retinol Efficacy Trial (CARET)** (Omenn et al, 1996) (#14,254 heavy smokers and 4,060 asbestos workers) (total #18,314)

18. **Cambridge Heart Antioxidant Study (CHAOS)** (Stephens et al., 1996) (#2,002 patients with coronary atherosclerosis)

19. **Physicians' Health Study (PHSI)** (Hennekens et al, 1996) (#22,071 US Physicians and Malignant Neoplasms or CVD)

20. **Dietary Antioxidant Vitamins and Death from Coronary Heart Disease in Postmenopausal Women** (Kushi et al, 1996) (#34,486 postmenopausal women with no cardiovascular disease)

21. **Mortality associated with low plasma concentration of beta carotene and the effect of oral supplementation** (Greenberg et al, 1996) (#1,720 men and women)

22. **The effect of antioxidant treatment on human spermatozoa and fertilization rate in an in vitro fertilization program** (Geva et al, 1996) (#Fifteen fertile normospermic male)
23. **Antioxidant Vitamin Effect on Traditional CVD Risk Factors** (Miller et al, 1997) (#297 retired teachers)
24. **ATBC Sub-Study Shows Increased CVD Deaths** (Rapola et al, 1997) (#1,862 men, with prior myocardial infarction)
25. **Effect of preoperative supplementation with alpha-tocopherol and ascorbic acid on myocardial injury in patients undergoing cardiac operations** (Westhuyzen et al, 1997) (#77 undergoing elective coronary artery bypass grafting)
26. **The influence of antioxidant nutrients on platelet function in healthy volunteers** (Calzada et al, 1997) (#40 healthy volunteers)
27. **The Multivitamins and Probucol Study** (Tardif et al, 1997) (#317 participants)
28. **Vitamin C intake and cardiovascular disease risk factors in persons with non-insulin-dependent diabetes mellitus** (Mayer-Davis et al, 1997) (#Insulin Resistance Atherosclerosis Study (IRAS, n = 520) **and from the San Luis Valley Diabetes Study (SLVDS, n = 422)** (total #942)
29. **Preformed Vitamin A Study Showed No Trend to Reduce Breast Cancer Risk.** (Longnecker, 1997) (#3,543 cases and 9,406 controls)
30. **Effect of Vitamin E and Beta Carotene on the Incidence of Primary Nonfatal Myocardial Infarction and Fatal Coronary Heart Disease** (Virtamo et al, 1998) (#27,271 Finnish male smokers)
31. **SU.VI.MAX** (Vasquez et al., 1998) (#13,017 French adults)
32. **A Sub-Study of SU.VI.MAX** (#1,162 subjects aged older than 50 years)
33. **The Nurses' Health Study and Folic Acid and Colon Cancer** (Giovannucci, 1998) (#88,756 women taking vitamin C and B-carotene, for 8 years)
34. **Effect of B-group vitamins and antioxidant vitamins on hyperhomocysteinemia** (Woodside, et al. 1998) (#101 men)
35. **Relationships of serum carotenoids, retinol, alpha-tocopherol, and selenium with breast cancer risk:**

results from a prospective study in Columbia, Missouri (United States). (Dorgan, 1998) (#105 cases of histologically confirmed breast cancer)

36. Incidence of cataract operations in Finnish male smokers unaffected by alpha tocopherol or beta carotene supplements. (Teikari, 1998) (#28,934 male smokers)

37. Effects of alpha-tocopherol and beta-carotene supplements on symptoms, progression, and prognosis of angina pectoris. (Rapola et al, 1998) (#1,795 male smokers aged 50–69 years who had angina pectoris)

38. The effects of antioxidant supplementation during Percoll preparation on human sperm DNA integrity (Hughes et al, 1998) (#150 patients)

39. GISSI-Prevention Trial (GISSI-Prevenzione Investigators;1999) (#11,324 patients with recent MI)

40. Women's Health Study (Lee et al., 1999) (#39,876 healthy women); 50 mg beta-carotene (alternate days)

41. The Health Professionals Follow-Up Study (Ascherio et al. 1999) (#43,738 men)

42. Familial hypercholesterolemia, intima-to-media thickness (FH IMT study) (Raal et al, 1999) (#15 with homozygous familial hypercholesterolemia)

43. Beta carotene supplementation in prevention of basal-cell and squamous-cell carcinomas of the skin (Green et al, 1999) (#1,383 participants)

44. Vitamins A, C and E and the risk of breast cancer: results from a case-control study in Greece, (Bohlke, 1999) (#830 patients with breast cancer plus 1,548 controls)

45. Dietary antioxidants and risk of myocardial infarction in the elderly: the Rotterdam Study. (Klipstein-Grobusch et al, 1999) (#4,802 participants of the Rotterdam Study aged 55–95 y who were free of MI)

46. A prospective study of vitamin supplement intake and cataract extraction among US women. (Chasan-Taber et al, 1999) (#47,152 female nurses)

47. Antioxidant treatment of patients with asthenozoospermia or moderate oligoasthenozoospermia with high-dose vitamin C and vitamin E: a randomized, placebo-

controlled, double-blind study (Rolf et al, 1999) (#31 without genital infection but with asthenozoospermia)

48. **Antioxidant supplementation in vitro does not improve human sperm motility** (Donnelly et al, Fertil Steril. 1999) (#60 patients)

49. **The effect of ascorbate and alpha-tocopherol supplementation in vitro on DNA integrity and hydrogen peroxide-induced DNA damage in human spermatozoa** (Donnelly et al, Mutagenesis. 1999) (#Semen samples with normozoospermic and asthenozoospermic profiles (n = 15 for each control and antioxidant group)

50. **Heart Outcome Prevention Evaluation Study (HOPE)** (Yusuf et al, 2000) (#9,541 patients at high risk for cardiovascular events or diabetes)

51. **Meta-Analysis of Vitamin E in CVD, Ischemic Heart Disease (IHD) and Mortality** (Dagenais et al. 2000) (#51,000 participants)

52. **Vitamin C and the risk of acute myocardial infarction.** (Riemersma et al, 2000) (#180 males with a first AMI and 177 healthy volunteers)

53. **The effects of combined conventional treatment, oral antioxidants and essential fatty acids on sperm biology in subfertile men** (Comhaire et al, 2000) (#27 infertile men)

54. **Dietary antioxidant vitamins, retinol, and breast cancer incidence in a cohort of Swedish women.** (Michels, 2001) (#59,036 women free of cancer)

55. **The secondary prevention HDL Atherosclerosis Treatment study (HATS)** (Brown et al., 2001) (#160 patients with coronary disease)

56. **The Perth Carotid Ultrasound Disease Assessment Study (CUDAS)** (McQuillan et al 2001) (#1,111 subjects)

57. **Randomized Trial of Supplemental ß-Carotene to Prevent Second Head and Neck Cancer** (Mayne et al, 2001) (#264 patients who had been curatively treated for a recent early-stage squamous cell carcinoma of the oral cavity, pharynx, or larynx.)

58. **Age-Related Eye Disease Study Research Group (AREDS)** (AREDS, 2001) (#4,757 participants)

59. **HDL Atherosclerosis Treatment study (HATS)** (Brown et al, 2001) (#160 participants)

60. **Vitamin C and Vitamin E Supplement Use and Colorectal Cancer Mortality in a Large American Cancer Society cohort. (Cancer Prevention Study II cohort - CPS-II)** (Jacobs, 2001) (#711,891 men and women in U.S.A.)

61. **Risk of Ovarian Carcinoma and Consumption of Vitamins A, C and E and Specific Carotenoids: a prospective analysis.** (Fairfield, 2001) (#80,326 women)

62. **Carotenoids, Alpha-tocopherols, and Retinol in Plasma and Breast Cancer Risk in Northern Sweden.** (Hulten, 2001) (#201 cases and 290 referents)

63. **The Vitamin E Atherosclerosis Prevention Study (VEAPS)** (Hodis et al, 2002) (#353 were randomized (176 placebo, 177 vitamin E)

64. **MRC/BHF** (MRC/BHF, 2002) (#20,536); (600 mg vitamin E, 250 mg vitamin C and 20 mg beta-carotene daily)

65. **Antioxidant Vitamins and US Physician CVD Mortality** (Muntwyler et al. 2002) (#83,639 male U.S.A. physicians)

66. **Women's Angiographic Vitamin and Estrogen (WAVE) Trial** (Waters et al, 2002) (#423 postmenopausal women, with at least one 15% to 75% coronary stenosis)

67. **Mega-dose vitamins and minerals in the treatment of non-metastatic breast cancer: an historical cohort study** (Lesperance et al, 2002) (#90 patients with non-metastatic breast cancer who received conventional treatment)

68. **The Roche European American Cataract Trial (REACT)** (Chylack et al. 2002) (#445 patients)

69. **Vitamin E supplementation and macular degeneration** (Taylor et al, 2002) (#1,193 subjects)

70. **Vitamin E on Cardiovascular and Microvascular Outcomes in High-Risk Patients With Diabetes. Results of the HOPE Study and MICRO-HOPE Substudy** (Lonn et al. 2002) (#3,654 with diabetes)

71. **Vitamin C and Vitamin E Supplement Use and Bladder Cancer Mortality in a Large Cohort of US Men and Women** (Cancer Prevention Study II (CPS-II) (Jacobs et al., 2002) (#991,522 US adults in the Cancer Prevention Study II (CPS-II) cohort.)

72. **Supplemental Vitamin C & E and Multivitamin use and Stomach cancer Mortality in U.S.A.** (Jacobs et al. Jan. 2002) (#1,045,923)

73. **Vitamin E and C Supplements and Risk of Dementia** (Laurin et al, 2002) (#3,734 Japanese men)

74. **Retinol intake and bone mineral density in the elderly: the Rancho Bernardo Study.** (Promislow et al, 2002) (#570 women and 388 men)

75. **Vitamin A intake and hip fractures among postmenopausal women.** (Feskanich et al, 2002) (#72,337 postmenopausal women)

76. **A prospective study on supplemental vitamin e intake and risk of colon cancer in women and men.** (Wu et al, 2002) (#87,998 females from the Nurses' Health Study and 47, 344 males from the Health Professionals Follow-up Study) (#135,332 total participants)

77. **The Collaborative Primary Prevention Project (PPP)** (Chiabrando et al., 2002) (#144 participants with CHD risk factors)

78. **Vitamins E & A fail to reduce incidence or mortality of lung cancer: Cochrane Database Syst Rev. 2003.** (Caraballoso et al., 2003) (#109,394 participants)

79. **Use of antioxidant vitamins for the prevention of cardiovascular disease: meta-analysis of randomized trials.** (Vivekananthan et al., 2003) (The vitamin E trials involved a total of #81,788 patients, and the beta-carotene trials involved #138,113)

80. **Antioxidant Vitamins Effect on Alzheimer's Disease: Washington Heights-Inwood Columbia Aging Project** (Luchsinger et al, 2003) (#980 elderly subjects)

81. **Neoplastic and Antineoplastic Effects of Beta Carotene on Colorectal Adenoma Recurrence: Results of a Randomized Trial** (Baron et al, 2003) (#864 subjects who had had an adenoma removed and were polyp-free)

82. **Routine Vitamin Supplementation To Prevent Cardiovascular Disease: A Summary of the Evidence for the U.S. Preventive Services Task Force** (Morris and Carson, 2003)

83. **Midlife Dietary Intake of Antioxidants and Risk of Late-Life Incident Dementia: The Honolulu-Asia Aging Study** (Laurin et al, 2003) (#2,459 men)

84. **Serum retinol levels and the risk of fracture.** (Michealsson, 2003) (#2,322 men)

85. **Impact of simvastatin, niacin, and/or antioxidants on cholesterol metabolism in CAD patients with low HDL.** (Matthan et al, 2003) (#123 HATS participants)

86. **A randomized trial of beta carotene and age-related cataract in US physicians.** (Christen et al, 2003) (#22,071 Male US physicians aged 40 to 84 years)

87. **Supplemental vitamin C increase cardiovascular disease risk in women with diabetes** (Lee et al, 2004) (#1,923 postmenopausal women who reported being diabetic)

88. **Cochrane Database Syst Rev. 2004: Vitamins E & A fail to reduce incidence or mortality of gastrointestinal cancer.** (Cochrane Database Syst Rev. G. Bjelakovic et al, 2004) (#170,525 participants)

89. **ATBC 6-year followup study (2004)** (Thornwall et al., 2004) (#29,133 male smokers)

90. **HOPE study of vitamin E on renal insufficiency (2004)** (Mann et al, 2004) (#993 people with a serum creatinine > or =1.4 to 2.3 mg/dL. And renal insufficiency)

91. **Randomized trials of vitamin E in the treatment and prevention of cardiovascular disease (2004)** (Eidelman et al., 2004) (7 large-scale randomized trials)

92. **Effect of supplemental vitamin E for the prevention and treatment of cardiovascular disease** (Shekelle et al, 2004) (#Eighty-four eligible trials)

93. **SU.VI.MAX Study (2004)** (Hercberg et al, 2004) (#A total of 13,017 French adults)

94. **Meta-analysis: high-dosage vitamin E supplementation may increase all-cause mortality** (Miller et al., 2004) (#135,967 subjects)

95. **The role of vitamin E in the prevention of coronary events and stroke. Meta-analysis of randomized controlled trials** (Alkhenizan and Al-Omran, 2004) (#80,645 subjects)

96. **Oats, Antioxidants and Endothelial Function in Overweight, Dyslipidemic Adults** (Katz et al, 2004) (#30) (16 males ≥age 35; 14 postmenopausal females)

97. **Vitamin C Worsens Coronary Atherosclerosis in Those with Two Copies of the Haptoglobin 2 Gene.** (Levy, 2004) (#299 postmenopausal women)

98. **Vitamin C for preventing and treating the common cold. Cochrane Database Syst Rev. 2004;(4):CD000980.** (Douglas, 2004) (#11,350 study participants)

99. **Vitamin E supplementation and cataract: randomized controlled trial.** (McNeil, 2004) (#1,193 eligible subjects with early or no cataract)

100. **Antioxidant vitamins and coronary heart disease risk: a pooled analysis of 9 cohorts.** (Knekt et al, 2004) (#293,172 subjects free of CHD at baseline)

101. **A review of the epidemiological evidence for the 'antioxidant hypothesis' by the British Nutrition Foundation (the Food Standards Agency).** (Stanner et al, 2004) (British Nutrition Foundation independent review)

102. **Impact of antioxidants, zinc, and copper on cognition in the elderly: a randomized, controlled trial.** (Yaffe et al, 2004) (#2,166 elderly persons)

103. **Use of multivitamins and prostate cancer mortality in a large cohort of US men.** (Stevens et al, 2005) (#475,726 men who were cancer-free)

104. **Vitamin A Supplementation for Reducing the Risk of Mother-to-child Transmission of HIV Infection.** (Wiysonge et al, 2005) (#3,033 females)

105. **The Alzheimer's Disease Cooperative Study (ADCS) Group** (Petersen et al, 2005) (#769 subjects)

106. **Vitamin E Supplementation in Alzheimer's Disease, Parkinson's Disease, Tardive Dyskinesia, and Cataract: Part 2** (Pham et al, 2005)

107. **Dementia and Alzheimer's Disease in Community-Dwelling Elders Taking Vitamin C and/or Vitamin E:** (Fillenbaum et al, 2005) (#626 elderly)

108. **HOPE-TOO Extension** (Lonn et al, 2005) (#3,994 original study enrollees)

109. **Women's Health Study (WHS)** (Lee et al, 2005) (#39,876 apparently healthy US women)
110. **A randomized trial of antioxidant vitamins to prevent second primary cancers in head and neck cancer patients** (Bairati et al, 2005 Apr 6) (#540 patients with stage I or II head and neck cancer treated by radiation therapy)
111. **Randomized trial of antioxidant vitamins to prevent acute adverse effects of radiation therapy in head and neck cancer patients** (Bairati et al, 2005 Aug 20) (#540 patients with stage I or II head and neck cancer treated by radiation therapy)
112. **Effect of intensive lipid lowering, with or without antioxidant vitamins, compared with moderate lipid lowering on myocardial ischemia** (Stone et al, 2005) (#300 patients with stable coronary disease)
113. **Vitamin C and vitamin E for Alzheimer's disease.** (Boothby and Doering, 2005)
114. **Vitamin-mineral supplementation and the progression of atherosclerosis** (Bleys et al, 2006) (searched the MEDLINE, EMBASE, and CENTRAL databases)
115. **Multivitamin/mineral supplements and prevention of chronic disease.** (Huang et al, 2006 May)
116. **The Efficacy and Safety of Multivitamin and Mineral Supplement Use To Prevent Cancer and Chronic Disease in Adults: A Systematic Review for a National Institutes of Health State-of-the-Science Conference.** (Huang et al, 2006 Sept)
117. **Antioxidants Vitamin C and Vitamin E for the Prevention and Treatment of Cancer** (Coulter et al, 2006) (Thirty-eight studies; participant # not available)
118. **Vitamin C levels in Type 2 diabetes and low vitamin C levels does not improve endothelial dysfunction or insulin resistance** (Chen et al, 2006) (#32 type 2 diabetics)
119. **Meta-analysis: antioxidant supplements for primary and secondary prevention of colorectal adenoma (2006)** (Bjelakovic et al., 2006) (#17,620 participants)
120. **Australian Collaborative Trial of Supplements (ACTS)** (Rumbold et al, 2006) (#1,877 subjects)

121. **The Antioxidants in Prevention of Cataracts Study (APC Study):   effects of antioxidant supplements on cataract progression in South India.** (Gritz, 2006) (#798)

122. **Vitamins in Pre-eclampsia (VIP) Trial Consortium** (Poston et al., 2006) (#2,410 women at increased risk for preeclampsia, analyzed 2,395)

123. **SU.VI.MAX (2006) Antioxidants do not affect fasting blood glucose** (Czernichow et al, 2006) (#3,146 subjects)

124. **Vitamin E and Risk of Type 2 Diabetes in the Women's Health Study** (Liu et al., 2006) (#38,716 apparently healthy U.S. women)

125. **Vitamin E supplementation and cognitive function in women: The Women's Health Study (2006)** (Kang et al., 2006) (#39,876 healthy US women)

126. **Supplemental and dietary vitamin E, beta-carotene, and vitamin C intakes and prostate cancer risk (PLCO Trial)** (Kirsh et al, 2006) (#29,361 men during up to 8 years of follow-up)

127. **Intakes of Vitamins A, C and E and Folate and Multivitamins and Lung Cancer: a pooled analysis of 8 prospective studies.** (Cho et al, 2006) (#430,281 persons over a maximum of 6-16 years in the studies)

128. **The Melbourne Atherosclerosis Vitamin E Trial (MAVET):   a study of high dose vitamin E in smokers.** (Magliano et al, 2006) (#409 male and female smokers)

129. **Mortality in Randomized Trials of Antioxidant Supplements for Primary and Secondary Prevention; Systematic Review and Meta-analysis** (Bjelakovic et al, 2007) (# 232,606 participants)

130. **Multivitamin Use and Risk of Prostate Cancer in the National Institutes of Health–AARP Diet and Health Study** (Lawson et al, 2007) (#295,344 men)

131. **A Randomized Factorial Trial of Vitamins C and E and Beta Carotene in the Secondary Prevention of Cardiovascular Events in Women: Results From the Women's Antioxidant Cardiovascular Study** (Cook et al. 2007) (#8,171 female health professionals at increased risk)

132. **Use of Supplements of Multivitamins, Vitamin C, and Vitamin E in Relation to Mortality** (Pocobelli et al, 2007) (#77,719 subjects aged 50–76 years)

133. **Health Professionals Follow-up Study (2007):**
Effect of vitamins C, E, A and carotenoids and the occurrence of oral pre-malignant lesions (Maserejian et al, 2007) (#42,340 men enrolled in the Health Professionals Follow-up Study) (#207 found with oral premalignant lesions)

134. **Antioxidant meta-analysis for the treatment of macular degeneration (2007)** (Chong et al, 2007) (#149,203 subjects)

135. **Effect of *RRR*-α-tocopherol supplementation on carotid atherosclerosis in patients with stable coronary artery disease (CAD)** (Devaraj et al, 2007) (#90 patients with CAD)

136. **Overview of the Women's Antioxidant Cardiovascular Study (WACS) (2007)** (Zaharris et al, 2007) (#8,171 women)

137. **Serum α-tocopherol, concurrent and past vitamin E intake, and mild cognitive impairment** (Dunn et al, 2007) (#526 subjects)

138. **The role of vitamin E in the prevention of cancer: a meta-analysis of randomized controlled trials.** (Alkhenizan and Hafez, 2007) (#167,025 subjects)

139. **Chemoprevention of Primary Liver Cancer: A Randomized, Double-Blind Trial in Linxian, China.** (Qu et al, 2007) (29,450 subjects)

140. **Risk of Mortality with Vitamin E Supplements: The Cache County Study.** (Hayden et al, 2007)

141. **Multivitamin-multimineral supplements and eye disease: age-related macular degeneration and cataract.** (Seddon, 2007) The Dietary Ancillary Study of the Eye Disease Case-Control Study (EDCCS)

142. **Antioxidant Supplementation Increases the Risk of Skin Cancers in Women but Not in Men.** (Hercberg et al, 2007) (#French adults, 7,876 women and 5,141 men. Total # = 13,017)

143. **Antioxidant Vitamin Supplement Use and Risk of Dementia or Alzheimer's Disease in Older Adults** (Gray et al, 2007) (#2,969)

144. **Antioxidant supplements for prevention of mortality in healthy participants and patients with various diseases.** (Bjelakovic, Nikolova, Gludd, Simonetti and Gludd, 2008 Apr) (#232,550 Cochrane Database Syst Rev.)

145. **Systematic review: primary and secondary prevention of gastrointestinal cancers with antioxidant supplements.** (Bjelakovic, Nikolova, Simonette and Gludd, 2008 Sept) (#211,818 participants)

146. **Vitamins E and C in the prevention of cardiovascular disease in men: the Physicians' Health Study II randomized controlled trial** (Sesso et al, 2008) (#14,641 US male physicians)

147. **Both {alpha}- and beta-Carotene, but Not Tocopherols and Vitamin C, Are Inversely Related to 15-Year Cardiovascular Mortality in Dutch Elderly Men** (Buijsse et al, 2008) (#559 men (mean age ~72 y) free of chronic diseases)

148. **Vitamin E and selenium supplementation and risk of prostate cancer in the Vitamins and lifestyle (VITAL) study cohort** (Peters et al, 2008) (#35,242 men)

149. **VITAL (VITamins And Lifestyle) study 2008** (Slatore et al, 2008) (#77,721 men and women)

150. **Vitamin E for Alzheimers and mild cognitive impairment. Cochrane Database Syst Rev. (2008)** (Isaac et al, 2008) (#769 participants)

151. **Efficacy of Antioxidant Supplementation in Reducing Primary Cancer Incidence and Mortality: Systematic Review and Meta-analysis** (Bardia et al, 2008) (#104,196 participants)

152. **Carotenoids and the risk of developing lung cancer: a systematic review.** (Gallicchio et al, 2008) (Six randomized clinical trials)

153. **Antioxidant enriched enteral nutrition and oxidative stress after major gastrointestinal tract surgery.** (van Stijn et al, 2008) (#21 undergoing major upper gastrointestinal tract surgery)

154. **Vitamin E supplementation may transiently increase tuberculosis risk in males who smoke heavily and have high dietary vitamin C intake.** (Hemila and Kaprio, 2008 Oct) (#29,023 males aged 50-69 years, smoking at baseline, with no tuberculosis)

155. **Vitamin E supplementation and pneumonia risk in males who initiated smoking at an early age: e f f e c t modification by body weight and dietary vitamin C.** (Hemila and Kaprio, 2008 Nov) (#21,657 ATBC Study participants who initiated smoking by the age of 20 years)

156. **Oral administration of vitamin C decreases muscle mitochondrial biogenesis and hampers training-induced adaptations in endurance performance.** (Gomez-Cabrera et al, 2008) (#14)

157. **Antioxidant vitamin and mineral supplements for preventing age-related macular degeneration.** (Evans and Henshaw, 2008) (#23,099 participants)

158. **Dietary antioxidants and the long-term incidence of age-related macular degeneration: the Blue Mountains Eye Study.** (Tan et al, 2008) (#2,454 Australian population-based cohort study)

159. **Multivitamin-multimineral supplement use and mammographic breast density.** (Berube et al, 2008) (#Premenopausal (777) and postmenopausal (783) women, total 1,560)

160. **Antioxidant supplements to prevent or slow down the progression of AMD: a systematic review and meta-analysis.** (Evans, 2008) (#23,099 people were randomized in three trials)

161. **Is there a role for supplemented antioxidants in the prevention of atherosclerosis?** (Katsiki and Manes, 2009)

162. **Plasma Carotenoids, Retinol, and Tocopherols and Postmenopausal Breast Cancer Risk in theMultiethnic Cohort Study:a nested case-control study.** (Epplein, 2009) (#286 incident postmenopausal breast cancer cases were matched to 535 controls)

163. **Vitamins E and C in the prevention of prostate and total cancer in men: the Physicians' Health Study II**

randomized controlled trial (2009) (Gaziano et al, 2009)
(#14,641 male physicians)

164. Vitamin E, vitamin C, beta carotene, and cognitive function among women with or at risk of cardiovascular disease: The Women's Antioxidant and Cardiovascular Study (2009) (Kang et al, 2009) (#2,824 participants)

165. Effects of vitamins C and E and beta-carotene on the risk of type 2 diabetes in women at high risk of cardiovascular disease: Women's Antioxidant Cardiovascular Study (2009) (Song et al, 2009) (#8,171 female health professionals)

166. Vitamins C and E and Beta Carotene Supplementation and Cancer Risk: Women's Antioxidant Cardiovascular Study (2009) (Lin et al, 2009) (#7,627 female health professionals)

167. Effect of selenium and vitamin E on risk of prostate cancer and other cancers: the Selenium and Vitamin E Cancer Prevention Trial (SELECT) (2009) (Lippman, 2009) (#35,533 men)

168. Multivitamin Use and Risk of Cancer and Cardiovascular Disease in the Women's Health Initiative Cohorts (Neuhouser et al, 2009) (#161,808 participants)

169. Effects of antioxidant supplements on cancer prevention: meta-analysis of randomized controlled trials (Myung et al, 2009) (#161,045 total subjects)

170. Decision Analysis Supports the Paradigm That Indiscriminate Supplementation of Vitamin E Does More Harm than Good (Dotan et al, 2009) (over 300,000 participants)

171. Effects of long-term antioxidant supplementation and association of serum antioxidant concentrations with risk of metabolic syndrome in adults (SU.VI.MAX) (Czernichow et al, 2009) (#5,220 adults)

172. Total and Cancer Mortality After Supplementation With Vitamins and Minerals: 10 year Follow-up of the Linxian General Population Nutrition Intervention Trial. (Qiao et al, 2009) (#29,584 adults)

173. Vitamin A and retinol intakes and the risk of fractures among participants of the Women's Health Initiative

Observational Study. (Caire-Juvera_et al. 2009) (#75,747 women from the Women's Health Initiative Observational Study)

174. **Modification of the effect of vitamin E supplementation on the mortality of male smokers by age and dietary vitamin C.** (Hemila and Kaprio, 2009 Apr) (#29,023 males aged 50-69 years, smoking at baseline, with no tuberculosis)

175. **Vitamin E supplement use and the incidence of cardiovascular disease and all-cause mortality in the Framingham Heart Study: Does the underlying health status play a role?** (Dietrich et al, 2009) (#4,270 Framingham study participants)

176. **Antioxidants prevent health-promoting effects of physical exercise in humans.** (Ristow et al, 2009) (#39 healthy adults)

177. **Long-term use of beta-carotene, retinol, lycopene, and lutein supplements and lung cancer risk: r e s u l t s from the VITamins And Lifestyle (VITAL) study.** (Satia et al, 2009) (#77,126 (VITAL) cohort Study in Washington State)

178. **Vitamin C supplements and the risk of age-related cataract: a population-based prospective cohort study in women.** (Rautiainen et al, 2010) (#24,593 women)

179. **Micronutrient concentrations and subclinical atherosclerosis in adults with HIV.** (Falcone et al, 2010) (#298 Nutrition for Healthy Living participants)

180. **Multivitamin use and breast cancer incidence in a prospective cohort of Swedish women.** (Larsson et al, 2010) (#35,329 cancer-free women)

181. **Vitamins C and E to prevent complications of pregnancy-associated hypertension** (Roberts et al, 2010) (#10,154)

Total of 181 studies with over 8,600,000 participants

CHAPTER FIVE:

Antioxidant Vitamin Studies (Expanded Data):

Negligible or failed studies and analysis reports

SUMMARY
R.M. Howes MD, PhD

RCTs (randomized, controlled trials) and cohort studies have complementary strengths and weaknesses and share problems and challenges. Considerable care is appropriate in observational studies to minimize potential biases such as residual confounding bias and measurement error bias. RCTs are costly and logistically require careful preliminary development that may consider multiple sources of information, including observational studies, trials with intermediate outcomes and basic science research. An RCT may be justified when the preliminary research is strong and the public health and safety implications are sufficiently great. Arguably, RCTs are considered the "gold standard" for evaluation of these types of studies.

The human diet is a very complex chemical mixture of foods and nutrients, with nearly countless interactive elements and studies attributing results to singular components of foods (such as fresh fruits and vegetables) must be viewed with caution. The dose of nutrients from diets and supplements can be highly influential and affect overall results of supplement studies. Extrapolation of results from one dose to another, and presumably from one agent to a mixture of agents, should be taken into account, along with all of the caveats I have already pointed out.

Studies with multivitamins, which contain the antioxidant vitamins, were also included.

This is a selective review of studies primarily showing marginal effectiveness, negligible effects, total ineffectiveness or the harmful potential and consequences of multivitamins and the antioxidant vitamins A, C and E.

Circa 1979

Failure of high-dose vitamin C (ascorbic acid) therapy to benefit patients with advanced cancer. A controlled trial. (Creagan et al , 1979) (#159 patients with advanced cancer) **One hundred and fifty patients with advanced cancer** participated in a controlled double-blind study to evaluate the effects of high-dose vitamin C on symptoms and survival. Patients were divided randomly into a group that **received vitamin C (10 g per day)** and one that received a comparably flavored lactose placebo. Sixty evaluable patients received vitamin C and 63 received a placebo. Both groups were similar in age, sex, site of primary tumor, performance score, tumor grade and previous chemotherapy. The two groups showed no appreciable difference in changes in symptoms, performance status, appetite or weight. The median survival for all patients was about seven weeks, and the survival curves essentially overlapped. In this selected group of patients, **we were unable to show a therapeutic benefit of high-dose vitamin C treatment.**

Circa 1985

High-dose vitamin C versus placebo in the treatment of patients with advanced cancer who have had no prior chemotherapy. A randomized double-blind comparison. (Moertel et al , 1985) (#100 patients with advanced colorectal cancer)

It has been claimed that high-dose vitamin C is beneficial in the treatment of patients with advanced cancer, especially patients who have had no prior chemotherapy. In a double-blind study **100 patients with advanced colorectal cancer** were randomly assigned to treatment with either **high-dose vitamin C (10 g daily**) or placebo. Overall, these patients were in very good general condition, with minimal symptoms. None had received any previous treatment with cytotoxic drugs. Vitamin C therapy showed no advantage over placebo therapy with regard to either the interval between the beginning of treatment and disease progression or patient survival. Among patients with measurable disease, none had objective improvement. On the basis of this and our previous randomized study, it can be concluded that **high-dose vitamin C therapy is not effective against advanced malignant disease regardless of whether the patient has had any prior chemotherapy.**

Circa 1990
Skin Cancer Prevention Study (Greenberg et al, 1990)
(#1,805 men and women with recent nonmelanoma skin cancer); "A clinical trial of beta carotene to prevent basal-cell and squamous-cell cancers of the skin. The Skin Cancer Prevention Study Group." a randomized, double-blind, placebo-controlled intervention; men and women with recent nonmelanoma skin cancer; beta-carotene; **No effect** on occurrence of new nonmelanoma skin cancers.

Circa 1992
Diet in the Epidemiology of Postmenopausal Breast Cancer in the New York State Cohort (Graham et al, 1992) (#18,586 postmenopausal women); **did not associate a greater vitamin E intake with a reduced risk of developing breast cancer.**

Women's Health Study (WHS) (Buring and Hennekens, 1992) (#39,876 healthy women); randomized, double-blind; placebo-controlled intervention; **600 IU of natural-source vitamin E taken every other day provided no overall benefit for major cardiovascular events or cancer, did not affect total mortality, and decreased cardiovascular mortality in healthy women. These data do not support recommending vitamin E supplementation for cardiovascular disease or cancer**

prevention among healthy women. The WHS data suggest that **vitamin E provides no protection against cancer in women.** In addition, **vitamin E offered no overall protection against CVD.**

Isotretinoin-Basal Cell Carcinoma Study Group

(Tangrea et al, 1992, 1993) (#981 patients with two or more previously treated basal cell carcinomas) randomly assigned; low-dose regimen of isotretinoin not only is **ineffective in reducing the occurrence of basal cell carcinoma at new sites** in patients with two or more previously treated basal cell carcinomas but *also is associated with significant adverse systemic effects.* The **toxicity associated with the long-term administration of isotretinoin, even at the low dose** (10 mg/day) **used in this trial, must be weighted in planning future prevention trials.** Isotretinoin is a modified vitamin A molecule used to treat severe _acne vulgaris._

(adverse mucocutaneous effects and serum triglyceride elevations)

Circa 1993

Prospective Study of the Intake of Vitamins C, E, and A and the Risk of Breast Cancer (Hunter et al, 1993)

(#89,494 women); prospective study; **Large intakes of vitamin C or E did not protect women in our study from breast cancer.** *A low intake of vitamin A may increase the risk of this disease.*

Serum micronutrients and the subsequent risk of cervical cancer in a population-based nested case-control study. (Batieha et al, 1993) (#15,161 women) A nested case-control study was conducted in Washington County, MD, to determine whether low serum micronutrients are related to the subsequent risk of cervical cancer. Among the **15,161 women** who donated blood for future cancer research during a serum collection campaign in 1974, **18 developed invasive cervical cancer and 32 developed carcinoma in situ** during the period January 1975 through May 1990. For each of these 50 cases, two matched controls were selected from the same cohort. The frozen sera of the cases and their matched controls were analyzed for a number of nutrients. The mean serum levels of total carotenoids, alpha-carotene, beta-carotene, cryptoxanthin, and lycopene were lower among cases than they

were among controls. **When examined by tertiles, the risk of cervical cancer was significantly higher among women in the lower tertiles of total carotenoids, alpha-carotene, and beta-carotene as compared to women in the upper tertiles and the trends were statistically significant.** Cryptoxanthin was significantly associated with a lower risk of cervical cancer when examined as a continuous variable. **Retinol, lutein, alpha- and gamma-tocopherol, and selenium were not related to cervical cancer risk.** Smoking was also strongly associated with cervical cancer. These findings are suggestive of a protective role for total carotenoids, alpha-carotene and beta-carotene in cervical carcinogenesis and possibly for cryptoxanthin and lycopene as well.

A randomized trial of vitamin A and vitamin E supplementation for retinitis pigmentosa. (Berson et al, 1993) (#601 patients aged 18 through 49 years with retinitis pigmentosa)

Objective. To determine whether supplements of vitamin A or vitamin E alone or in combination affect the course of retinitis pigmentosa. Design. Randomized, controlled, double-masked trial with 2x2 factorial design and duration of 4 to 6 years. Electroretinograms, visual field area, and visual acuity were measured annually. Setting. Clinical research facility. Patients. 601 patients aged 18 through 49 years with retinitis pigmentosa meeting preset eligibility criteria. Ninety-five percent of the patients completed the study. There were no adverse reactions. Intervention. Patients were assigned to one of four treatment groups receiving 15 000 IU/d of vitamin A, 15 000 IU/d of vitamin A plus 400 IU/d of vitamin E, trace amounts of both vitamins, or 400 IU/d of vitamin E. Main Outcome Measure. Cone electroretinogram amplitude. Results. The two groups receiving 15 000 IU/d of vitamin A had on average a slower rate of decline of retinal function than the two groups not receiving this dosage (*P*=.01). Among 354 patients with higher initial amplitudes, the two groups receiving 15 000 IU/d of vitamin A were 32% less likely to have a decline in amplitude of 50% or more from baseline in a given year than those not receiving this dosage (*P*=.01), while the two groups receiving 400 IU/d of vitamin E were 42% more likely to have a decline in amplitude of 50% or more from baseline than those not receiving this dosage (*P*=.03). While not statistically significant, similar trends were observed for rates of decline of visual field area. Visual acuity declined about 1 letter per year in all groups. Conclusions. **These results support a beneficial effect of 15 000 IU/d of vitamin A and suggest an adverse effect of 400 IU/d of vitamin E on** the course of retinitis pigmentosa. Supplementation with 400 IU/day of vitamin E has been found to accelerate the progression of retinitis pigmentosa that is not associated with vitamin E deficiency.

Circa 1994

Alpha-tocopherol, Beta-Carotene Cancer Prevention Study (ATBC study) (Heinonen et al, 1994) (#29,133 men); randomized, double-blind, placebo-controlled intervention; no effect of vitamin E on lung cancer. Men with known coronary artery disease given 50 mg of a synthetic vitamin E **had no reduction in fatal heart attacks.** *50% increase in hemorrhagic stroke deaths among vitamin E group; 11% increase in ischemic heart disease deaths among* beta-carotene *group; 18% increase in lung cancer among* beta-carotene *group.*

This study was stopped 21 months earlier than planned.

The incidence of lung cancer was 18% higher among men who took the beta-carotene supplement and *eight percent more men in this group died, as compared to those receiving other treatments or placebo.* (Albanes et al, 1996)

The negative (and harmful) results of the 2 beta carotene intervention trials were completely **unexpected and counterintuitive**, according to predominant thinking of the time, which was based totally on the free radical theory.

However, results from the **Alpha-Tocopherol Beta Carotene Prevention Study** (Heinonen et al, 1994) and the **Carotene and Retinol Efficiency Trial (CARET)** (Omenn et al, 1996) **showed an increase in lung cancer** among smokers or asbestos-exposed workers after beta carotene supplementation. **The Physician's Health Study**, in which only a small percentage of subjects were smokers (11%), showed no significant effect of beta carotene supplementation on lung cancer (Hennekens et al, 1996).

Polyp Prevention Study (Greenberg et al, 1994) (#864); randomized, double-blind, placebo-controlled intervention; **There was no evidence that either beta carotene or vitamins C and E reduced the incidence of adenomas.** CONCLUSION. The lack of efficacy of these

vitamins argues against the use of supplemental beta carotene and vitamins C and E to prevent colorectal cancer.

Circa 1995

Effect of vitamin C supplementation on lipoprotein cholesterol, apolipoprotein, and triglyceride concentrations (Jaques et al, 1995) (#139); **the overall results of this trial were negative.**

The effect of high-dose ascorbate supplementation on plasma lipoprotein(a) levels in patients with premature coronary heart disease (Bostom et al, 1995) (#44 patients with premature CHD); findings do not support a clinically important lowering effect of high-dose ascorbate on plasma Lp(a) in patients with premature CHD.

Cholesterol Lowering Atherosclerosis Study (CLAS) (1995) (Hodis et al, 1995) (#156 men); a randomized, placebo-controlled, serial angiographic clinical trial; Supplementary and dietary vitamin E and C intake (nonrandomized) in association with cholesterol-lowering diet and either colestipol-niacin or placebo (randomized). Result: Overall, subjects with supplementary vitamin E intake of 100 IU per day or greater **demonstrated less coronary artery lesion progression** than did subjects with supplementary vitamin E intake less than 100 IU per day for all lesions and for mild/moderate lesions. Within the drug group, benefit of supplementary vitamin E intake was found for all lesions and mild/moderate lesions. Within the placebo group, benefit of supplementary vitamin E intake was not found. **No benefit was found for use of supplementary vitamin C exclusively or in conjunction with supplementary vitamin E, use of multivitamins, or increased dietary intake of vitamin E or vitamin C.**

Yet, they concluded that, "These results indicate an association between supplementary vitamin E intake and angiographically demonstrated reduction in coronary artery lesion progression." But this was only true in the group also receiving colestipol-niacin. **Otherwise, neither vitamins E nor C had a positive effect.** (Hodis et al, 1995).

Effects of Vitamin E on susceptibility of low-density lipoprotein and low-density lipoprotein subfractions to oxidation and on protein glycation in NIDDM.

(Reaven et al, 1995) (#21 men with NIDDM) To evaluate the effect of vitamin E supplementation on the susceptibility of low-density lipoprotein (LDL) and LDL subfractions to oxidation and on protein glycation in non-insulin-dependent diabetes mellitus (NIDDM). RESEARCH DESIGN --**Twenty-one men with NIDDM** (HbA1c = 6-10%), ages 50-70, were randomly assigned to either 1,600 IU/day of vitamin E or placebo for 10 weeks after a 4-week placebo period. LDL and LDL subfractions were isolated after 4 weeks of placebo and after 6 and 10 weeks of therapy. Susceptibility of LDL to copper-mediated oxidation was measured by conjugated diene formation (lag time) and formation of thiobarbituric acid-reactive substances (TBARS). Fasting serum glucose, mean weekly blood glucose, HbA1c, and glycated plasma protein concentrations were also determined at these time points. RESULTS--Vitamin E content in plasma and LDL increased 4.0- and 3.7-fold, respectively, in the vitamin E-treated group. Vitamin E decreased the susceptibility of LDL to oxidation in comparison with placebo. Vitamin E content also increased significantly in both buoyant and dense LDL subfractions, and their oxidation was dramatically reduced. The lag time of LDL oxidation correlated well with the content of vitamin E in both LDL and its subfractions. Glycemic indexes did not change significantly in either group during the study. **Protein glycation, including glycated hemoglobin, glycated albumin, glycated total plasma proteins, and glycated LDL were unchanged in the vitamin E group.** CONCLUSIONS--Supplementation of vitamin E in NIDDM leads to enrichment of LDL and LDL subfractions and reduced susceptibility to oxidation. **Despite a greater percentage increase in vitamin E content in small dense LDL, it remained substantially more susceptible to oxidation than was buoyant LDL.** This suggests that dense, LDL may gain less protection against oxidation from antioxidant supplementation than does larger, more buoyant LDL. **In contrast to previous reports, vitamin E supplementation did not reduce glycation of intracellular or plasma proteins.**

Excretion of alpha-tocopherol into human seminal plasma after oral administration (Moilanen

and Hovatta, 1995) (#15 unselected male volunteers) In this open controlled study, we investigated the blood and seminal plasma concentrations of alpha-tocopherol in **15 unselected male volunteers**, who received either 600, 800 or 1200 mg d-alpha-tocopherol per day for 3 weeks. During the intervention, both the blood and seminal plasma vitamin E concentrations increased significantly, although the increase did not correlate with the dose administered. The highest median blood and seminal plasma concentrations were achieved with 800 mg vitamin E per day, but the differences between the group medians were not significant, except in the blood plasma concentration after the first week of treatment between men receiving 600 and 800 mg per day (P < 0.05). **No significant improvement was noted in the movement characteristics of spermatozoa, hypo-osmolar swelling of spermatozoa, or the velocity of deterioration in the parameters mentioned above**. The seminal plasma vitamin E concentrations achieved during the treatment remained low (< 1 mumol l-1) compared to the concentrations found effective in protecting spermatozoa from peroxidative damage in vitro.

Circa 1996

The Beta-Carotene and Retinol Efficacy Trial (CARET) (Omenn et al, 1996) (#14,254 heavy smokers and 4,060 asbestos workers) (total #18,314 men and women); randomized, double-blind, placebo-controlled intervention; Duration of Treatment Years: 4; Daily Dose: 30 mg beta-carotene, 25,000 IU retinol (as retinyl palmitate); *28% increase in lung cancer; 26% increase in CVD (nonsignificant); 17% increase in total mortality* among treatment group. This study was stopped 21 months earlier than planned.

RMH Note: A 6-year follow-up of a large, randomized trial in people with a history of smoking has found that the overall harm associated with beta-carotene supplementation on cardiovascular disease mortality disappeared quickly after participants stopped taking the supplements. However, the risk of lung cancer may persist, especially in females and former smokers, according to the study in the December 1, 2004 issue of the Journal of the National Cancer Institute. Gary E. Goodman, M.D., of the Fred Hutchinson Cancer Research Center in Seattle, and colleagues followed the more than 18,000 participants in CARET for 6 years after the trial was stopped, until the end of 2001.**The increased risk of cardiovascular disease mortality quickly disappeared after participants stopped taking the supplements.** However, *women had a higher risk of death from cardiovascular disease or from any cause than men. In addition,* **the incidence of lung cancer and deaths from all causes decreased but did not disappear completely after the supplementation ceased.** The excess risk of lung cancer was restricted primarily to females and former smokers.

"When chemoprevention agents are administered to large, healthy populations, it is necessary to document long-term safety, efficacy and, importantly, the duration of the beneficial (or adverse) effect," the authors write. "**This is especially true when the basic underlying molecular and genetic mechanism of the agent is unclear.** The results of CARET and ATBC emphasize that chemoprevention trials require careful monitoring of all disease endpoints ... even after the study intervention is discontinued." (Goodman et al, 2004).

Based on the free radical theory, beta carotene was known to be an effective antioxidant and a precursor of vitamin A, and was therefore believe to be a plausible mechanism to block lung cancer. However, a series of beta carotene intervention trials were conducted that **categorically dispelled the notion that supplemental beta carotene could effectively reduce lung cancer risk** (Hennekens et al, 1996) (Heinonen et al, 1994) (Omenn et al, NEJM. 1996).

The lessons from the beta-carotene **studies in relation to chronic disease include the possibility that antioxidants may have surprising short and long term health consequences**, even if generally regarded as safe, which could be important in determining the balance of benefits and risks for the individual.

Cambridge Heart Antioxidant Study (CHAOS)

(Stephens et al., 1996) (#2,002 patients with coronary atherosclerosis); randomized, double-blind, placebo-controlled intervention; patients with coronary atherosclerosis; in patients with angiographically proven symptomatic coronary atherosclerosis, alpha-tocopherol treatment substantially reduces the rate of non-fatal MI, with beneficial effects apparent after 1 year of treatment (**77% decrease in risk of subsequent nonfatal MI); no benefit on cardiovascular mortality,** *even though paralleled by a not significant 22% increase in all deaths.*

This landmark study was begun in the fall of 1982 to test the benefits and risks of aspirin and beta carotene in the primary prevention of cardiovascular disease and cancer. The original randomized trial, the Physicians' Health Study-I, ended in 1995. Its finding that daily low-dose aspirin decreased the risk of a first myocardial infarction by 44% helped focus on the role of aspirin in primary prevention of coronary heart disease. In 1996, it also **showed no benefit or harm from beta carotene**.

Physicians' Health Study (PHSI) (Hennekens et al, 1996) (#22,071 US Physicians and Malignant Neoplasms or CVD); randomized, double-blind, placebo-controlled intervention; beta-carotene in US Physicians and Malignant Neoplasms or CVD; among healthy men, 12 years of supplementation with **beta carotene produced neither benefit nor harm in terms of the incidence of malignant neoplasms, cardiovascular disease, or death from all causes.**

Dietary Antioxidant Vitamins and Death from Coronary Heart Disease in Postmenopausal Women (Kushi et al, 1996) (#34,486 postmenopausal women with no cardiovascular disease); completed a questionnaire that assessed, among other factors, their intake of vitamins A, E, and C from food sources and supplements; vitamin E consumption appeared to be inversely associated with the risk of death from coronary heart disease. This association was particularly striking in the subgroup of 21,809 women who did not consume vitamin supplements.

There was little evidence that the intake of vitamin E from supplements was associated with a decreased risk of death from coronary heart disease, but the effects of high-dose supplementation and the duration of supplement use could not be definitively addressed. **Intake of vitamins A and C did not appear to be associated with the risk of death from coronary heart disease.**

Mortality associated with low plasma concentration of beta carotene and the effect of oral supplementation (Greenberg et al, 1996) (#1,720 men and women) **Cohort study** of plasma concentrations; randomized, controlled clinical trial of supplementation. A # **1,720 total of 1188 men and 532 women** with mean age of 63.2 years. Beta carotene, 50 mg per day for a median of 4.3 years. **Patients randomly assigned to beta carotene**

supplementation showed no reduction in relative mortality rates from all causes or from cardiovascular disease. CONCLUSION: These analyses provide no support for a strong effect of supplemental beta carotene in reducing mortality from cardiovascular disease or other causes.

The following study by Clark et al, 1996 is included because of the studies claiming the antioxidant properties of selenium. No vitamins A, C or E were in this study and it is not part of the numbered studies.

The Nutritional Prevention of Cancer Trial (Clark et al. 1996) (#1,312 men and women with a history of basal or squamous cell carcinoma) A multicenter, double-blind, randomized, placebo-controlled cancer prevention trial. **Selenium treatment did not protect against development of basal or squamous cell carcinomas of the skin.**

The effect of antioxidant treatment on human spermatozoa and fertilization rate in an in vitro fertilization program (Geva et al, 1996) (#Fifteen fertile normospermic male) Investigators studied the possible influence of antioxidant treatment on human spermatozoa and the fertilization rate in an IVF program. DESIGN: Prospective study. SETTING: In Vitro Fertilization Unit, Serlin Maternity Hospital, and the Laboratory of Male Fertility, Bar-Ilan University, Ramat-Gan, Israel. PATIENTS: **Fifteen fertile normospermic male** volunteers who had low fertilization rates in their previous IVF cycles. INTERVENTIONS: Vitamin E (alpha-tocopherol) 200 mg daily by mouth for 3 months. MAIN OUTCOME MEASURES: Lipid peroxidation potential (amount of malondialdehyde [MDA]), quantitative ultramorphologic analysis of spermatozoa, and fertilization rate per cycle. RESULTS: The high MDA levels significantly decreased from 12.6 +/- 9.4 nmol/10(8) spermatozoa to normal levels of 7.8 +/- 4.2 nmol/10(8) spermatozoa after 1 month of treatment. The fertilization rate per cycle increased significantly from 19.3 +/- 23.3 to 29.1 +/- 22.2 after 1 month of treatment. No additional effects on MDA levels and fertilization rate were observed after completion of treatment. **With regard to the quantitative ultramorphologic analysis, none of the sperm cell subcellular organelles were affected significantly by vitamin E treatment.** CONCLUSION: Vitamin E may improve the fertilization rate of fertile normospermic males with low fertilization rates after 1 month of treatment, possibly by reducing the lipid peroxidation potential, and with no change of the quantitative ultramorphologic analysis of subcellular organelles.

Circa 1997

Antioxidant Vitamin Effect on Traditional CVD Risk Factors (Miller et al, 1997) (#297 retired teachers); **the combined antioxidant supplement of vitamin C, E and beta carotene had no significant effect on the systolic and diastolic blood pressures, fasting serum lipids (total cholesterol, high-density lipoprotein cholesterol, and LDL cholesterol) and fasting glucose, with unadjusted and adjusted analyses.**

ATBC Sub-Study Shows Increased CVD Deaths (Rapola et al, 1997) (#1,862 men, with prior myocardial infarction); there **were no significant differences** in major coronary events but *significantly more deaths from fatal coronary heart disease.* **There were no significant differences in the number of major coronary events between any supplementation group and the placebo group. There were *significantly more deaths from fatal coronary heart disease in the beta-carotene and combined alpha-tocopherol and beta-carotene groups* than in the placebo group. *The risk of fatal coronary heart disease increased in the groups that received either beta-carotene or the combination of alpha-tocopherol and beta-carotene.* They do not recommend the use of alpha-tocopherol or beta-carotene supplements in this group of patients.**

Effect of preoperative supplementation with alpha-tocopherol and ascorbic acid on myocardial injury in patients undergoing cardiac operations (Westhuyzen et al, 1997) (#77 undergoing elective coronary artery bypass grafting) **There were no significant differences between the groups with respect to release of creatine kinase MB isoenzyme over 72 hours, nor in the reduction of the myocardial perfusion defect determined by thallium 201 uptake. Electrocardiography provided no evidence of a benefit from antioxidant supplementation. Thus the supplementation regimen provided no measurable reduction in myocardial injury after the operation.**

The influence of antioxidant nutrients on platelet function in healthy volunteers (Calzada et al, 1997) (#40 healthy volunteers) **Supplementation of healthy volunteers with *vitamin E decreased platelet function* whereas supplementation with vitamin c or beta-carotene had no significant effects.**

The Multivitamins and Probucol Study (Tardif et al, 1997) (#317 participants); (Beta carotene 30 000 IU, vitamin C 500 mg and E 700 IU); the **combination of vitamins C and E and beta carotene had no effect in reducing the rate of restenosis in patients after angioplasty.**

Probucol reduced restenosis rates from 38.9% to 20.7% and rates of repeated PTCA from 24.4% to 11.2%; multivitamins alone had no effect. *Probucol has been pulled off the market due harmful effects and the likelihood of cardiac arrhythmias.*

Vitamin C intake and cardiovascular disease risk factors in persons with non-insulin-dependent diabetes mellitus (Mayer-Davis et al, 1997) (#Insulin Resistance Atherosclerosis Study (IRAS, n = 520) **and from the San Luis Valley Diabetes Study (SLVDS, n = 422) (total #942); across a wide range of intake, vitamin C does not appear to be associated with improved CVD risk factor status among community-dwelling persons with diabetes.**

Preformed Vitamin A Study Showed No Trend to Reduce Breast Cancer Risk. (Longnecker, 1997) (#3,543 cases and 9,406 controls) Intake of fruits, vegetables, vitamin A, and related compounds are associated with a decreased **risk of breast cancer** in some studies, but additional data are needed. To estimate intake of beta-carotene and vitamin A, the authors included nine questions on food and supplement use in a population-based case-control study of breast cancer risk conducted in Maine, Massachusetts, New Hampshire, and Wisconsin in 1988-1991. Multivariate-adjusted models were fit to data for **3,543 cases and 9,406 controls**. Eating carrots or spinach more than twice weekly, compared with no intake, was associated with an odds ratio of 0.56 (95% confidence interval 0.34-0.91). **Estimated intake of preformed vitamin A from all evaluated foods and supplements showed no trend or monotonic decrease in risk across categories of intake.** These data

do not allow us to distinguish among several potential explanations for the protective association observed between intake of carrots and spinach and risk of breast cancer. The findings are, however, consistent with a diet rich in these foods having a modest protective effect.

The majority of epidemiological studies have failed to find significant associations between retinol intake and breast cancer risk in women.

Circa 1998

In 1998, The Medical Letter concluded: (Medical letter, 1998)
- The benefits of taking high doses of vitamin E remain to be established.
- There is no convincing evidence that taking supplements of vitamin C prevents any disease.
- No one should take beta carotene supplements

A second randomized trial, the Physician's Health Study-II, was started in 1997 to test the balance of benefits and risks of three other widely used, but as yet unproven, supplements for the primary prevention of cardiovascular disease, cancer, age-related eye disease, and cognitive decline--vitamin E, vitamin C, and a multivitamin. **The vitamin C and vitamin E components, which ended as planned in 2007, found that these vitamin supplements do not prevent major cardiovascular events or cancer.**

Nutritional Prevention of Cancer Study (Clark et al, 1996) (#1,312 men and women with a history of basal or squamous cell carcinoma); Daily Dose: 200 pg **selenium**; Primary Disease Outcome: Skin cancer, prostate cancer; Results: **No effect on incidence of skin cancer**; 63% reduction in prostate cancer incidence; reduction in total cancer mortality and total cancer incidence. *Reference to this particular study was included, even though it did not test vitamins A, C or E, due to the antioxidant claims of selenium.*

RMH Note: **Intakes of dietary or supplemental antioxidants were not associated with a decreased risk of prostate cancer among men in the Prostate (CaP), Lung, Colorectal, and Ovarian (PLCO) Cancer Screening Trial**, according to a study in the February 15, 2006 issue of the *Journal of the National Cancer Institute.* Kirsh and Hayes, at the National

Cancer Institute, and colleagues assessed the risk of prostate cancer for **29,361 men ages** 55 to 74 enrolled in the PLCO Cancer Screening Trial, based on their daily intake of beta-carotene, vitamin E, and vitamin C. The researchers looked at intake of antioxidants from both dietary sources and from supplements. The authors found that, **overall, dietary or supplemental intake of vitamin E, vitamin C, or beta-carotene was not associated with prostate cancer incidence** in this group of PLCO trial participants. **In short,** in the 29,361 men in the trial, 1,338 cases of CaP were identified over the 8 years of follow-up. In general, **there was no clear CaP risk reduction resulting from dietary or supplemental intake of vitamins E and C or b-carotene** (Kirsh et al, 2006).

Effect of Vitamin E and Beta Carotene on the Incidence of Primary Nonfatal Myocardial Infarction and Fatal Coronary Heart Disease

(Virtamo et al, 1998) (#27,271 Finnish male smokers) effect of vitamin E (alpha tocopherol) and beta carotene supplementation on major coronary events in the Alpha-Tocopherol, Beta-Carotene Cancer Prevention Study. The incidence of primary major coronary events decreased 4% among recipients of vitamin E and increased 1% among recipients of beta carotene compared with the respective nonrecipients. Neither agent affected the incidence of nonfatal myocardial infarction. Supplementation with vitamin E decreased the incidence of fatal coronary heart disease by 8%, but beta carotene had no effect on this end point. **CONCLUSION: Supplementation with a small dose of vitamin E has only marginal effect on the incidence of fatal coronary heart disease in male smokers with no history of myocardial infarction, but no influence on nonfatal myocardial infarction. Supplementation with beta carotene has no primary preventive effect on major coronary events.**

SUVIMAX (Vasquez et al, 1998) (#13,017 French adults); take either a daily capsule containing 120 milligrams of ascorbic acid, 30 milligrams of vitamin E, six milligrams of beta carotene, 100 micrograms of selenium, and 20 milligrams of zinc; or a placebo capsule; researchers found **no differences between the antioxidant and placebo group in terms of cancer incidence, or in cardiovascular disease incidence, or all-cause death.**

A Sub-Study of SUVIMAX (#1,162 subjects aged older than 50 years); results suggest **no beneficial effects of long-term daily** low-dose supplementation of antioxidant vitamins and minerals on carotid atherosclerosis and arterial stiffness.

The Nurses' Health Study and Folic Acid and Colon Cancer (Giovannucci et al, 1998) (#88,756 women taking vitamin C and B-carotene, for 8 years); **No benefit with respect to colon cancer after 4 years of use and had no significant risk reductions after 5 to 9 or 10 to 14 years of use. Long-term use of over 15 years of multivitamins may substantially reduce risk for colon cancer.** This effect may be related to the folic acid contained in multivitamins.

Dr. Andy Ness, of Bristol University, reported in the British Medical Journal in Dec. 2004, that there is the **possibility of increased risk of breast cancer in women taking folic acid supplements throughout pregnancy.** The researchers followed up **2,928 pregnant women** who had taken part in a supplemental trial in the 1960s. **The risk of death from breast cancer was much higher in women who had received high doses of the supplement than in those who had been given a placebo.** However, Godfrey Oakley and Jack Mandel, of Emory University, said other research studies indicate that more folic acid is likely to prevent breast cancer rather than cause it. **This is another glaring example of the contradictory and dangerous nature of the vitamin studies.**

Effect of B-group vitamins and antioxidant vitamins on hyperhomocysteinemia (Woodside, et al, 1998) (#101 men); **8-wk B-group vitamins with antioxidant vitamins, or placebo intervention. Homocysteine concentrations had significant decreases in both groups receiving B-group vitamins either with or without antioxidants. The effect of B-group vitamins alone over 8 wk was a reduction in homocysteine concentrations,** whereas **antioxidants alone produced a nonsignificant increase.**

Relationships of serum carotenoids, retinol, alpha-tocopherol, and selenium with breast cancer risk: results from a prospective study in Columbia, Missouri (United States). (Dorgan et al, 1998) (#105 cases of histologically confirmed breast cancer) To evaluate relationships of serum carotenoids, alpha-tocopherol, selenium, and retinol with breast cancer prospectively, we conducted a case-control study nested in a cohort from the Breast Cancer Serum Bank in Columbia, Missouri (United States).

Women free of cancer donated blood to this bank in 1977-87. **During up to 9.5 years of follow-up** (median = 2.7 years), **105 cases of histologically confirmed breast cancer** were diagnosed. For each case, two women alive and free of cancer at the age of the case's diagnosis and matched on age and date of blood collection were selected as controls. A nonsignificant gradient of decreasing risk of breast cancer with increasing serum beta-cryptoxanthin was apparent for all women. Serum lycopene also was associated inversely with risk, and among women who donated blood at least two years before diagnosis, a significant gradient of decreasing breast cancer risk with increasing lycopene concentration was evident. A marginally significant gradient of decreasing risk with increasing serum lutein/zeaxanthin also was apparent among these women. **They did not observe any evidence for protective effects of alpha- and beta-carotene, alpha-tocopherol, retinol, or selenium for breast cancer.** Results of this study suggest that the carotenoids beta-cryptoxanthin, lycopene, and lutein/zeaxanthin may protect against breast cancer.

Two prospective studies did not observe significant associations between blood retinol levels and subsequent risk of developing breast cancer, i.e., Hulten and Dorgan.

Incidence of cataract operations in Finnish male smokers unaffected by alpha tocopherol or beta carotene supplements. (Teikari et al, 1998) (#28,934 male smokers) Invesitgators examined the effect of alpha tocopherol and beta carotene supplementation on the incidence of age related cataract extraction. SETTING: The **Alpha-tocopherol Beta-carotene (ATBC) Study** was a randomised, double blind, placebo controlled, 2 x 2 factorial trial conducted in south western Finland. The cataract surgery study population of **28,934 male smokers 50-69 years** of age at the start. INTERVENTION: Random assignment to one of four regimens: alpha tocopherol 50 mg per day, beta carotene 20 mg per day, both alpha tocopherol and beta carotene, or placebo. Follow up continued for five to eight years (median 5.7 years) with a total of 159,199 person years. OUTCOME MEASURE: Cataract extraction, ascertained from the National Hospital

Discharge Registry. RESULTS: 425 men had cataract surgery because of senile or presenile cataract during the follow up. Of these, 112 men were in the alpha tocopherol alone group, 112 men in the beta carotene alone group, 96 men in the alpha tocopherol and beta carotene group, and 105 men in the placebo group. When supplementation with alpha tocopherol and with beta carotene were introduced to a Cox proportional hazards model with baseline characteristics (age, education, history of diabetes, body mass index, alcohol consumption, number of cigarettes smoked daily, smoking duration, visual acuity, and total cholesterol), **neither alpha tocopherol nor beta carotene supplementation affected the incidence of cataract surgery.** CONCLUSION: **Supplementation with alpha tocopherol or beta carotene does not affect the incidence of cataract extractions among male smokers.**

Effects of alpha tocopherol **and** beta carotene**supplements on symptoms, progression, and prognosis of angina pectoris.** (Rapola et al, 1998) (#1,795

Male smokers aged 50–69 years who had angina pectoris) They evaluated the effects of alpha tocopherol and beta carotenesupplements on recurrence and progression of angina symptoms, and incidence of major coronary events in men with angina pectoris. Design: Placebo controlled clinical trial. The Finnish alpha tocopherol beta carotenecancer prevention study primarily undertaken to examine the effects of alpha tocopherol and beta caroteneon cancer. Male smokers aged 50–69 years who had angina pectoris in the Rose chest pain questionnaire at baseline (n = **1795**). Interventions: alpha tocopherol (vitamin E) 50 mg/day, beta carotene20 mg/day or both, or placebo in 2 × 2 factorial design. Main outcome measures: Recurrence of angina pectoris at annual follow up visits when the questionnaire was readministered; progression from mild to severe angina; incidence of major coronary events (non-fatal myocardial infarction and fatal coronary heart disease). **Results:** There were 2513 recurrences of angina pectoris during follow up (median 4 years). Compared to placebo, the odds ratios for recurrence in the active treatment groups were:alpha tocopherol only 1.06, alpha tocopherol and beta carotene1.02, beta caroteneonly 1.06. **There were no significant differences in progression to severe angina among the groups given supplements or placebo.** Altogether 314 major coronary events were observed during follow up (median 5.5 years) and the risk for them did not differ significantly among the groups given supplements or placebo. **Conclusions: There was no evidence of beneficial effects for**

alpha tocopherol or beta carotene supplements in male smokers with angina pectoris, indicating no basis for therapeutic or preventive use of these agents in such patients.

The effects of antioxidant supplementation during Percoll preparation on human sperm DNA integrity (Hughes et al, 1998) (#150 patients) The integrity

of sperm DNA is crucial for the maintenance of genetic health. A major source of damage is reactive oxygen species (ROS) generation; therefore, antioxidants may afford protection to sperm DNA. The objectives of the study were, first, to measure the effects of antioxidant supplementation in vitro on endogenous DNA damage in spermatozoa using the single cell gel electrophoresis (comet) assay and, second, to assess the effect of antioxidant supplementation given prior to X-ray irradiation on induced DNA damage. Spermatozoa from **150 patients** were prepared by Percoll centrifugation in the presence of **ascorbic acid (300, 600 microM), alpha tocopherol (30, 60 microM), urate (200, 400 microM), or acetyl cysteine (5, 10 microM).** DNA damage was induced by 30 Gy X-irradiation. DNA strand breakage was measured using the comet assay. **Sperm DNA was protected from DNA damage by ascorbic acid (600 microM), alpha tocopherol (30 and 60 microM) and urate (400 microM).** These antioxidants provided protection from subsequent DNA damage by X-ray irradiation. *In contrast, acetyl cysteine or ascorbate and alpha tocopherol together induced further DNA damage to human sperm.* Supplementation in vitro with the antioxidants ascorbate, urate and alpha tocopherol separately has beneficial effects for sperm DNA integrity.

Circa 1999

GISSI-Prevention Trial (GISSI-Prevenzione Investigators;1999)
(#11,324 patients with recent MI); **No benefit from vitamin E**; 15% decrease in risk of death, nonfatal MI, and stroke from omega-3 PUFA.

With the release in 1999 of the Gruppo Italiano per lo Studio della Sopravvivenza nell'Infarto miocardico **(GISSI)** and the Heart Outcomes Prevention Evaluation **(HOPE)**, the role of antioxidants for secondary prevention was **again in doubt**. The **HOPE** study reported **no reduction in heart attack, stroke, or death in patients with heart disease or** diabetes after use of vitamin E supplements for more than 4 years. Similarly, the **GISSI trial, which followed 11,324 patients** with recent heart attacks, **showed no benefit from use of vitamin E supplements for up to 2 years.**

The lack of benefit with vitamin E, however, was corroborated by the results of the HOPE trial and therefore the refutation of the 'antioxidant hypothesis' was at hand. (Marchioli and Valagussa, 2000).

Women's Health Study (Lee et al., 1999) (#39,876 healthy women); 50 mg beta-carotene (alternate days); **No effect on incidence of cancer, CVD, or total mortality; no benefit or harm from beta-carotene supplementation after a median of 4.1 years on the incidence of cancer and of cardiovascular disease.**

The beta-carotene part of the study was **stopped early,** in 1996, when other studies showed no protection and even a possible risk of cancer.

A study by Lee et al in the Nov. 2004 issue of American Journal of Clinical Nutrition, found that *such supplements may actually promote the clogging of arteries.* They evaluated cardiovascular disease in **1,923 post-menopausal women with diabetes,** part of the **Iowa Women's Health Study**, which collected data in 1986 about diets and vitamin C consumption in nearly **35,000 recruits.** The researchers found that **women with diabetes consuming at least 300 milligrams of vitamin C per day faced** *2.3 times the risk of death from stroke and 2 times the risk of dying from coronary artery disease* as did diabetic women who took in less of the vitamin C.

A recent study showed that **mega-doses of vitamin C might actually speed up hardening of the arteries.** Researchers from the University of Southern California studied **573** outwardly healthy middle-aged men and women. About 30% of them regularly took various vitamins. The study found no clear-cut sign that getting lots of vitamin C from food or a daily multivitamin does any harm. But *those taking vitamin C pills had accelerated thickening of the walls of the big arteries in their necks. The more they took, the faster the buildup.*

The Health Professionals Follow-Up Study (Ascherio et al. 1999) (#43,738 men); followed for 8 years. Vitamin E and vitamin C supplements and specific carotenoids **did not substantially reduce risk for stroke** in this cohort with 8 year followup.

Familial hypercholesterolemia, intima-to-media thickness (FH IMT study) (Raal et al, 1999) (#15 with homozygous familial hypercholesterolemia); *homozygous familial hypercholesterolemia, intima-to-media thickness (FH IMT study) increased with vitamin E supplements (400 mg/day) for 2 years,* but decreased when subjects received statin therapy. **Vitamin E supplementation fails to slow (or inhibit) the progression of intima-to-media thickness in healthy men and women at low risk for cardiovascular disease.**

At about this time in 1999, researcher Rudolph Salganik, PhD, of the University of North Carolina research team stated, "The truth is we don't know how useful vitamins are for us." In the experiments by Salganik they found that mice that were deprived of all but the smallest traces of vitamins A and E had tumors that were 17 percent smaller than those with normal amounts of the vitamins in their diet. **The vitamin-deficient mice also had five times the number of dying cells in their tumors.** Their work suggested that using vitamins can backfire, actually helping the cancer spread more quickly. Salganik said, "If you suppress free radicals (with antioxidants), you suppress programmed cell death." (Salganik et al, 2000) (Albright et al, 2003).

Beta carotene supplementation in prevention of basal-cell and squamous-cell carcinomas of the skin (Green et al, 1999) (#1,383 participants) **There was no beneficial or harmful effect on the rates of either type of skin cancer, as a result of beta carotene supplementation.**

Vitamins A, C and E and the Risk of Breast Cancer: results from a case-control study in Greece. (Bohlke et al, 1999) (#820 patients with breast cancer plus 1,548 controls) Although several dietary compounds are hypothesized to have anticarcinogenic properties, the role of specific micronutrients in the development of breast cancer remains unclear. To address this issue, they assessed intake of retinol, β-carotene, vitamin C and vitamin E in relation to breast cancer risk in a case–control study in Greece. **Eight hundred and twenty women with histologically confirmed breast cancer were compared with 1548 control women.** Dietary data were collected through a 115-item semiquantitative food frequency questionnaire. Data were modelled by logistic regression, with adjustment for total energy intake and established breast cancer risk factors, as well as mutual adjustment among the micronutrients. **Among post-menopausal women, there was no association between any of the micronutrients evaluated and risk of breast cancer.**

Among premenopausal women, β-carotene, vitamin C and vitamin E were each inversely associated with breast cancer risk, but after mutual adjustment among the three nutrients only β-carotene remained significant; the odds ratio (OR) for a one-quintile increase in β-carotene intake was 0.84. The inverse association observed with β-carotene intake, however, is slightly weaker than the association previously observed with vegetable intake in these data, raising the possibility that the observed β-carotene effect is accounted for by another component of vegetables.

Dietary antioxidants and risk of myocardial infarction in the elderly: the Rotterdam Study.

(Klipstein-Grobusch et al, 1999) (#4,802 participants of the Rotterdam Study aged 55–95 y who were free of MI) Epidemiologic studies have shown dietary antioxidants to be inversely correlated with ischemic heart disease. They investigated whether dietary ß-carotene, vitamin C, and vitamin E were related to the risk of myocardial infarction (MI) in an elderly population. **Design:** The study sample consisted of **4,802 participants of the Rotterdam Study** aged 55–95 y who were free of MI at baseline and for whom dietary data assessed by a semiquantitative food frequency questionnaire were available. During a **4-y follow-up** period, 124 subjects had an MI. The association between energy-adjusted ß-carotene, vitamin C, and vitamin E intakes and risk of MI was examined by multivariate logistic regression. **Results:** Risk of MI for the highest compared with the lowest tertile of ß-carotene intake was 0.55, adjusted for age, sex, body mass index, pack-years, income, education, alcohol intake, energy-adjusted intakes of vitamin C and E, and use of antioxidative vitamin supplements. **When ß-carotene intakes from supplements were considered, the inverse relation with risk of MI was slightly more pronounced. Stratification by smoking status indicated that the association was most evident in current and former smokers.** No association with risk of MI was observed for dietary vitamin C and vitamin E. **Conclusion:** The results of this **observational study** in the elderly population of the Rotterdam Study support the hypothesis that **high dietary ß-carotene** intakes may protect against cardiovascular disease. However, they did not observe an association between vitamin C or vitamin E and MI.

A prospective study of vitamin supplement intake and cataract extraction among US women.

(Chasan-Taber et al, 1999) (#47,152 female nurses) We prospectively examined the association between vitamin supplement intake and the incidence of cataract extraction during 12 years of follow-up in a cohort of **47,152 female nurses**. Women were 45 years or older and free of diagnosed cancer in 1980; others were added as they reached 45 years of age, for a total of 73,956 women. During years of follow-up, 1,377 senile cataracts were diagnosed and extracted. **Those who used multivitamins or separate supplements of vitamin C, E, or A did not have decreased risks of cataract as compared with nonusers even for use of 10 or more years.** After adjusting for cataract risk factors, including cigarette smoking, body mass index, and diabetes mellitus, users of vitamin C supplements for 10 or more years had a relative risk (RR) of 0.95. Associations were stronger among long-term vitamin C supplement users who were never-smokers and less than 60 years of age. These findings suggest that **there is little overall benefit of long-term use of vitamin supplements for risk of cataracts requiring extraction.**

Antioxidant treatment of patients with asthenozoospermia or moderate oligoasthenozoospermia with high-dose vitamin C and vitamin E: a randomized, placebo-controlled, double-blind study (Rolf et al, 1999) (#31 without genital

infection but with asthenozoospermia) In a **randomized, placebo-controlled, double-blind study** we investigated whether high-dose oral treatment with vitamins C and E for 56 days was able to improve semen parameters of infertile men. Ejaculate parameters included semen volume, sperm concentration and motility, and sperm count and viability. **Thirty-one patients** without genital infection but with asthenozoospermia (< 50% motile spermatozoa) and normal or only moderately reduced sperm concentration (> 7 x 10(6) spermatozoa/ml) (according to WHO criteria) were examined. To investigate the influence of the epididymal storage period on semen parameters, the patients were asked to deliver two semen samples with abstinence times of 2 and 7 days both before and at the end of vitamin treatment. After randomization, the **patients received either 1000 mg vitamin C and 800 mg vitamin E (n = 15) or identical placebo capsules** (n = 16). **No changes in semen parameters were observed during treatment**, and no pregnancies were initiated during the treatment period. **Combined high-dose antioxidative treatment with vitamins C and E did not improve conventional semen parameters or the 24-h sperm survival rate.** Prolonged abstinence time increased ejaculate volume, sperm count, sperm concentration and the total number of motile spermatozoa.

Antioxidant supplementation in vitro does not improve human sperm motility (Donnelly et al, Fertil Steril. 1999) (#60 patients) Investigators determined the effects of supplementation of preparation media with ascorbate and alpha-tocopherol on subsequent sperm motility and reactive oxygen species production. DESIGN: **Prospective study** to analyze postpreparation human sperm motility parameters and reactive oxygen species production following antioxidant supplementation. SETTING: Andrology Laboratory, Royal Maternity Hospital, Belfast, Northern Ireland. PATIENT(S): **Sixty patients** attending the Andrology Laboratory for semen analysis. INTERVENTION(S): Normozoospermic and asthenozoospermic semen samples (n = 10 for each control and antioxidant group) were prepared by Percoll density centrifugation in **media supplemented with ascorbate or alpha-tocopherol to different concentrations within physiologic levels.** Controls were included that were not exposed to antioxidant. OUTCOME: Sperm motility parameters were assessed using computer-assisted semen analysis. The generation of reactive oxygen species was determined using luminol-dependent chemiluminescence. RESULT(S): **The production of reactive oxygen species by sperm was reduced by supplementation in vitro with ascorbate and alpha-tocopherol. However, *progressive motility, average path velocity, curvilinear velocity, straight-line velocity, and linearity were decreased significantly, with the greatest inhibition observed with the highest concentrations of antioxidants.*** CONCLUSION(S): **Supplementation of preparation media with ascorbate and alpha-tocopherol, either singly or in combination, is not beneficial to sperm motility. In short, *sperm motility was significantly decreased by antioxidants vitamin C and alpha-tocopherol.***

The effect of ascorbate and alpha-tocopherol supplementation in vitro on DNA integrity and hydrogen peroxide-induced DNA damage in human spermatozoa (Donnelly et al, Mutagenesis. 1999)

(#Semen samples with normozoospermic and asthenozoospermic profiles (n = 15 for each control and antioxidant group) The aim of this study was to determine the effects of **supplementation with ascorbate and alpha-tocopherol, both singly and in combination**, during sperm preparation on subsequent sperm DNA integrity, induced DNA damage and reactive oxygen species (ROS) generation. Semen samples with normozoospermic and asthenozoospermic profiles (n = 15 for each control and antioxidant group) were prepared by Percoll density centrifugation where the medium had been supplemented with these antioxidants to a number of different concentrations, all within physiological levels. Controls were included which had no ascorbate or alpha-tocopherol added. DNA damage was induced using hydrogen peroxide (H_2O_2) and DNA integrity was determined using a modified alkaline single cell gel electrophoresis (Comet) assay, while ROS generation was measured using chemiluminescence. Addition of ascorbate to sperm preparation medium did not affect baseline DNA integrity but did provide sperm with complete protection against H_2O_2-induced DNA damage. Generation of H_2O_2-induced ROS was also significantly reduced after treatment with ascorbate, although baseline levels were unaffected by this antioxidant. Supplementation of sperm preparation medium with alpha-tocopherol did not influence baseline DNA integrity but provided sperm with dose-dependent protection against H_2O_2-induced DNA damage. Generation of H_2O_2-induced ROS was significantly reduced after treatment with alpha-tocopherol, although baseline ROS levels were unaffected by this antioxidant. **Addition of *both ascorbate and alpha-tocopherol in combination to sperm preparation medium actually induced DNA damage and intensified the damage induced by H_2O_2,*** however, **H_2O_2-induced ROS production was significantly reduced in a dose-dependent manner by supplementation with both vitamins.**

Circa 2000

Heart Outcome Prevention Evaluation Study (HOPE) (Yusuf et al, 2000) (#9,541 patients at high risk for cardiovascular events or diabetes) Dose: 400 IU (268 mg) *a*-tocopherol; patients at high risk for cardiovascular events or diabetes, **treatment with vitamin E for a mean of 4.5 years had no apparent effect on cardiovascular outcomes.** There were no significant differences in the numbers of deaths from cardiovascular causes, myocardial infarction, or stroke. There were no significant differences in the incidence of secondary cardiovascular outcomes or in death from any cause.

Meta-Analysis of Vitamin E in CVD, Ischemic Heart Disease (IHD) and Mortality (Dagenais et al. 2000) (#51,000 participants); a meta-analysis of the four randomized trials done in Europe and America involving a total of **51,000** participants allocated to vitamin E or placebo for 1.4 to 6 years, **did not demonstrate a reduction in cardiovascular and IHD mortality and nonfatal myocardial infarction**. In 1999-2000, there were no data to support the use of these vitamins to reduce the risk of cardiovascular events.

This same data is discussed at the following reference:
Dagenais GR, Marchioli R, Yusuf S, Tognoni G. Beta-carotene, vitamin C, and vitamin E and cardiovascular diseases. Curr Cardiol Rep. 2000 Jul;2(4):293-9.

In contrast, four large randomized trials did not reveal a reduction in cardiovascular events with beta-carotene use, and *may, in fact, increase IHD and total mortality in male smokers.*

Vitamin C and the Risk of Acute Myocardial Infarction. (Riemersma et al, 2000) (#180 males with a first AMI and 177 healthy volunteers) Low-fat soluble-antioxidant status is associated with an increased risk of heart disease. The aim of this study was to examine whether low plasma concentrations of vitamin C confer an independent risk of acute myocardial infarction (AMI). **Design:** Male patients (*n* = **180**) aged <65 y **with a first AMI and without an existing diagnosis of angina** (>6 mo) who were admitted within 12 h after onset of symptoms were compared with apparently healthy volunteers (*n* = 177). Plasma concentrations and dietary intakes of vitamin C were determined during hospitalization and 3 mo later. **Results:** Compared with the control

subjects, **the patients had higher total cholesterol and lower HDL-cholesterol concentrations and more of them smoked**. The relative risk of AMI for the lowest compared with the highest quintile of plasma vitamin C during hospitalization was 8.37 after adjustment for classic risk factors. At 3 mo, mean (±SEM) plasma vitamin C concentrations in patients had increased significantly, from 19.6 ± 1.2 to 35.1 ± 1.9 µmol/L and no longer conferred a risk of AMI. Habitual dietary vitamin C intake of patients (before AMI) did not differ significantly from that of control subjects. The increase in plasma vitamin C after recovery from the infarction could not be explained by a similarly large increase in dietary vitamin C. **Conclusions:** **A low plasma concentration of vitamin C was not associated with an increased risk of AMI, irrespective of smoking status**. The apparent risk of AMI due to a low plasma vitamin C concentration was distorted by the acute phase response.

The effects of combined conventional treatment, oral antioxidants and essential fatty acids on sperm biology in subfertile men (Comhaire et al, 2000) (#27 infertile men)

They evaluated the effects of combined conventional treatment, oral antioxidants **(N-acetyl-cysteine or vitamins A plus E)** and essential fatty acids (FA) on sperm biology in an open prospective study including 27 infertile men. The evaluation included sperm characteristics, seminal reactive oxygen species (ROS), FA of sperm membrane phospholipids, sperm oxidized DNA (8-OH-dG), and induced acrosome reaction (AR). **Treatment did not improve sperm motility and morphology, nor decrease the concentration of round cells and white blood cells in semen**. Sperm concentration increased in oligozoospermic men. Treatment significantly reduced ROS and 8-OH-dG. Treatment increased the AR, the proportion of polyunsaturated FA of the phospholipids, and sperm membrane fluidity. The overall pregnancy rate was 4.5% in 134 months. The per month pregnancy rate tended to be higher in partners of (ex)-smokers than in never-smokers.

Circa 2001

Dietary antioxidant vitamins, retinol, and breast cancer incidence in a cohort of Swedish women.

(Michels et al, 2001) (#59,036 women free of cancer) Dietary antioxidant vitamins and retinol have been proposed to be protective against breast cancer on the basis of their ability to reduce oxidative DNA damage and their role in cell differentiation. Epidemiologic studies have not been convincing in supporting this hypothesis, but women with high exposure to free radicals and oxidative processes have not been specifically considered. They explored these issues in the Swedish Mammography Screening Cohort, a large population-based prospective cohort study in Sweden that comprised **59,036 women**, 40-76 years of age, who were free of cancer at baseline and who had answered a validated 67-item food frequency questionnaire. During 508,267 person-years of follow-up, 1,271 cases of invasive breast cancer were diagnosed. **There was no overall association between intake of ascorbic acid, beta-carotene, retinol or vitamin E and breast cancer incidence.** High intake of ascorbic acid was inversely related to breast cancer incidence among overweight women and women with high consumption of linoleic acid (HR=0.72; 95% Cl 0.52-1.02, for highest quintile of ascorbic acid intake and average consumption of more than 6 grams of linoleic acid per day). Among women with a body mass index of 25 or below, the hazard ratio for breast cancer incidence was 1.27, comparing the highest to the lowest quintile of ascorbic acid intake. Consumption of foods high in ascorbic acid may convey protection from breast cancer among women who are overweight and/or have a high intake of linoleic acid.

The secondary prevention HDL Atherosclerosis Treatment study (HATS) (Brown et al., 2001) (#160 patients

with coronary disease); alpha tocopherol, vitamin E, beta carotene, and selenium. Compared with no treatment, only simvastatin/niacin significantly lowered stenosis progression rate and favorably altered plasma lipid profiles. **Antioxidant supplementation alone had no significant effect on clinical end points** but, notably, *when used in combination with simvastatin/niacin, antioxidants negated the benefit of the latter on plasma lipid profile and stenosis progression.*

The Perth Carotid Ultrasound Disease Assessment Study (CUDAS) (McQuillan et al 2001) (#1,111

subjects); antioxidant vitamins (vitamins A, C and E, lycopene and alpha- and beta-carotene) were independently associated with common carotid artery intima-media (wall) thickness (IMT) or focal plaque, or both. This study provided limited support for the hypothesis that increased dietary intake of vitamin E and increased plasma lycopene may decrease the risk of atherosclerosis. **No benefit was demonstrated for supplemental antioxidant vitamin use.**

Previous observational reports of subclinical atherosclerosis evaluated by carotid IMT and antioxidant vitamins have also generally yielded quite confusing and often conflicting results. For example, a report from the **Atherosclerosis Risk In Communities (ARIC)** group found individuals with **the highest carotid IMT to have lower levels of plasma carotenoids but higher alpha-tocopherol and retinol levels compared to controls** (Iribarren et al, 1997).

Randomized Trial of Supplemental ß-Carotene to Prevent Second Head and Neck Cancer (Mayne et al, 2001) (#264 patients who had been curatively treated for a recent early-stage squamous cell carcinoma of the oral cavity, pharynx, or larynx.); randomized, placebo-controlled, double-blinded clinical trial; 50 mg of ß-carotene per day; After a median follow-up of 51 months, there **was no difference between the two groups** in the time to failure [second primary tumors plus local recurrences. **Supplemental ß-carotene had no significant effect on second head and neck cancer or lung cancer.** Whereas none of the effects were statistically significant, the *point estimates suggested a possible decrease in second head and neck cancer risk but a possible increase in lung cancer risk.*

Age-Related Eye Disease Study Research Group (AREDS) (AREDS, 2001) (#4,757 participants); a high-dose formulation of vitamin C, vitamin E, and beta carotene in **4,757** participants, relatively well-nourished older adult cohort, had **no apparent effect on the 7-year risk of development or progression of age-related lens opacities or visual acuity loss.**

Meagher et al, **found no effect of vitamin E supplements on biochemical markers of lipid peroxidation in 30** healthy men and women, aged 18-60 years in an 8 wk. study. Garret A. FitzGerald and Emma Meagher, University of Pennsylvania Medical Center, said, "**There are no large-scale controlled trials indicating that healthy people derive any benefit from vitamin E supplements**. It would seem therapeutically judicious and economically prudent for such individuals to abstain from vitamin E consumption and await the evidence." (Meagher et al. 2001).

HDL Atherosclerosis Treatment study (HATS)

(Brown et al, 2001) (#160 participants); an antioxidant cocktail (vitamin E, ß-carotene, vitamin C, and selenium) had a 0.7% progression in stenosis after 3 years, compared with 0.4% regression in the group on only simvastatin/ niacin. Thus, *antioxidant supplements may have interfered with the efficacy of statin-plus-niacin therapy.* **No clinical or angiographically measurable benefit from antioxidants was found.**

Brown et al. conclude that antioxidant vitamins E and C and ß-carotene, alone or in combination, do not protect against cardiovascular disease. Their use for this purpose may create a diversion away from proven therapies. Because these vitamins blunt the protective HDL2 cholesterol response to HDL cholesterol–targeted therapy, they are potentially harmful in this setting. We conclude that they should rarely, if ever, be recommended for cardiovascular protection (Brown et al., 2002).

Thus, in agreement with many in the field, **it was concluded that the existing scientific database does not justify routine use of antioxidant supplements for the prevention and treatment of CVD** i.e., the Nutrition Committee of the American Heart Association Council on Nutrition, Physical Activity, and Metabolism. Antioxidant Vitamin Supplements and Cardiovascular Disease; the American College of Cardiology/ American Heart Association 2002 Guideline Update; American College of Cardiology/American Heart Association Task Force on Practice Guidelines. Committee on the Management of Patients With Chronic Stable Angina. ACC/AHA 2002 guideline update for the management of patients with chronic stable angina.

Additionally, "Evidence-Based Guidelines for Cardiovascular Disease Prevention in Women" concluded that **antioxidant vitamin supplements should not be used to prevent CVD, pending the results of ongoing trials (Class III, Level A Evidence).**

Even in 2001, the thrust of the data was turning against the overly-hyped antioxidant supplements as evidenced in an article entitled, "Antioxidant supplements to prevent heart disease: Real hope or empty hype?" (Tran et al, 2001).

Vitamin C and Vitamin E Supplement Use and Colorectal Cancer Mortality in a large American Cancer Society cohort. (Cancer Prevention Study

II cohort - CPS-II) (Jacobs, 2001) (#711,891 men and women in U.S.A.)

Some recent epidemiological studies have suggested that use of vitamin C or vitamin E supplements, both of which are important antioxidants, may substantially reduce the risk of colon or colorectal cancer. They examined the association between colorectal cancer mortality and use of individual vitamin C and E supplements in the American Cancer Society's Cancer Prevention Study II cohort. We used proportional hazards modeling to estimate rate ratios among **711,891 men and women** in the United States who completed a self-administered questionnaire at study enrollment in 1982, had no history of cancer, and were followed for mortality through 1996. During the 14 years of follow-up, 4404 deaths from colorectal cancer occurred. After adjustment for multiple colorectal cancer risk factors, regular use of vitamin C or E supplements, even long-term use, was not associated with colorectal cancer mortality. The combined-sex rate ratios were 0.89 for 10 or more years of vitamin C use and 1.08) for 10 or more years of vitamin E use. In subgroup analyses, use of vitamin C supplements for 10 or more years was associated with decreased risk of colorectal cancer mortality before age 65 years (rate ratio = 0.48; 95% CI, 0.28-0.81) and decreased risk of rectal cancer mortality at any age (rate ratio = 0.40; 95% CI, 0.20-0.80). **Our results do not support a substantial effect of vitamin C or E supplement use on overall colorectal cancer mortality.**

Risk of Ovarian Carcinoma and Consumption of Vitamins A, C and E and Specific Carotenoids: a prospective analysis. (Fairfield et al, 2001) (#80,326 women)

Antioxidant vitamins may decrease risk of cancer by limiting oxidative DNA damage leading to cancer initiation. Few prospective studies have assessed relations between antioxidant vitamins and ovarian carcinoma. METHODS: The authors prospectively assessed consumption of vitamins A, C, and E and specific carotenoids, as well as fruit and vegetable intake, in relation to ovarian carcinoma risk among Women reported on **known and suspected ovarian carcinoma risk 80,326 participants in the Nurses' Health Study who had no history of cancer other than nonmelanoma skin carcinoma.** factors including reproductive factors, smoking, and use of vitamin supplements on biennial mailed questionnaires from 1976 to 1996. Food frequency questionnaires were included in 1980, 1984, 1986, and 1990. The authors confirmed 301 incident cases of invasive epithelial ovarian carcinoma during 16 years of dietary follow-up (1980-1996). Pooled logistic regression was used to control for age, oral contraceptive use, body mass index, smoking history, parity, and tubal ligation. RESULTS: The authors observed no association between ovarian carcinoma risk and antioxidant vitamin consumption from foods, or foods and supplements together. The multivariate relative risks (95% confidence intervals [CIs]) for ovarian carcinoma among women in the highest versus lowest quintile of intake were 1.04 for vitamin A from foods and supplements; 1.01 for vitamin C; 0.88 for vitamin E; and 1.10 for beta-carotene. **Among users of vitamin supplements, the authors found no evidence of an association between dose or duration of any specific vitamin and ovarian carcinoma risk,** although the authors had limited power to assess these relations. **No specific fruits or vegetables were associated significantly with ovarian carcinoma risk. The authors found no association between ovarian carcinoma and consumption of total fruits or vegetables, or specific subgroups including cruciferous vegetables, green leafy vegetables, legumes, or citrus fruits. Women who consumed at least 2.5 total servings of fruits and vegetables as adolescents had a 46% reduction in ovarian carcinoma risk** (relative risk, 0.54, 95% CI, 0.29-1.03; P value for trend 0.04). CONCLUSIONS: **These data do not support an important relation between consumption of antioxidant vitamins from foods or supplements, or intake of fruits and vegetables, and incidence of ovarian carcinoma in this cohort.** However, modest associations cannot be excluded, and the authors' finding of an inverse association for total fruit and vegetable intake during adolescence raises the possibility that the pertinent exposure period may be much earlier than formerly anticipated.

As of 2010, new studies may be exposing another "medical myth." Investigators, writing in the Journal of the National Cancer Institute, are now telling us that **fruits and vegetables do not dramatically lower the risk of common diseases, including cancer.** Since the early 1980s, the dietary guidelines for Americans, published jointly by the USDA and the DHHS, have reflected the accumulated scientific research concerning diet and health. Early 1980 guidelines pertaining to nutrition and cancer were to "eat a variety of foods" and "eat foods with adequate starch and fiber." In 1990, "eat a variety of foods" remained a guideline but "choose a diet with plenty of vegetables, fruits, and grain products" replaced the starch and fiber reference. This mirrored the growing data suggesting a lowered risk of cancer with increased vegetable and fruit consumption. But, in 1995, grain products were placed ahead of vegetables and fruit in the guidelines to better reflect the structure of the USDA food pyramid. Other recommendations included the 1989 National Research Council *Diet and Health* report supporting consumption of 5 fruit and vegetable servings per day and the 1991 National Cancer Institute–DHHS sponsorship of the 5-A-Day Program. Public health guidelines for food oriented toward high vegetable and fruit consumption continued up to the present. This scenario led to the rising popularity of vitamin supplements from the 1980s until today, but there have been huge problems with these trends. First, the vitamin supplements were shown to lack the effect of vitamins acquired through the diet and second, vitamins A (beta carotene) and E (alpha tocopherol) were shown to have particularly harmful potential. Yet, recommendations promoting vegetable and fruit consumption remained a center piece, until now. A study of 500,000 Europeans joins a growing body of evidence undermining the high hopes that pushing "five-a-day" might slash Western cancer rates and it estimated that only around 2.5% of cancers could be averted by increasing fruit and vegetable intake. In short, **research has failed to substantiate the suggestion that as many as 50% of cancers could be prevented by boosting the public's consumption of fruit and vegetables.**

This latest study, which analyzed recruits from 10 countries to the highly-regarded **European Prospective Investigation into Cancer and Nutrition, confirms that the association between fruit and vegetable intake and reduced cancer risk is indeed weak.** The team, led by researchers from the Mount Sinai School of Medicine, in New York, calculated for lifestyle factors such as smoking and exercise before drawing their conclusions.

Carotenoids, Alpha-tocopherols, and Retinol in Plasma and Breast Cancer Risk in Northern Sweden.

(Hulten et al, 2001) (#201 cases and 290 referents) Using a nested case-referent design we evaluated the relationship between plasma levels of six carotenoids, alpha-tocopherol, and retinol, sampled before diagnosis, and later breast cancer risk. **Methods:** In total, 201 cases and 290 referents were selected from three population-based cohorts in northern Sweden, where all subjects donated blood samples at enrollment. All blood samples were stored at -80 degreesC. Cases and referents were matched for age, age of blood sample, and sampling centre. Breast cancer cases were identified through the regional and national cancer registries. **Results:** Plasma concentrations of carotenoids were positively intercorrelated. In analysis of three cohorts as a group **none of the carotenoids was found to be significantly related to the risk of developing breast cancer. Similarly, no significant associations between breast cancer risk and plasma levels of alpha -tocopherol or retinol were found.** However, **in postmenopausal women from a mammography cohort with a high number of prevalent cases, lycopene was significantly associated with a decreased risk of breast cancer.** A significant trend of an inverse association between lutein and breast cancer risk was seen in premenopausal women from two combined population-based cohorts with only incident cases. A non-significant reduced risk with higher plasma alpha -carotene was apparent throughout all the sub-analyses. **Conclusion: No significant associations were found between plasma levels of carotenoids, alpha -tocopherol or retinol and breast cancer risk in analysis of three combined cohorts.** However, results from stratified analysis by cohort membership and menopausal status suggest that lycopene and other plasma-carotenoids may reduce the risk of developing breast cancer and that menopausal status has an impact on the mechanisms involved.

Circa 2002

The Vitamin E Atherosclerosis Prevention Study (VEAPS) (Hodis et al, 2002) (#353 were randomized (176 placebo, 177 vitamin E) Epidemiological studies have demonstrated an inverse relationship between vitamin E intake and cardiovascular disease (CVD) risk. In contrast, randomized controlled trials have reported conflicting results as to whether vitamin E supplementation reduces atherosclerosis progression and CVD events. METHODS AND RESULTS: T h e study population consisted of men and women > or =40 years old with an LDL cholesterol level > or =3.37 mmol/L (130 mg/dL) and no clinical signs or symptoms of CVD. Eligible participants were randomized to DL-alpha-tocopherol 400 IU per day or placebo and followed every 3 months for an average of 3 years. A mixed effects model using all determinations of IMT was used to test the hypothesis of treatment differences in IMT change rates. Compared with placebo, alpha-tocopherol supplementation

significantly raised plasma vitamin E levels (P<0.0001), reduced circulating oxidized LDL (P=0.03), and reduced LDL oxidative susceptibility (P<0.01). However, **vitamin E supplementation did not reduce the progression of IMT over a 3-year period compared with subjects randomized to placebo.** CONCLUSIONS: The results are consistent with previous randomized controlled trials and **extend the null results of vitamin E supplementation to the progression of IMT in healthy men and women at low risk for CVD.**

MRC/BHF (MRC/BHF, 2002) (#20,536); (600 mg vitamin E, 250 mg vitamin C and 20 mg beta-carotene daily) It has been suggested that increased intake of various antioxidant vitamins reduces the incidence rates of vascular disease, cancer, and other adverse outcomes. METHODS: **20,536 UK adults (aged 40-80) with coronary disease, other occlusive arterial disease, or diabetes** were randomly allocated to receive antioxidant vitamin supplementation (600 mg vitamin E, 250 mg vitamin C, and 20 mg beta-carotene daily) or matching placebo. Intention-to-treat comparisons of outcome were conducted between all vitamin-allocated and all placebo-allocated participants. Allocation to this vitamin regimen approximately doubled the plasma concentration of alpha-tocopherol, increased that of vitamin C by one-third, and quadrupled that of beta-carotene. FINDINGS: **There were no significant differences in all-cause mortality or in deaths due to vascular causes. Nor were there any significant differences in the numbers of participants having non-fatal myocardial infarction or coronary death, non-fatal or fatal stroke, or coronary or non-coronary revascularization.** For the first occurrence of any of these "major vascular events", there were no material differences either or in any of the various subcategories considered. There were no significant effects on cancer incidence or on hospitalization for any other non-vascular cause. INTERPRETATION: Among the high-risk individuals that were studied, these antioxidant vitamins appeared to be safe. But, **although this regimen increased blood vitamin concentrations substantially, it did not produce any significant reductions in the 5-year mortality from, or incidence of, any type of vascular disease, cancer, or other major outcome.**

Antioxidant Vitamins and US Physician CVD

Mortality (Muntwyler et al. 2002) (#83,639 male U.S.A. physicians); use of supplements (**vitamin E, vitamin C, and multivitamin supplements was reported by 29% of the participants (16,727 patients). US male**

physicians self-selected supplementation with vitamin E, vitamin C or multivitamins was not associated with a significant decrease in total CVD or CHD mortality.

Women's Angiographic Vitamin and Estrogen (WAVE) Trial (Waters et al, 2002) (#423 postmenopausal women, with at least one 15% to 75% coronary stenosis); **neither HRT nor antioxidant vitamin supplements (vitamins C & E) provided any cardiovascular benefit.** Instead, *a potential for harm was suggested there is some **evidence of potentially adverse effects of antioxidant supplements on CVD as assessed by angiographic end points.*** In the Women's Angiographic Vitamin and Estrogen Study, *postmenopausal women with coronary disease on hormone replacement therapy given vitamin E plus vitamin C had an unexpected significantly higher all-cause mortality rate and a trend for an increased cardiovascular mortality rate* compared with the vitamin placebo women.

Mega-dose vitamins and minerals in the treatment of non-metastatic breast cancer: a n historical cohort study (Lesperance et al, 2002) (#90 patients with non-metastatic breast cancer who received conventional treatment) a historical cohort of 90 patients with non-metastatic breast cancer who received conventional treatment (eg, surgery, chemotherapy, radiation therapy, and hormonal therapy) either alone or in combination with high doses of beta-carotene, vitamin C, niacin, selenium, coenzyme Q10, and/ or zinc. **Breast cancer–specific survival (ie, patients censored only at death from breast cancer) and** *disease-free survival were shorter in the nutrient-supplemented group* **than in the non-supplemented group,** but the differences were not statistically significant.

Investigators stated that, "**It is troubling that both (Lesperance et al, 2002 and Ferreira et al, 2004) reported results suggesting poorer survival with concurrent administration of antioxidants and cytotoxic therapy.**"

The Roche European American Cataract Trial (REACT) (Chylack et al. 2002) (#445 patients); followed for 3 years after treatment with oral Vitamins E, C and beta-carotene. After two

years of treatment, there was **a small positive treatment effect in U.S.** patients. There was **no statistically significant benefit** of treatment in the U.K. group.

RMH Note: Long-term supplementation with alpha-tocopherol or beta-carotene was studied for an association with cataract prevalence and severity. An end-of-trial random sample of **1,828** participants from the randomized, double-blind, placebo-controlled clinical trial the alpha-tocopherol, beta-carotene cancer prevention study. Supplementation with alpha-tocopherol or beta-carotene for 5 to 8 years does not influence the cataract prevalence among middle-aged, smoking men (Teikari et al, 1997).

Vitamin E supplementation and macular degeneration (Taylor et al, 2002) (#1,193 subjects); Vitamin E 500 IU or placebo daily for four years; Daily supplement with **vitamin E supplement does not prevent the development or progression of early or later stages of age related macular degeneration.**

Vitamin E on Cardiovascular and Microvascular Outcomes in High-Risk Patients With Diabetes. Results of the HOPE Study and MICRO-HOPE Substudy (Lonn et al. 2002) (#3,654 with diabetes); people with diabetes in a randomized clinical trial with a 2 x 2 factorial design, which evaluated the effects of vitamin E and of ramipril in patients at high risk for CV events. The **daily administration of 400 IU vitamin E for an average of 4.5 years to middle-aged and elderly people with diabetes and CV disease** and/or additional coronary risk factor(s) has **no effect on CV outcomes or nephropathy.**

Vitamin C and Vitamin E Supplement Use and Bladder Cancer Mortality in a Large Cohort of US Men and Women (Cancer Prevention Study II (CPS-II) (Jacobs et al., 2002) (#991,522 US adults in the Cancer Prevention Study II (CPS-II) cohort.); CPS-II participants completed a self-administered questionnaire at enrollment in 1982 and were followed regarding mortality through 1998. Regular vitamin C supplement use (≥15 times per month) was not associated with bladder cancer mortality, regardless of duration. Regular vitamin E supplement use for ≥10 years

was associated with a reduced risk of bladder cancer mortality, but regular use of shorter duration was not. **Subjects who regularly consumed a vitamin E supplement for longer than 10 years had a reduced risk of death from bladder cancer. No benefit was seen from vitamin C supplements.**

Supplemental Vitamin C & E and Multivitamin use and Stomach Cancer Mortality in U.S.A. (Cancer Prevention Study II cohort - CPS-II)

(Jacobs et al. Jan. 2002) (#1,045,923 in U.S.A.) Supplementation with antioxidant vitamins has been associated with decreased risk of stomach cancer or regression of precancerous lesions in high-risk areas of China and Colombia. We examined the association between stomach cancer mortality and regular use (> or =15 times per month) of individual vitamin C supplements, individual vitamin E supplements, and multivitamins among **1,045,923 United States adults in the Cancer Prevention Study II (CPS-II) cohort.** CPS-II participants completed a questionnaire at enrollment in 1982 and were followed for mortality through 1998. During follow-up, there were 1,725 stomach cancer deaths (1,127 in men and 598 in women). After adjustment for multiple potential stomach cancer risk factors, **vitamin C use at enrollment was associated with reduced risk of stomach cancer mortality.** However, this reduction in risk was observed only among participants with short duration use at enrollment. **There was no association between stomach cancer mortality and regular use of vitamin E or multivitamins, regardless of duration of use.** Our results suggest that **the use of vitamin C, vitamin E, or multivitamin supplements may not substantially reduce risk of stomach cancer mortality in North American** populations in which stomach cancer rates are relatively low. Our results do not rule out effects of vitamin supplementation in areas in which stomach cancer rates are high and stomach cancer etiology may differ.

As in any observational study, the effects of potential confounding factors need to be considered, which is particularly true in analyses of vitamin supplement use because regular vitamin users are generally more likely to practice "health-conscious" behaviors. **At this time researchers cannot confidently recommend vitamin E supplements for the prevention of cancer because the evidence on this issue is inconsistent and limited.**

As of 2002, according to M.A. Moyad, "Some evidence for the use of these supplements exists, but **serious embellishment of study findings may be leading to an inappropriate use of these supplements** [selenium and vitamin E] **in a clinical setting**." Moyad et al had published an article entitled, "Selenium and vitamin E supplements for prostate cancer: evidence or embellishment?" (Moyad et al, 2002).

Vitamin E and C Supplements and Risk of Dementia
(Laurin et al, 2002) (#3,734 Japanese men) Honolulu-Asia Aging Study (HAAS), Intake of supplemental vitamins E and C was assessed from data collected in the 1988 mailed questionnaire and at the 1991 through 1993 asessment. **Men using both vitamin E and vitamin C (either for long or short term) were not at reduced risk for dementia or for the AD, AD with CVD, or VaD subtypes. No association was noted for supplements taken separately.** CONCLUSION: **we did not find a significant association of vitamin E or vitamin C supplement use and incident dementia**. Our results are based on incident cases and a longer period between the 1988 report of supplement use and assessment of dementia. Our data suggest that **supplemental intake of both vitamins E and C does not alter the risk for dementia.**

Retinol intake and bone mineral density in the elderly: the Rancho Bernardo Study.
(Promislow et al, 2002) (#570 women and 388 men) **Retinol is involved in bone remodeling, and excessive intake has been linked to bone demineralization**, yet its role in osteoporosis has received little evaluation. We studied the associations of retinol intake with bone mineral density (BMD) and bone maintenance in an ambulatory community-dwelling cohort of 570 women and 388 men, aged 55-92 years at baseline. Regression analyses, adjusted for standard osteoporosis covariates, showed an inverse U-shaped association of retinol, assessed by food-frequency questionnaires in 1988-1992, with baseline BMD, BMD measured 4 years later, and BMD change. Supplemental retinol use, reported by 50% of women and 39% of men, was an effect modifier in women; **the associations of log retinol with BMD and BMD change were negative for supplement users and positive for nonusers at the hip, femoral neck, and spine. At the femoral neck, for every unit increase in log retinol intake, supplement users had 0.02 g/cm^2 (p = 0.02) lower BMD and 0.23% (p = 0.05) greater annual bone loss, and nonusers had 0.02 g/cm^2 (p = 0.04) greater BMD and 0.22% (p =**

0.19) greater bone retention. However, among supplement users, retinol from dietary and supplement sources had similar associations with BMD, suggesting total intake is more important than source. In both sexes, *increasing retinol became negatively associated with skeletal health at intakes not far beyond the recommended daily allowance (RDA), intakes reached predominately by supplement users.* This study suggests **there is a delicate balance between ensuring that the elderly consume sufficient vitamin A and simultaneously cautioning against excessive retinol supplementation.**

Vitamin A intake and hip fractures among postmenopausal women. (Feskanich et al, 2002) (#72,337

postmenopausal women) Ingestion of toxic amounts of vitamin A affects bone remodeling and can have adverse skeletal effects in animals. The possibility has been raised that long-term high vitamin A intake could contribute to fracture risk in humans. **Objective** To assess the relationship between high vitamin A intake from foods and supplements and risk of hip fracture among postmenopausal women. **Design** Prospective analysis begun in 1980 with 18 years of follow-up within the Nurses' Health Study. **Setting** General community of registered nurses within 11 US states. **Participants** A total of 72,337 postmenopausal women aged 34 to 77 years. **Main Outcome Measures** Incident hip fractures resulting from low or moderate trauma, analyzed by quintiles of vitamin A intake and by use of multivitamins and vitamin A supplements, assessed at baseline and updated during follow-up. **Results** From 1980 to 1998, 603 incident hip fractures resulting from low or moderate trauma were identified. After controlling for confounding factors, *women in the highest quintile of total vitamin A intake (≥3000 µg/d of retinol equivalents [RE]) had a significantly elevated relative risk (RR) of hip fracture* compared with women in the lowest quintile of intake (<1250 µg/d of RE). *This increased risk was attributable primarily to retinol.* **The association of high retinol intake with hip fracture was attenuated among women using postmenopausal estrogens.** Beta carotene did not contribute significantly to fracture risk. Women currently taking a specific vitamin A supplement had a nonsignificant 40% increased risk of hip fracture compared with those not taking that supplement, and, among women not taking supplemental vitamin A, retinol from food was significantly associated with fracture risk. **Conclusions** *Long-term intake of a diet high in retinol may promote the development of osteoporotic hip fractures in women.* The amounts of retinol in fortified foods and vitamin supplements may need to be reassessed.

A prospective study on supplemental vitamin e intake and risk of colon cancer in women and men.

(Wu et al, 2002) (#87,998 females from the Nurses' Health Study and 47, 344 males from the Health Professionals Follow-up Study) (#135,332 total participants) They conducted a prospective study on the association between supplemental vitamin E and colon cancer in **87,998 females from the Nurses' Health Study and 47, 344 males from the Health Professionals Follow-up Study.** There was some suggestion that men with supplemental vitamin E intake of 300 IU/day or more may be at lower risk for colon cancer when compared with never users [multivariate relative risk (RR), 300-500 IU/day versus never users, 0.73; >or=600 IU/day versus never users = 0.70, but CIs included 1. **In women, there was no evidence for an inverse association between vitamin E supplementation and risk of colon cancer. Our findings do not provide consistent support for an inverse association between supplemental vitamin E and colon cancer risk.** Considering the paucity of epidemiological data on this association, further studies of vitamin E and colon cancer are warranted.

The Collaborative Primary Prevention Project

(PPP) (Chiabrando et al., 2002) (#144 participants with CHD risk factors); vitamin E (300 mg/day for about three years); reassess critically the role of vitamin E in CVD prevention; **Prolonged vitamin E supplementation did not reduce lipid peroxidation in subjects with major cardiovascular risk factors.**

Circa 2003

Vitamins E & A fail to reduce incidence or mortality of lung cancer: Cochrane Database Syst Rev.

2003. (Caraballoso et al., 2003) (#109,394 participants);**The electronic databases MEDLINE (1966-july 2001), EMBASE (1974-july 2001) and the Cochrane Controlled Trial Register (CENTRAL, Issue 3/2001) and bibliographies were searched. Duration of treatment varied from 2 to 12 years and follow-up was from two to five years.** When beta-carotene was combined with retinol, data from a single study showed that there was a statistically significant, **increased risk of lung cancer incidence and mortality** in people with risk factors for lung cancer who took both vitamins. **There is currently no evidence to support recommending vitamins such as alpha-tocopherol, beta-carotene or retinol, alone or in combination, to prevent lung cancer. A harmful effect was found for beta-carotene with retinol at pharmacological doses in people with risk factors for lung cancer.**

Use of antioxidant vitamins for the prevention of cardiovascular disease: meta-analysis of randomized trials.

(Vivekananthan et al., 2003) (The vitamin E trials involved a total of #81,788 patients, and the beta-carotene trials involved #138,113); **Vitamin E did not provide any benefit in lowering mortality compared to control treatments, and it did not significantly decrease the risk of cardiovascular death or stroke** ("cerebrovascular accident"). **The lack of any beneficial effect was seen consistently regardless of the doses of vitamins used and the diversity of the patient populations.** Therefore, **the CCF (Cleveland Clinic) researchers conclude that this study does "not support the routine use of vitamin E."**

Beta carotene led to small but statistically significant increase in all-cause mortality and a slight increase in cardiovascular death.

The researchers call their findings *"especially concerning"* because beta carotene doses are commonly included in over-the-counter vitamin supplements and multivitamin supplements that have been advocated for widespread use.

The study says that using vitamin supplements that contain beta carotene should be "actively discouraged" because of the increase in the risk of death. They also *recommend discontinuing study of beta carotene supplements because of their risk.*

Despite the negative findings of most of the clinical trials, **manufacturers continue to promote antioxidants as though they have been proven beneficial "wonder drugs."** Many also hype mixtures of beta-carotene and other carotenoids, which, they suggest, may provide the same benefits as fruits and vegetables, which they know is not true. **The FDA will not permit any of these substances to be labeled or marketed with claims that they can prevent disease.** The increased death rate from lung cancer in smokers who took beta carotene is evidence enough that high doses of vitamins and minerals are not necessarily harmless and may be fatal.

Two studies examined effects of *dietary* antioxidant intake on incidence of Alzheimer's disease. One found protective effects of E and C (Engelhart et al, 2002); the other only for E (Morris et al, 2002). **Neither found a benefit from vitamin supplements.** A third study found **no effect** of dietary carotenes, vitamin C, or vitamin E, nor effects of vitamin C or E supplements (Luchsinger et al. (2003).

Antioxidant Vitamins Effect on Alzheimer's Disease: Washington Heights-Inwood Columbia Aging Project (Luchsinger et al, 2003) (#980 elderly subjects)

relationship between AD and the intake of carotenes, vitamin C, and vitamin E in 980 elderly subjects in the Washington Heights-Inwood Columbia Aging Project who were free of dementia at baseline and were followed for a mean time of 4 years. CONCLUSION: **Neither dietary, supplemental, nor total intake of carotenes and vitamins C and E was associated with a decreased risk of AD in this study.**

Neoplastic and Antineoplastic Effects of Beta Carotene on Colorectal Adenoma Recurrence: Results of a Randomized Trial (Baron et al, 2003) (#864

subjects who had had an adenoma removed and were polyp-free); the effect of beta carotene supplementation on colorectal adenoma recurrence among subjects in a multicenter double-blind, placebo-controlled clinical trial of antioxidants for the prevention of colorectal adenomas. Results: **Among subjects who neither smoked cigarettes nor drank alcohol, beta-carotene was associated with a marked decrease in the risk of one or more recurrent adenomas, but beta carotene supplementation conferred a modest increase in the risk of recurrence among those who smoked. *For participants who smoked cigarettes and also drank more than one alcoholic drink per day, beta carotene doubled the risk of adenoma recurrence.***

Routine Vitamin Supplementation To Prevent Cardiovascular Disease: A Summary of the Evidence for the U.S. Preventive Services Task Force

(Morris and Carson, 2003); **Data Sources:** Cochrane Controlled Trials Registry and MEDLINE (1966 to September 2001), reference lists, and experts. **Conclusions:** Some good-quality cohort studies have reported an association between the use of vitamin supplements and lower risk for cardiovascular disease. **Randomized, controlled trials of specific supplements, however, have failed to demonstrate a consistent or significant effect of any single vitamin or combination of vitamins on incidence of or death from cardiovascular disease.**

In 2003, the **U.S. Preventive Services Task Force** (an independent panel sponsored by the Agency for Healthcare Research and Quality) concluded that **"the evidence is insufficient to recommend for or against the use of supplements of vitamins A, C, or E; multivitamins with folic acid; or antioxidant combinations for the prevention of cancer or cardiovascular disease."**

An **American Heart Association Science Advisory statement** (Circulation 110, 637-641 (2004)) concluded, **"At this time, the scientific data do not justify the use of antioxidant vitamin supplements for CVD risk reduction."**

Midlife Dietary Intake of Antioxidants and Risk of Late-Life Incident Dementia: The Honolulu-Asia Aging Study (Laurin et al, 2003) (#2,459 men) Data were obtained from the Honolulu-Asia Aging Study, a prospective community-based study of Japanese-American men. Analysis included 2,459 men with complete dietary data who were dementia-free at the first assessment. CONCLUSION: **Intakes of beta-carotene, flavonoids, and vitamins E and C were not associated with the risk of dementia or its subtypes.** This analysis suggests that **midlife dietary intake of antioxidants does not modify the risk of late-life dementia or its most prevalent subtypes.**

Serum retinol levels and the risk of fracture.
(Michealsson et al, 2003) (#2,322 men) Although studies in animals and epidemiologic studies have indicated that a high vitamin A intake is associated with increased bone fragility, no biologic marker of vitamin A status has thus far been used to assess the risk of fractures in humans. **Methods:** We enrolled 2,322 men, 49 to 51 years of age, in a population-based, longitudinal cohort study. Serum retinol and beta carotene were analyzed in samples obtained at enrollment. Fractures were documented in 266 men during 30 years of follow-up. Cox regression analysis was used to determine the risk of fracture according to the serum

retinol level. **Results:** *The risk of fracture was highest among men with the highest levels of serum retinol.* Multivariate analysis of the risk of fracture in the highest quintile for serum retinol (>75.62 µg per deciliter [2.64 µmol per liter]) as compared with the middle quintile (62.16 to 67.60 µg per deciliter [2.17 to 2.36 µmol per liter]) showed that the rate ratio was 1.64 (95 percent confidence interval, 1.12 to 2.41) for any fracture and 2.47 (95 percent confidence interval, 1.15 to 5.28) for hip fracture. *The risk of fracture was further increased within the highest quintile for serum retinol. Men with retinol levels in the 99th percentile (>103.12 µg per deciliter [3.60 µmol per liter]) had an overall risk of fracture that exceeded the risk among men with lower levels by a factor of seven* (P<0.001). The level of serum beta carotene was not associated with the risk of fracture. **Conclusions:** Our findings, which are consistent with the results of studies in animals, as well as in vitro and epidemiologic dietary studies, suggest that **current levels of vitamin A supplementation and food fortification in many Western countries may need to be reassessed.**

Impact of simvastatin, niacin, and/or antioxidants on cholesterol metabolism in CAD patients with low HDL.

(Matthan et al, 2003) (#123 HATS participants) The HDL Atherosclerosis Treatment Study (HATS) demonstrated a clinical benefit in coronary artery disease patients with low HDL cholesterol (HDL-C) levels treated with simvastatin and niacin (S-N) or S-N plus antioxidants (S-N+A) compared with antioxidants alone or placebo. Angiographically documented stenosis regressed in the S-N group but progressed in all other groups. To assess the mechanism(s) responsible for these observations, surrogate markers of cholesterol absorption and synthesis were measured in a subset of **123 HATS participants** at 24 months (on treatment) and at 38 months (off treatment). Treatment with S-N reduced desmosterol and lathosterol levels (cholesterol synthesis indicators) 46% and 36%, respectively, and elevated campesterol and ß-sitosterol levels (cholesterol absorption indicators) 70% and 59%, respectively, relative to placebo and antioxidant but not S-N+A. **Treatment with antioxidants alone had no significant effect.** Combining S-N with antioxidants reduced desmosterol and lathosterol by 37% and 31%, and elevated campesterol and ß-sitosterol levels by 54% and 46%, but differences did not attain significance.

A randomized trial of beta carotene and age-related cataract in US physicians. (Christen et al, 2003)

(#22,071 Male US physicians aged 40 to 84 years) OBJECTIVE:
To examine the development of age-related cataract in a trial of beta carotene supplementation in men. DESIGN: **Randomized, double-masked, placebo-controlled trial**. METHODS: **Male US physicians** aged 40 to 84 years (n = 22 071) were randomly assigned to receive either beta carotene (50 mg on alternate days) or placebo for 12 years. MAIN OUTCOME MEASURES: Age-related cataract and extraction of age-related cataract, defined as an incident, age-related lens opacity, responsible for a reduction in best-corrected visual acuity to 20/30 or worse, based on self-report confirmed by medical record review. RESULTS: There was no difference between the beta carotene and placebo groups in the overall incidence of cataract or cataract extraction. In subgroup analyses, the effect of beta carotene supplementation appeared to be modified by smoking status at baseline (P =.02). Among current smokers, there were 108 cases of cataract in the beta carotene group and 133 in the placebo group. Among current nonsmokers, there was no significant difference in the number of cases in the 2 treatment groups. The results for cataract extraction appeared to be similarly modified by baseline smoking status (P =.05). CONCLUSIONS: **Randomized trial data from a large population of healthy men indicate no overall benefit or harm of 12 years of beta carotene supplementation on cataract or cataract extraction**. However, among current smokers at baseline, beta carotene appeared to attenuate their excess risk of cataract by about one fourth.

Circa 2004

There has been evidence of adverse effects of antioxidant supplements on cardiovascular disease (CVD) as assessed by angiographic end points. In the Women's Angiographic Vitamin and Estrogen Study (2002), postmenopausal women with coronary disease on hormone replacement therapy given vitamin E plus vitamin C had an unexpected significantly higher all-cause mortality rate and a trend for an increased cardiovascular mortality rate compared with the vitamin placebo women. Similarily, in the HDL-Atherosclerosis Treatment Study (2001), subjects with angiographically demonstrated coronary artery disease on simvastatin/

niacin and an antioxidant cocktail (vitamin E, ß-carotene, vitamin C, and selenium) had a 0.7% progression in stenosis after 3 years, compared with 0.4% regression in the group on only simvastatin/niacin. Thus, antioxidant supplements may have interfered with the efficacy of statin-plus-niacin therapy. Further evaluation of data showed that the addition of the antioxidant vitamins blunted the expected rise in the protective HDL-2 cholesterol and apolipoprotein A1 subfractions of HDL. Overall, the studies showing either positive or adverse effects (especially for vitamins E, vitamins E and C, and the antioxidant cocktails) are much smaller studies than the larger clinical trials that consistently have not shown any beneficial effects of antioxidant supplements on several CVD end points. The existing scientific database, as of 2004, does not justify routine use of antioxidant supplements for the prevention and treatment of CVD.

Supplemental vitamin C increase cardiovascular disease risk in women with diabetes (Iowa Women's Health study) (Lee et al, 2004) (#1,923 postmenopausal women who reported being diabetic) When dietary and supplemental vitamin C were analyzed separately, only supplemental vitamin C showed a positive association with mortality endpoints. CONCLUSION: *A high vitamin C intake from supplements is associated with an increased risk of cardiovascular disease mortality in postmenopausal women with diabetes.*

Cochrane Database Syst Rev. 2004: Vitamins E & A fail to reduce incidence or mortality of gastrointestinal cancer. (Cochrane Database Syst Rev.) (Bjelakovic et al, 2004) (#170,525 participants); **14 randomized trials (170,525 participants), assessing beta-carotene (9 trials), vitamin A (4 trials), vitamin C (4 trials), vitamin E (5 trials), and selenium (6 trials). Neither the fixed effect nor random effects meta-analyses showed significant effects of supplementation with antioxidants on the incidences of gastrointestinal cancers.**

Among the seven high-quality trials reporting on mortality (131,727 participants), the fixed effect unlike the random effects meta-analysis showed that *antioxidant supplements significantly increased mortality. Beta-carotene and vitamin A and beta-carotene and vitamin E significantly increased mortality,* while beta-carotene alone only tended to do so. **Selenium showed significant beneficial effect on gastrointestinal cancer incidences.** *When the selenium trials* *were excluded, both analyses showed a statistically significant increase in mortality, which was particularly strong in patients taking beta carotene and vitamin A.*

No single antioxidant or combination of antioxidants significantly reduced the incidence of esophageal, gastric, colorectal, pancreatic, or hepatic cancer.

CONCLUSIONS: **They could not find evidence that antioxidant supplements prevent gastrointestinal cancers. On the contrary, they seem to increase overall mortality.**

ATBC 6-year followup study (2004) (Thornwall et al., 2004) (#29,133 male smokers); evaluated the 6-year post-trial effects of α-tocopherol and ß-carotene supplementation on coronary heart disease (CHD) in the α-tocopherol, ß-carotene cancer prevention (ATBC) study.

ß-Carotene seemed to increase the post-trial risk of first-ever non-fatal MI but there is no plausible mechanism to support it. Among men with pre-trial myocardial infarction, **no effects were observed** in post-trial risk of major coronary event.

HOPE study of vitamin E on renal insufficiency (2004) (Mann et al, 2004) (#993 people with a serum creatinine > or =1.4 to 2.3 mg/dL. And renal insufficiency); In people with mild-to-moderate renal insufficiency at high cardiovascular risk, vitamin E at a dose of 400 IU/day had **no apparent effect on cardiovascular outcomes.**

Randomized trials of vitamin E in the treatment and prevention of cardiovascular disease (2004) (Eidelman et al., 2004) (7 large-scale randomized trials) **Six of the 7 trials showed no significant effect of vitamin E on cardiovascular disease. In an overview, vitamin E had neither a statistically significant nor a clinically important effect on any important cardiovascular event or its components: nonfatal myocardial infarction or cardiovascular death.**

A point of emphasis is that, **"The use of agents of proven lack of benefit, especially those easily available over the counter, may contribute to underuse of agents of proven benefit and failure to adopt healthy lifestyles."**

Effect of supplemental vitamin E for the prevention and treatment of cardiovascular disease

(Shekelle et al, 2004) (#Eighty-four eligible trials) 84 trials were identified. For the outcomes of all-cause mortality, cardiovascular mortality, fatal or nonfatal myocardial infarction, and blood lipids, **neither supplements of vitamin E alone nor vitamin E given with other agents yielded a statistically significant beneficial or adverse pooled relative risk for all-cause mortality, cardiovascular mortality, and nonfatal myocardial infarction,** respectively. CONCLUSIONS: **There is good evidence that vitamin E supplementation does not beneficially or adversely affect cardiovascular outcomes.**

SU.VI.MAX Study (2004) (Hercberg et al, 2004) (#A total
of 13,017 French adults (7,876 women aged 35-60 years and 5141 men aged 45-60 years); All participants took a single daily capsule of a combination of 120 mg of ascorbic acid, 30 mg of vitamin E, 6 mg of beta carotene, 100 mug of selenium, and 20 mg of zinc, or a placebo. Median follow-up time was 7.5 years. RESULTS: **No major differences were detected between the groups in total cancer incidence, ischemic cardiovascular disease incidence or all-cause mortality.** However, unexplainably, after 7.5 years, low-dose antioxidant supplementation lowered total cancer incidence and all-cause mortality in men but not in women.

Meta-analysis: high-dosage vitamin E supplementation may increase all-cause mortality
(Miller et al., 2004) (#135,967 subjects); **Meta-analysis, including more than 135,000 subjects, concluded that *high doses of vitamin E increased mortality*.** Researchers said the current **U.S. dietary guidelines do not recommend vitamin E supplementation.** As a result, you will never see beta carotene supplements recommended again," Miller said.

Further, in January 2005, Gullar, Hanley and Miller et al. published a dose–response meta-analysis showing that high-dosage (≥400 IU/d) vitamin E supplementation was associated with a small but statistically significant increased risk for mortality (relative risk, 1.04 [95% CI, 1.01 to 1.07]) (1). The precise dosage of vitamin E at which the relative risk for mortality exceeded 1 and the magnitude of the risk increase were uncertain. However, the analysis showed that high-dosage vitamin E supplementation was likely to be harmful (Gullar et al, 2005).

Also, a 2004 study found vitamin E did not reduce onset of Alzheimer's.

Five studies included **102,735 patients** taking various doses of **vitamin C but showed no effect on cardiovascular disease mortality** (Morris and Carson, 2003).

Therefore, vitamin E (alpha-tocopherol) alone in doses of 400 units is of questionable value, and larger doses may cause intracranial hemorrhage or interact negatively with lipid-lowering drugs. Vitamin E should not be used in patients who have bleeding disorders or patients on anticoagulants or acetylsalicylic acid (ASA).

The role of vitamin E in the prevention of coronary events and stroke. Meta-analysis of randomized controlled trials (Alkhenizan and Al-Omran, 2004) (#80,645 subjects) a meta-analysis, using the Cochrane Group Methodology, of all available randomized controlled trials (RCTs) to evaluate the role of vitamin E in the prevention of CVD. Nine studies met inclusion criteria. **Vitamin E supplementation was not associated with a reduction in total mortality or total CVD mortality**, but it was associated with a small statistically significant reduction in non-fatal myocardial infarction in patients with pre-existing coronary artery disease.

Oats, Antioxidants and Endothelial Function in Overweight, Dyslipidemic Adults (Katz et al, 2004) (#30) (16 males ≥age 35; 14 postmenopausal females) were assigned, in random order, to oats (60 g oatmeal), vitamin E (400 IU) plus vitamin C (500 mg), the combination of oats and vitamins, or placebo; brachial artery reactivity scans (BARS) following a single dose of each treatment, and again following 6 weeks of daily ingestion, with 2-week washout periods. CONCLUSION: **The direction of effect was negative for vitamins C and E and the oat/vitamin combination with both acute and sustained treatment.**

Vitamin C worsens coronary atherosclerosis in those with two copies of the haptoglobin 2 gene.
(Levy et al, 2004) (#299 postmenopausal women) Antioxidant trials have not demonstrated efficacy in slowing cardiovascular disease but could not rule out benefit for specific patient subgroups. Antioxidant therapy reduces LDL oxidizability in haptoglobin 1 allele homozygotes (Hp 1-1), but not in individuals with the haptoglobin 2 allele (Hp 2-1 or Hp 2-2).

They therefore hypothesized that haptoglobin type would be predictive of the effect of vitamin therapy on coronary atherosclerosis as assessed by angiography.

They tested this hypothesis in the Women's Angiographic Vitamin and Estrogen (WAVE) trial, a prospective angiographic study of vitamins C and E with or without hormone replacement therapy (HRT) in postmenopausal women. Haptoglobin type was determined in **299 women** who underwent baseline and follow-up angiography. The annualized change in the minimum luminal diameter (MLD) was examined in analyses stratified by vitamin use, haptoglobin type, and diabetes status.

RESULTS—They found a significant benefit on the change in MLD with vitamin therapy as compared with placebo in Hp 1-1 subjects (0.079 ± 0.040 mm, $P = 0.049$). This benefit was more marked in diabetic subjects (0.149 ± 0.064 mm, $P = 0.021$). On the other hand, there was a trend toward a more rapid decrease in MLD with vitamin therapy in Hp 2-2 subjects, which was more marked in diabetic subjects (0.128 ± 0.057 mm, $P = 0.027$). HRT had no effect on these outcomes.

CONCLUSIONS—**The relative benefit or harm of vitamin therapy on the progression of coronary artery stenoses in women in the WAVE study was dependent on haptoglobin type.** This influence of haptoglobin type seemed to be stronger in women with diabetes. When the results of one randomized controlled trial were reanalyzed based on haptoglobin genotype, **antioxidant therapy (1,000 mg/day of vitamin C + 800 IU/day of vitamin E) was associated with improvement of coronary atherosclerosis in diabetic women with two copies of the haptoglobin 1 gene** *but worsening of coronary atherosclerosis in those with two copies of the haptoglobin 2 gene.*

Vitamin C for preventing and treating the common cold. Cochrane Database Syst Rev. 2004;(4):CD000980. (Douglas et al, 2004) (#11,350 study

participants) The role of vitamin C (ascorbic acid) in the prevention and treatment of the common cold has been a subject of controversy for 60 years, but is widely sold and used as both a preventive and therapeutic agent. OBJECTIVES: To discover whether oral doses of 0.2 g or more daily of vitamin C reduces the incidence, duration or severity of the common cold when used either as continuous prophylaxis or after the onset of symptoms. SEARCH STRATEGY: We   searched the Cochrane Central Register of Controlled Trials (CENTRAL) (The

Cochrane Library Issue 4, 2006); MEDLINE (1966 to December 2006); and EMBASE (1990 to December 2006). SELECTION CRITERIA: Papers were excluded if a dose less than 0.2 g per day of vitamin C was used, or if there was no placebo comparison. DATA COLLECTION AND ANALYSIS: Two review authors independently extracted data and assessed trial quality. 'Incidence' of colds during prophylaxis was assessed as the proportion of participants experiencing one or more colds during the study period. 'Duration' was the mean days of illness of cold episodes. MAIN RESULTS: Thirty trial comparisons involving **11,350 study participants** contributed to the meta-analysis on the relative risk (RR) of developing a cold whilst taking prophylactic vitamin C. The pooled RR was 0.96. A subgroup of six trials involving a total of 642 marathon runners, skiers, and soldiers on sub-arctic exercises reported a pooled RR of 0.50. Thirty comparisons involving 9676 respiratory episodes contributed to a meta-analysis on common cold duration during prophylaxis. A consistent benefit was observed, representing a reduction in cold duration of 8% for adults and 13.6% for children. Seven trial comparisons involving 3294 respiratory episodes contributed to the meta-analysis of cold duration during therapy with vitamin C initiated after the onset of symptoms. **No significant differences from placebo were seen.** Four trial comparisons involving 2,753 respiratory episodes contributed to the meta-analysis of cold severity during therapy and **no significant differences from placebo were seen.** CONCLUSIONS: **The failure of vitamin C supplementation to reduce the incidence of colds in the normal population indicates that routine mega-dose prophylaxis is not rationally justified for community use.** But evidence suggests that it could be justified in people exposed to brief periods of severe physical exercise or cold environments. **A meta-analysis of 30 placebo-controlled prevention trials found that vitamin C supplementation in doses up to 2 grams/day did not decrease the incidence of colds.**

Vitamin E supplementation and cataract: randomized controlled trial. (McNeil et al, 2004) (#1,193

eligible subjects with early or no cataract) Investigators determined whether treatment with vitamin E (500 IU daily) reduces either the incidence or rate of progression of age-related cataracts. DESIGN: A prospective, randomized, double-masked, placebo-controlled clinical trial entitled the Vitamin E, Cataract and Age-Related Maculopathy Trial. PARTICIPANTS: Of 1906 screened volunteers, **1,193 eligible subjects**

with early or no cataract, aged 55 to 80 years, were enrolled and followed up for 4 years. INTERVENTION: Subjects were assigned randomly to receive either **500 IU of natural vitamin E** in soybean oil encapsulated in gelatin or a placebo with an identical appearance. MAIN OUTCOME MEASURES: The incidence and progression rates of age-related cataract were assessed annually with both clinical lens opacity gradings and computerized analysis of Scheimpflug and retroillumination digital lens images obtained with a Nidek EAS-1000 lens camera. The analysis was undertaken using data from the eye with the more advanced opacity for each type of cataract separately and for any cataract changes in each individual. RESULTS: Overall, **87% of the study population completed the 4 years of follow-up**, with 74% of the vitamin E group and 76% of the placebo group continuing on their randomized treatment allocation throughout this time. For cortical cataract, the 4-year cumulative incidence rate was 4.5% among those randomized to vitamin E and 4.8% among those randomized to placebo. For nuclear cataract, the corresponding rates were 12.9% and 12.1%. For posterior subcapsular cataract, the rates were 1.7% and 3.5%, whereas for any of these forms of cataract, they were 17.1% and 16.7%, respectively. Progression of cortical cataract was seen in 16.7% of the vitamin E group and 18.4% of the placebo group. Corresponding rates for nuclear cataract were 11.4% and 11.9%, whereas those of any cataract were 16.5% and 16.7%, respectively. **There was no difference in the rate of cataract extraction between the 2 groups.** Lens characteristics of the participants withdrawn from the randomized medications were not different from those who continued. CONCLUSIONS: **Vitamin E given for 4 years at a dose of 500 IU daily did not reduce the incidence of or progression of nuclear, cortical, or posterior subcapsular cataracts. These findings do not support the use of vitamin E to prevent the development or to slow the progression of age-related cataracts.**

Antioxidant vitamins and coronary heart disease risk: a pooled analysis of 9 cohorts. (Knekt et al, 2004)

(#293,172 subjects free of CHD at baseline) Epidemiologic studies have suggested a lower risk of coronary heart disease (CHD) at higher intakes of fruit, vegetables, and whole grain. Whether this association is due to antioxidant vitamins or some other factors remains unclear. They studied the relation between the intake of antioxidant vitamins and CHD risk. **Design:** A **cohort study pooling 9 prospective studies** that included information on intakes of **vitamin E, carotenoids, and vitamin C** and that met specific criteria was carried out. During a **10-y follow-up**, 4647 major incident CHD events occurred in **293,172 subjects** who were free of CHD at baseline. **Results: Dietary intake of antioxidant vitamins was only weakly related to a reduced CHD risk after adjustment for potential nondietary and dietary confounding factors.** Compared with subjects in the lowest dietary intake quintiles for vitamins E and C, those in the highest intake quintiles had relative risks of CHD incidence of 0.84 and 1.23, respectively, and the relative risks for subjects in the highest intake quintiles for the various carotenoids varied from 0.90 to 0.99. **Subjects with higher supplemental vitamin C intake had a lower CHD incidence.** Compared with subjects who did not take supplemental vitamin C, those who took >700 mg supplemental vitamin C/d had a relative risk of CHD incidence of 0.75. **Supplemental vitamin E intake was not significantly related to reduced CHD risk. Conclusions:** The results suggest a reduced incidence of major CHD events at high supplemental vitamin C intakes. **The risk reductions at high vitamin E or carotenoid intakes appear small.**

A review of the epidemiological evidence for the 'antioxidant hypothesis' by the British Nutrition Foundation (the Food Standards Agency). (Stanner et

al, 2004) (British Nutrition Foundation independent review) The British Nutrition Foundation was recently commissioned by the Food Standards Agency to conduct a review of the government's research programme on Antioxidants in Food. Part of this work involved an independent review of the scientific literature on the role of antioxidants in chronic disease prevention, which is presented in this paper. BACKGROUND: There is consistent evidence that diets rich in fruit and vegetables and other plant foods are associated with moderately lower overall mortality rates and lower death rates from cardiovascular disease and some types of cancer. The 'antioxidant hypothesis' proposes that vitamin C, vitamin E, carotenoids and other antioxidant nutrients afford protection against chronic diseases by decreasing oxidative damage. RESULTS: Although scientific rationale and observational studies have been convincing, **randomized primary and secondary intervention trials have failed to show any consistent benefit from the use of antioxidant supplements on cardiovascular disease or cancer risk, with some trials even suggesting possible harm in certain subgroups.** These trials have usually involved the administration of single antioxidant nutrients given at relatively high doses. The results of trials investigating the effect of a balanced combination of antioxidants at levels achievable by diet are awaited. CONCLUSION: **The suggestion that antioxidant supplements can prevent chronic diseases has not been proved or consistently supported by the findings of published intervention trials.** Further evidence regarding the efficacy, safety and appropriate dosage of antioxidants in relation to chronic disease is needed. The most prudent public health advice remains to increase the consumption of plant foods, as such dietary patterns are associated with reduced risk of chronic disease.

Impact of antioxidants, zinc, and copper on cognition in the elderly: a randomized, controlled trial. (Yaffe et al, 2004) (#2,166 elderly persons) Participants in the Age-Related Eye Disease Study were randomly assigned to receive daily antioxidants (vitamin C, 500 mg; vitamin E, 400 IU; beta carotene, 15 mg), zinc and copper (zinc, 80 mg; cupric oxide, 2 mg), antioxidants plus zinc and copper, or placebo. A cognitive battery was administered to **2,166 elderly persons** after a median of 6.9 years of treatment. Treatment groups did not differ on any of the six cognitive tests (p > 0.05 for all). **These results do not support a beneficial or harmful effect of antioxidants or zinc and copper on cognition in older adults.**

Circa 2005

Use of multivitamins and prostate cancer mortality in a large cohort of US men. (Stevens et al, 2005) (#475,726 men who were cancer-free) Investigators assessed the association between the use of multivitamins and prostate cancer mortality. METHODS: A total of 5585 deaths from prostate cancer were identified during 18 years of follow-up of 475,726 men who were cancer-free and provided complete information on multivitamin use at enrollment in the Cancer Prevention Study II (CPS-II) cohort in 1982. Cox proportional hazards modeling was used to measure the association between multivitamin use at baseline and death from prostate cancer and to adjust for potential confounders. RESULTS: **The death rate from prostate cancer was marginally higher among men who took multivitamins regularly** (> or =15 times/ month) **compared to non-users; this risk was statistically significant only for those multivitamin users who used no additional (vitamin A,**

C, or E) supplements. In addition, risk was greatest during the initial four years of follow-up. CONCLUSIONS: *Regular multivitamin use was associated with a small increase in prostate cancer death rates* in our study, and this association was limited to a subgroup of users.

Vitamin A Supplementation for Reducing the Risk of Mother-to-child Transmission of HIV Infection: Cochrane systematic review 2005.

(Wiysonge et al, 2005) (#3,033 females) Mother-to-child transmission (MTCT) of HIV is the dominant mode of acquisition of HIV infection for children, currently resulting in more than 2000 new pediatric HIV infections each day worldwide. Observational studies have found significant associations between low serum vitamin A levels and increased risk of MTCT of HIV. We systematically reviewed currently available randomized controlled trials (RCTs) to evaluate the efficacy of vitamin A supplementation in preventing MTCT of HIV and other adverse pregnancy outcomes.

RCTs published between January 1980 and September 2005 were identified by searching the Cochrane Controlled Trials Register, PubMed, EMBASE, AIDSearch and conference proceedings, and contacting researchers. At least two authors independently assessed trial eligibility, and quality, and extracted data. We conducted meta-analysis using a fixed effects method, assessed heterogeneity between study results using the X^2 test of homogeneity, and used Higgins' I^2 to quantify the heterogeneity.

Four trials, involving **3,033 participants**, met the inclusion criteria. There was no evidence of an effect of vitamin A supplementation on MTCT of HIV infection. However, there was evidence of heterogeneity between the three trials with information on MTCT of HIV. **While the trials conducted in South Africa and Malawi did not find evidence that the effect of Vitamin A supplementation was different from that of placebo,** *the trial in Tanzania found evidence that vitamin A supplementation increased the risk of MTCT of HIV* compared with placebo and multivitamins (excluding vitamin A).

However, **synthesis of the currently available data does not show evidence of an effect of vitamin A supplementation on the risk of MTCT of HIV**, though there is an indication that vitamin A supplementation improves birth weight. The data suggest that the association between low serum vitamin A levels and increased risk of MTCT of HIV, seen in observational studies, could have alternative explanations, for example, low serum vitamin A levels may be a marker of advanced HIV infection and not causally related to MTCT of HIV.

The Alzheimer's Disease Cooperative Study (ADCS) Group (Petersen et al, 2005) (#769 subjects); Neither vitamin E nor donepezil delays progression from amnestic mild cognitive impairment to Alzheimer's disease in 769 subjects over 3 years.

Vitamin E Supplementation in Alzheimer's Disease, Parkinson's Disease, Tardive Dyskinesia, and Cataract: Part 2 (Pham et al, 2005); Using the MeSH terms alpha-tocopherol, tocopherols, vitamin E, Parkinson disease, tardive dyskinesia, Alzheimer disease, cataract, and clinical trials, a literature review was conducted to identify peer-reviewed articles in MEDLINE (1966-July 2005). RESULT: The clinical studies demonstrated contradicting results regarding the benefits of vitamin E in Parkinson's disease, tardive dyskinesia, and cataract. There is enough evidence from large, well-designed studies to discourage the use of vitamin E in Parkinson's disease, cataract, and Alzheimer's disease.

Dementia and Alzheimer's Disease in Community-Dwelling Elders Taking Vitamin C and/or Vitamin E: (Fillenbaum et al, 2005) (#626 elderly) a subgroup from the Duke Established Populations for Epidemiologic Studies of the Elderly; a longitudinal study. Information gathered during in-home interviews included sociodemographic characteristics, health status, health service use, and vitamin use. Neither use of any vitamins C and/or E (used by 8% of subjects at baseline) nor high-dose use reduced the time to dementia or AD. CONCLUSION: In this community in the southeastern US where vitamin supplement use is low, use of vitamins C and/or E did not delay the incidence of dementia or AD.

HOPE-TOO Extension (Lonn et al, 2005) (#3,994 original study enrollees) The Heart Outcomes Prevention Evaluation (HOPE) investigators report an extension of the 9,541-patient HOPE Vitamin E trial. In the 2.5-year extension of HOPE (HOPE-TOO) 174 of the original 267 centers continued an extended follow-up. From these centers, 3,994 of the 7,030 original study enrollees who were still alive elected to

continue the randomized vitamin E/placebo drug assignment. **After a mean of 7.2 years of follow-up, vitamin E did not significantly reduce the relative risk (RR) of total cancer incidence, of cancer death, or a composite of cardiovascular events including cardiovascular death, nonfatal myocardial infarction, and stroke, or of individual components of this composite end point. These findings of lack of benefit from vitamin E (natural source, 400 IU α-tocopheryl acetate) during the extended study are consistent with the original HOPE report and with recent meta-analyses of** Vivekananthan and Miller. *Another subgroup finding in HOPE-TOO was a vitamin E–associated* **increased risk of heart failure incidence** *that appeared in a secondary end point analysis in the 4.5-year report and persisted in the 7-year extended follow-up, as did the risk of hospitalization for heart failure.*

An increased risk of heart failure was associated with vitamin E supplementation in multiple analyses, including a 19% increased risk of all heart failure events and a 40% increase in the risk of hospital admission due to heart failure.

CONCLUSION: **In patients with vascular disease or diabetes mellitus, long-term vitamin E supplementation does not prevent cancer or major cardiovascular events and may increase the risk for heart failure.**

Patients in *the vitamin E group had a higher risk of heart failure and hospitalization for heart failure.* Similarly, among patients enrolled at the centers participating in the HOPE-TOO trial, **there were no differences in cancer incidence, cancer deaths, and major cardiovascular events, but** *higher rates of heart failure and hospitalizations for heart failure.*

The National Cancer Institute (NCI) issued a statement following the HOPE-TOO study as follows: **"NCI has never recommended that people take vitamin E outside a clinical trial for the prevention of cancer."**

In 2005, **the evidence for a relationship between vitamin E and heart disease and selenium and cancer was reviewed by the U.S. FDA. It was determined that there was insufficient evidence to permit a qualified health claim for vitamin E and cancer**, whereas there was some evidence for permitting a qualified health claim for selenium and cancer. The FDA also concluded that the primary prevention studies did not provide evidence for the relationship between vitamin E and reduced risk of CVD (Trombo, 2005).

The British Medical Journal reported on 8/05/05 that **multivitamins and minerals do not prevent respirator, stomach, skin or other infections in the elderly**. An estimated 10% of elderly over 70 years are thought to have vitamin and mineral deficiencies, which may lead to poor immune responses and increased infections. Dr. Avenell studied 900 elderly and **found no benefit in preventing infections with the use of multivitamins and mineral supplements.**

Recent attempts the validate the teachings of the free radical theory, in the prevention of cardiovascular disease and cancer have failed, as demonstrated with vitamin E and beta carotene. Data on hundreds of thousands of patients have resulted in antioxidant failure and ineffectiveness in the prevention of disease. Moreover, **previously unrecognized risks caused by nutrient toxicity and nutrient interactions have surfaced during intervention studies.** (Lichtenstein and Russell, 2005).

Women's Health Study (WHS) (Lee et al, 2005) (#39,876 apparently healthy US women); "Vitamin E in the Primary Prevention of Cardiovascular Disease and Cancer" **600 IU of natural-source vitamin E taken every other day provided no overall benefit for major cardiovascular events or cancer, did not affect total mortality, and decreased cardiovascular mortality in healthy women.** These **data do not support recommending vitamin E supplementation for cardiovascular disease or cancer prevention among healthy women.**

Randomized controlled trials like the WHS are considered the gold standard in medical research and provide the most reliable results.

A randomized trial of antioxidant vitamins to prevent second primary cancers in head and neck cancer patients (Bairati et al, 2005 Apr 6) (#540 patients with stage I or II head and neck cancer treated by radiation therapy) 540 patients with stage I or II head and neck cancer treated by radiation therapy. Supplementation with alpha-tocopherol (400 IU/day) and beta-carotene (30 mg/day). In the course of the trial, **beta-carotene supplementation was discontinued after 156 patients had enrolled because of ethical concerns.** Compared with patients receiving placebo, *patients receiving alpha-tocopherol supplements had a higher rate of second primary cancers during the supplementation period* but a lower rate after supplementation was discontinued. Similarly, *the rate of having a recurrence or second primary cancer was higher during* but lower after supplementation with alpha-tocopherol. The proportion of participants free of second primary cancer overall after 8 years of follow-up was similar in both arms. CONCLUSIONS: *alpha-Tocopherol supplementation produced unexpected adverse effects on the occurrence of second primary cancers and on cancer-free survival.*

Note: Patients taking an antioxidant were 1.65 times more likely to suffer a return of their original cancer during the three years they were on the supplement. The risk was highest among those taking only vitamin E (1.86 times higher). Five years after they stopped taking the supplement, their recurrence risk had fallen to the same level as those in the placebo group. Although suggestive of harm, these results were not statistically significant.

Randomized trial of antioxidant vitamins to prevent acute adverse effects of radiation therapy in head and neck cancer patients (Bairati et al, 2005 Aug 20) (#540 patients with stage I or II head and neck cancer treated

by radiation therapy) A randomized trial was conducted to determine whether supplementation with antioxidant vitamins could reduce the occurrence and severity of acute adverse effects of radiation therapy and improve quality of life without compromising treatment efficacy. During the course of the trial, *supplementation with beta-carotene was discontinued because of ethical concerns.* **Quality of life was not improved by the supplementation.** *The rate of local recurrence of the head and neck tumor tended to be higher in the supplement arm* of the trial. CONCLUSION: Supplementation with high doses of alpha-tocopherol and beta-carotene during radiation therapy could reduce the severity of treatment adverse effects. However, **this trial suggests that use of high doses of antioxidants as adjuvant therapy might compromise radiation treatment efficacy.**

Note: Researchers were concerned to find that the rate of local recurrence (that is, a return of the original cancer) was 54 percent higher among patients on the combination pill than those on placebo. There was a smaller but still worrisome increase among those on vitamin E only.

NCI COMMENT: "This is a large, well-done study with good compliance from the participants," said Eva Szabo, M.D., of the National Cancer Institute's Division of Cancer Prevention. "The results demonstrate that the use of vitamin E supplementation is not beneficial to patients with stage I or II head and neck cancer, either as a chemoprevention agent or to enhance quality of life during radiation therapy."

At about this point in 2005, the followers of the free radical theory were scrambling to explain the repeated RCT failures. **Despite overwhelming evidence on the damaging consequences of oxidative stress and its role in experimental diabetes, large scale clinical trials with classic antioxidants failed to demonstrate any benefit for diabetic patients** (Johansen et al, 2005).

Effect of intensive lipid lowering, with or without antioxidant vitamins, compared with moderate lipid lowering on myocardial ischemia (Stone et al, 2005) (#300 patients with stable coronary disease); **randomized, double-blind, placebo-controlled trial; antioxidant vitamins C (1000 mg/d) and E (800 mg/d); Angina frequency decreased in each group. There was no incremental effect of supplemental vitamins C and E on any ischemia outcome.** CONCLUSIONS: **Intensive lipid lowering with atorvastatin to an LDL level of 80 mg/dL, with or without antioxidant vitamins, does not provide any further benefits in ambulatory ischemia, exercise time to onset of ischemia, and angina frequency than moderate lipid lowering with diet and low-dose lovastatin to an LDL level of <120 mg/dL.**

Vitamin C and vitamin E for Alzheimer's disease.

(Boothby and Doering, 2005) To evaluate the literature on supplemental vitamin C and vitamin E therapy in the prevention and treatment of Alzheimer's disease (AD). DATA SOURCES: Literature retrieval was accessed through MEDLINE (1966-March 2005) using the key words antioxidants, vitamin C, vitamin E, Alzheimer's disease, and dementia. International Pharmaceutical Abstracts (1970-March 2005), Current Contents (1996-March 2005), Cochrane Database of Systematic Reviews (1994-March 2005), and Ebsco's Academic Search Elite (1975-March 2005) were searched with the same key words. STUDY SELECTION AND DATA EXTRACTION: Articles related to the objective that were identified through PubMed were included. DATA SYNTHESIS:
Oral supplementation of vitamin C (ascorbic acid) and vitamin E (D-alfa-tocopherol acetate) alone and in combination have been shown to decrease oxidative DNA damage in animal studies in vivo, in vitro, and in situ.

Recent results of a prospective observational study (n = **4,740**) **suggest that the combined use of vitamin E 400 IU daily and vitamin C 500 mg daily for at least 3 years was associated with the reduction of AD prevalence** and incidence. **Contradicting this is a previous prospective observational study (n = 980) evaluating the relationship between 4 years of vitamin C and E intake and the incidence of AD, which detected no difference in the incidence of AD during the 4-year follow-up. Recent meta-analysis results suggest that doses of vitamin E > or =400 IU daily for more than one year are associated with increased all-cause mortality. Mega-trial results suggest that vitamin E doses > or =400 IU daily for 6.9 years in patients with preexisting vascular disease or diabetes mellitus increase the incidence of heart failure, with no other outcome benefits noted.** CONCLUSIONS: In   the absence of prospective, randomized, controlled clinical trials documenting benefits that outweigh recently documented morbidity and mortality risks, **vitamin E supplements should not be recommended for primary or secondary prevention of AD**. Although the risks of taking high doses of vitamin C are lower than those with vitamin E, the lack of consistent efficacy data for vitamin C in preventing or treating AD should discourage its routine use for this purpose.

An Interesting Case of "Supplement Nephropathy"

A 48-year-old Japanese woman previously in good health was found to have severe proximal tubular dysfunction with a high serum level of ascorbic acid (57.3 microg/ml, reference range: 1.9 - 15.0 microg/ml). Renal biopsy specimen showed marked tubulointerstitial damage, i.e. tubular atrophy, dilatation of tubular lumen with flattened tubular epithelial cells, vacuolization of proximal and distal tubular epithelial cells, and severe interstitial fibrosis with mild infiltration of mononuclear cells. Calcified lesions, which caused tubular obstruction or stenosis, were also seen in interstitial area adjacent to degenerated proximal tubuli. Hypokalemic nephropathy, probably due to long-term use of laxatives, was clearly shown. However, **calcified lesions seemed to be caused by inappropriate excessive daily ingestion of ascorbic acid (6,000 mg/day),** calcium lactate, and vitamin D because of the patient's misunderstanding that these supplements could keep her in a good health. This condition may be clinically called "supplement nephropathy" (Ohtake et al, 2005).

Circa 2006

Vitamin-mineral supplementation and the progression of atherosclerosis (Bleys et al, 2006) (searched the MEDLINE, EMBASE, and CENTRAL databases); a meta-analysis of randomized controlled trials; meta-analysis showed **no evidence of a protective effect of antioxidants** (vitamins E and C, ß-carotene, or selenium) **or B vitamin supplements on the progression of atherosclerosis.**

Also in 2006, there was "The Efficacy and Safety of Multivitamin and Mineral Supplement Use To Prevent Cancer and Chronic Disease in Adults: A Systematic Review for a National Institutes of Health State-of-the-Science Conference by Huang et al. They concluded that the **evidence was insufficient to prove the presence or absence of benefits from use of multivitamin and mineral supplements to prevent cancer and chronic disease** (Huang et al, 2006).

Multivitamin/mineral supplements and prevention of chronic disease. (Huang et al, 2006 May) OBJECTIVES: To review and synthesize published literature on the efficacy of multivitamin/mineral supplements and certain single nutrient supplements in the primary prevention of chronic disease in the general adult population, and on the safety of multivitamin/mineral supplements and certain single nutrient supplements, likely to be included in multivitamin/mineral supplements, in the general population of adults and children. DATA SOURCES: All articles published through February 28, 2006, on MEDLINE, EMBASE, and the Cochrane databases. REVIEW METHODS: Each article underwent double reviews on title, abstract, and inclusion eligibility. Two reviewers performed data abstraction and quality assessment. **Differences in opinion were resolved through consensus adjudication.** RESULTS: Few trials have addressed the efficacy of multivitamin/mineral supplement use in chronic disease prevention in the general population of the United States. One trial on poorly nourished Chinese showed supplementation with combined Beta-carotene, vitamin E and selenium reduced gastric cancer incidence and

mortality, and overall cancer mortality. In a French trial, combined vitamin C, vitamin E, Beta-carotene, selenium, and zinc reduced cancer risk in men but not in women. No cardiovascular benefit was evident in both trials. **Multivitamin/mineral supplement use had no benefit for preventing cataract.** Zinc/antioxidants had benefits for preventing advanced age-related macular degeneration in persons at high risk for the disease. **With few exceptions, neither Beta-carotene nor vitamin E had benefits for preventing cancer, cardiovascular disease, cataract, and age-related macular degeneration.** *Beta-carotene supplementation increased lung cancer risk in smokers and persons exposed to asbestos.* **Folic acid alone or combined with vitamin B12 and/or vitamin B6 had no significant effects on cognitive function.** Selenium may confer benefit for cancer prevention but not cardiovascular disease prevention. Calcium may prevent bone mineral density loss in postmenopausal women, and may reduce vertebral fractures, but not non-vertebral fractures. The evidence suggests dose-dependent benefits of vitamin D with/without calcium for retaining bone mineral density and preventing hip fracture, non-vertebral fracture and falls. **We found no consistent pattern of increased adverse effects of multivitamin/mineral supplements except for skin yellowing by Beta-carotene.** CONCLUSIONS: Multivitamin/mineral supplement use may prevent cancer in individuals with poor or suboptimal nutritional status. The heterogeneity in the study populations limits generalization to United States population. **Multivitamin/mineral supplements conferred no benefit in preventing cardiovascular disease or cataract**, and may prevent advanced age-related macular degeneration only in high-risk individuals. The overall quality and quantity of the literature on the safety of multivitamin/mineral supplements is limited.

The Efficacy and Safety of Multivitamin and Mineral Supplement Use To Prevent Cancer and Chronic Disease in Adults: A Systematic Review for a National Institutes of Health State-of-the-Science Conference. (Huang et al, 2006 Sept)

BACKGROUND: Multivitamin and mineral supplements are the most commonly used dietary supplements in the United States. PURPOSE: To synthesize studies on the efficacy and safety of multivitamin/mineral supplement use in primary prevention of cancer and chronic disease in the general population. DATA SOURCES: English-language literature search of the MEDLINE, EMBASE, and Cochrane databases through February 2006 and hand-searching of pertinent journals and articles. STUDY SELECTION: **Randomized, controlled trials** in adults were reviewed to assess efficacy, and **randomized, controlled trials and observational studies in adults or children were reviewed to assess safety.** DATA EXTRACTION: Paired reviewers extracted data and independently assessed study quality. DATA SYNTHESIS: 12 articles from 5 randomized, controlled trials that assessed efficacy and 8 articles from 4 randomized, controlled trials and 3 case reports on adverse effects were identified. Study quality was rated fair for the studies on cancer, cardiovascular disease, cataracts, or age-related macular degeneration and poor for the studies on hypertension. **In a poorly nourished Chinese population, combined supplementation with beta-carotene, alpha-tocopherol, and selenium reduced the incidence of and mortality rate from gastric cancer and the overall mortality rate from cancer by 13% to 21%. In a French trial, combined supplementation with vitamin C, vitamin E, beta-carotene, selenium, and zinc reduced the rate of cancer by 31% in men but not in women. Multivitamin and mineral supplements had no significant effect on cardiovascular disease or cataracts**, except that combined beta-carotene, selenium, alpha-tocopherol, retinol, and zinc supplementation reduced the mortality rate from stroke by 29% in the Linxian study and that a combination of 7 vitamins and minerals stabilized visual acuity loss in a small trial. **Combined zinc and antioxidants slowed the progression of advanced age-related macular degeneration in high-risk persons.** No consistent adverse effects of multivitamin and mineral supplements were evident. LIMITATIONS: Only randomized, controlled trials were considered for efficacy assessment. Special nutritional needs, such as use of folic acid by pregnant women to prevent birth defects, were not addressed. Findings may not apply to use of commercial multivitamin supplements by the general U.S. population. CONCLUSIONS: **Evidence is insufficient to prove the presence or absence of benefits from use of multivitamin and mineral supplements to prevent cancer and chronic disease.**

Antioxidants Vitamin C and Vitamin E for the Prevention and Treatment of Cancer (Coulter et al, 2006)

(Thirty-eight studies); **The systematic review of the literature does not** support the hypothesis that the use of supplements of vitamin C or vitamin E in the doses tested helps prevent and/or treat cancer in the populations tested. The findings from randomized clinical trials were generally negative.

Vitamin C levels in Type 2 diabetes and low vitamin C levels does not improve endothelial dysfunction or insulin resistance (Chen et al, 2006) (#32 type 2 diabetics); randomized, double-blind, placebo-controlled study of vitamin C (800 mg/day for 4 wk; CONCLUSION: **high-dose oral vitamin C therapy**, resulting in incomplete replenishment of vitamin C levels, is **ineffective at improving endothelial dysfunction and insulin resistance in Type 2 diabetes.**

Meta-analysis: antioxidant supplements for primary and secondary prevention of colorectal adenoma (2006) (Bjelakovic et al., 2006) (#17,620 participants); eight randomized trials (**17,620 participants**). **Neither fixed-effect nor random-effect model meta-analyses showed statistically significant effects of supplementation with beta-carotene, vitamins A, C, E and selenium alone or in combination.** They found no convincing evidence that antioxidant supplements have significant beneficial effect on primary or secondary prevention of colorectal adenoma.

Australian Collaborative Trial of Supplements (ACTS) (Rumbold et al, 2006) (#1,877 pregnant women); Supplementation with vitamin C (1,000 mg) and vitamin E (400 IU) **during pregnancy does not reduce the risk of pre-eclampsia in nulliparous women, the risk of intrauterine growth restriction, or the risk of death or other serious outcomes in their infants. Certain adverse maternal outcomes were more common in the antioxidant group than in the placebo group, but these findings could be explained by chance alone.**

This is **the second major report in a month to find no apparent benefit for the supplements in preventing pre-eclampsia.** These results followed closely similar findings reported in the March 30, 2006 issue of *The Lancet* by researchers at Kings College London. In that **randomized study of high-risk women, not only did these vitamins fail to reduce the pre-eclampsia risk,** but *the rate of low-birth-weight babies was* *higher and the rate for gestational hypertension was higher for women in the vitamin group.*

There were no significant differences between the groups for death or serious outcomes among the infants. The vitamins were not associated with any primary benefits for the infants. Although vitamin therapy reduced the risk of respiratory distress syndrome in the infants, the downside of the therapy for the women was an increased risk of hospitalization for hypertension and the use of anti-hypertensive medication.

Of concern, there was a downside for the women taking vitamins. *Women in the vitamin group had an increased risk of being hospitalized antenatally for hypertension and having to take antihypertensive medication.* In addition, *a subgroup of women in the vitamin group had a higher frequency of abnormal liver-function tests.*

"Until more data are available, given the scant evidence of benefit and the potential for harm, supplemental antioxidant therapy for the prevention of pre-eclampsia should be limited to women enrolled in randomized trials and should not be prescribed as part of routine practice."

The Antioxidants in Prevention of Cataracts Study (APC Study): effects of antioxidant supplements on cataract progression in South

India. (Gritz et al, 2006) (#798 subjects) (supplementation with beta carotene, vitamins C and E) To determine if antioxidant supplements (beta carotene and vitamins C and E) can decrease the progression of cataract in rural South India. METHODS: The **Antioxidants in Prevention of Cataracts (APC) Study** was a 5 year, randomized, triple masked, placebo controlled, field based clinical trial to assess the ability of interventional antioxidant supplements to slow cataract progression. The primary outcome variable was change in nuclear opalescence over time. Secondary outcome variables were cortical and posterior subcapsular opacities and nuclear color changes; best corrected visual acuity change; myopic shift; and failure of treatment. Annual examinations were performed for each subject by three examiners, in a masked fashion. Multivariate modeling using a general estimating equation was used for analysis of results, correcting for multiple measurements over time. RESULTS: Initial enrollment was **798 subjects**. Treatment groups were comparable at baseline. There was high compliance with follow up and study medications. **There was progression in cataracts. There was no significant difference between placebo and active treatment groups for either the primary or secondary outcome variables.** CONCLUSION: **Antioxidant supplementation with beta carotene, vitamins C and E did not affect cataract progression in a population with a high prevalence of cataract whose diet is generally deficient in antioxidants.**

Vitamins in Pre-eclampsia (VIP) Trial Consortium (Poston et al., 2006) (#2,410 women at increased risk

for preeclampsia, analyzed 2,395) 1000 mg of vitamin C and 400 IU vitamin E; Concomitant supplementation with vitamin C and vitamin E does not prevent pre-eclampsia in women at risk, but *does increase the rate of babies born with a low birth weight.* "As such, use of these high-dose antioxidants is not justified in pregnancy." Thus, vitamin C and vitamin E supplementation are not helpful for woman with preeclampsia and may be harmful to the fetus

Drs Lindheimer and Sibai write. **"It appears surprising that administration of vitamins in amounts that did not exceed maximum daily tolerable allowances should be associated with adverse effects,** but the VIP data are not the first time that vitamin or nutrient supplements administered to populations already consuming considerable amounts of the supplement's content in their diets have had adverse effects.

SU.VI.MAX (2006) Antioxidants do not affect fasting blood glucose (Czernichow et al, 2006) (#3,146 subjects);

a daily capsule containing 120 mg vitamin C, 30 mg vitamin E, 6 mg ß-carotene, 100 µg Se, and 20 mg Zn or a placebo. Observational data suggest a protective effect of several antioxidants on fasting plasma glucose (FPG) and type 2 diabetes. However, randomized trials have yielded inconsistent results. **Supplementation with antioxidants at nutritional doses for 7.5 y had no effect on FPG** in men or women who followed a balanced diet. An inverse association of baseline ß-carotene dietary intake and plasma concentrations with FPG was found, probably because ß-carotene is an indirect marker of fruit and vegetable intakes.

Full title for Czernichow et al. 2006 article: A n t i o x i d a n t supplementation does not affect fasting plasma glucose in the Supplementation with Antioxidant Vitamins and Minerals (SU.VI.MAX) study in France: association with dietary intake and plasma concentrations.

Vitamin E and Risk of Type 2 Diabetes in the Women's Health Study (Liu et al., 2006) (#38,716 apparently healthy U.S. women); efficacy of vitamin E supplements for primary prevention of type 2 diabetes among apparently healthy women. **In this large trial with 10-year follow-up, alternate-day doses of 600 IU vitamin E provided no significant benefit for type 2 diabetes in initially healthy women.**

Because of repeated failures of antioxidant vitamins, the Harvard School of Public Health posted the following: **"The evidence accumulated so far isn't promising. Randomized trials of vitamin C, vitamin E, and beta-carotene haven't revealed much in the way of protection from heart disease, cancer, or aging-related eye diseases." (Harvard School of Public Health, website accessed 2/09/06).**

Vitamin E supplementation and cognitive function in women: The Women's Health Study (2006) (Kang et al., 2006) (#39,876 healthy US women); **There were no differences in global score between the vitamin E and placebo groups at the first assessment (5.6 years** after randomization) **or at the last assessment (9.6 years** of treatment). CONCLUSION: **Long-term use of vitamin E supplements did not provide cognitive benefits among generally healthy older women.**

Supplemental and dietary vitamin E, beta-carotene, and vitamin C intakes and prostate cancer risk (PLCO Trial) (Kirsh et al, 2006) (#29,361 men during up to 8 years of follow-up); the screening arm of the Prostate, Lung, Colorectal, and Ovarian Cancer Screening Trial; Overall, **there was no association between prostate cancer risk and dietary or supplemental intake of vitamin E, beta-carotene, or vitamin C.** CONCLUSIONS: **Our results do not provide strong support for population-wide implementation of high-dose antioxidant supplementation for the prevention of prostate cancer.** However, vitamin E supplementation in male smokers and beta-carotene supplementation in men with low dietary beta-carotene intakes were associated with reduced risk of this disease.

Intakes of vitamins A, C and E and folate and multivitamins and lung cancer: a pooled analysis

of 8 prospective studies. (Cho et al, 2006) (#430,281 persons over a maximum of 6-16 years in the studies)

Intakes of vitamins A, C and E and folate have been hypothesized to reduce lung cancer risk. We examined these associations in a pooled analysis of the primary data from 8 prospective studies from North America and Europe. Baseline vitamin intake was assessed using a validated food-frequency questionnaire, in each study. We calculated study-specific associations and pooled them using a random-effects model. During follow-up of 430,281 persons over a maximum of 6-16 years in the studies, 3,206 incident lung cancer cases were documented. Vitamin intakes were inversely associated with lung cancer risk in age-adjusted analyses; the associations were greatly attenuated after adjusting for smoking and other risk factors for lung cancer. The pooled multivariate relative risks, comparing the highest vs. lowest quintile of intake from food-only, were 0.96 for vitamin A, 0.80 for vitamin C, 0.86 for vitamin E and 0.88 for folate. The association with vitamin C was not independent of our previously reported inverse association with beta-cryptoxanthin. Further, **vitamin intakes from foods plus supplements were not associated with a reduced risk of lung cancer in multivariate analyses, and use of multivitamins and specific vitamin supplements was not significantly associated with lung cancer risk.** The results generally did not differ across studies or by sex, smoking habits and lung cancer cell type. In conclusion, **these data do not support the hypothesis that intakes of vitamins A, C and E and folate reduce lung cancer risk.**

In discussing the role of micronutrients, Shenkin said, "Micronutrients play a central role in metabolism and in the maintenance of tissue function, but effects in preventing or treating disease which is not due to micronutrient deficiency cannot be expected from increasing the intake. **Provision of excess supplements to individuals who do not need them may be harmful.** Clinical benefit is most likely in those individuals who are severely depleted and at risk of complications, and is unlikely if this is not the case. Much more research is needed to characterize better markers of micronutrient status both in terms of metabolic effects and antioxidant effects (Shenkin, 2006).

The Melbourne Atherosclerosis Vitamin E Trial (MAVET): a study of high dose vitamin E in smokers. (Magliano et al, 2006) (#409 male and female smokers) Their

aim was to evaluate whether vitamin E (500 IU) slowed the progression of carotid atherosclerosis in a population of chronic smokers over 4 years as measured by ultrasound determination of carotid intima-media thickness (IMT) and systemic arterial compliance (SAC). Methods: The Melbourne Atherosclerosis Vitamin E Trial (MAVET) was **a randomized, double-blind, placebo-controlled trial** in which **409 male and female smokers** aged 55 years and over were randomized to receive 500 IU per day of natural vitamin E or placebo. The primary endpoint was progression of carotid atherosclerosis determined by intima-media thickness of the right common carotid artery. Secondary outcomes were change in systemic arterial compliance and low-density lipoprotein (LDL) oxidative susceptibility over time. Results: *The mean increase in intima-media thickness over time in the vitamin E group was 0.0041 mm/year faster than placebo* (95% confidence interval -0.0021 to 0.0102 mm/year, *P*=0.20). Similarly, a non-significant difference between vitamin E and placebo was found for rate of change in systemic arterial compliance (*P*=0.11). Vitamin E supplementation did, however, significantly reduce LDL oxidative susceptibility (*P*<0.001). Conclusion: **Vitamin E supplementation is ineffective in reducing the progression of carotid atherosclerosis as measured by intima-media thickness in chronic smokers. This finding extends our knowledge of lack of effectiveness of vitamin E supplementation in populations with high oxidant stress.**

An interesting overview was offered by Siekmeier and Marz in 2006 in the following abstract: **Can antioxidants prevent atherosclerosis?**

In vitro studies have shown that antioxidants (e. g. beta-carotene, vitamin C and vitamin E) can interfere with some pathomechanisms of atherosclerosis and therefore might have a protective effect. From the investigated antioxidants vitamin E showed the best effect. Some animal and epidemiological studies confirmed such a protective effect in vivo especially after administration of high doses of vitamin E. However, **most of the placebo-controlled studies for primary or secondary prevention failed to show a protective effect even after administration of high doses.** In addition, **other studies demonstrated a risk for adverse effects due to antioxidant supplementation (beta-carotene and vitamin E).** Our review summarizes the principle of antioxidant supplementation and a number of relevant epidemiological and clinical studies for prevention of atherosclerosis. The obtained results suggest that **supplementation of antioxidants cannot be recommended for the normal population** (Siekmeier and Marz, 2006).

In 2007, they said," The protective effect of antioxidants on atherosclerotic pathomechanisms has been confirmed in vitro, but only in some animal studies. Various epidemiological and observational studies have produced conflicting results on the protective effect of antioxidants. **Most studies of primary or secondary prevention failed to show a protective effect of antioxidants against atherosclerosis** (Siekmeier and Marz, 2007).

Circa 2007

Mortality in Randomized Trials of Antioxidant Supplements for Primary and Secondary Prevention; Systematic Review and Meta-analysis

(Bjelakovic et al, 2007) (#232,606 participants); 68 randomized trials with 232,606 participants (385 publications. In 47 low-bias trials with 180,938 participants, the antioxidant supplements significantly increased mortality. In low-bias risk trials, after exclusion of selenium trials, **beta carotene, vitamin A, and vitamin E, singly or combined, significantly increased mortality.** Vitamin C and selenium had no significant effect on mortality. **Bjelakovic's analysis found no evidence that taking beta-carotene, vitamin A or vitamin E extends life span.** Conservatively, *the supplements increase the likelihood of dying by about 5 percent. When looked at separately, they found that Vitamin A increased death risk by 16 per cent, beta carotene by 7 per cent and Vitamin E by 4 per cent.*

Vitamin C gave contradictory results, but when given singly or in combination with other vitamins in good-quality trials, increased the death rate by 6 per cent. Selenium was the only supplement to emerge with any credit. It appears to cut death rates by 10 per cent when given on its own or with other supplements in high-quality trials, but the result is **not statistically significant**.

In 2007, Dr. Kristine Yaffe of the San Francisco Veterans Affairs Medical Center and University of California at San Francisco stated, **"For the clinician, there is no convincing justification to recommend** the use of antioxidant dietary supplements to maintain cognitive performance in cognitively normal adults or in those with mild cognitive impairment." (Nov. 2007 Archives of Internal Medicine)

Multivitamin Use and Risk of Prostate Cancer in the National Institutes of Health–AARP Diet and Health Study (Lawson et al, 2007) (#295,344 men); investigated the association between multivitamin use and prostate cancer risk; *use of multivitamins more than seven times per week, when compared with never use, was associated with a doubling in the risk of fatal prostate cancer* (The study of Lawson et al. is observational, and therefore confounding by indication and other confounding cannot be excluded. But the sample studied is very large, which reduces random errors, and the study seems well conducted.) **According to Victoria Stevens of the American Cancer Society, "There certainly is no evidence in healthy, relatively well-nourished people that vitamins or anti-oxidants protect against chronic diseases."**

The results are in accord with the results of systematic reviews and meta-analyses of randomized clinical trials (Vivekananthan et al., 2003) (Bjelakovic et al, Cochrane Database Syst Rev. 2004) (Stevens et al, 2005) (Bjelakovic et al, 2007) (Caraballoso et al., 2003).

This study of Lawson et al is so disturbing that I have expanded it in the section, "Where are the bodies?"

A Randomized Factorial Trial of Vitamins C and E and Beta Carotene in the Secondary Prevention of Cardiovascular Events in Women: R e s u l t s From the Women's Antioxidant Cardiovascular Study (Cook et al. 2007) (#8,171 female health professionals at increased risk); ascorbic acid (500 mg/d), vitamin E (600 IU every other day), and beta carotene (50 mg every other day) on the combined outcome of myocardial infarction, stroke, coronary revascularization, or CVD. **There was no overall effect of ascorbic acid, vitamin E, or beta carotene on the primary combined end point or on the individual secondary outcomes of myocardial infarction, stroke, coronary revascularization, or CVD death. There were no overall effects of ascorbic acid, vitamin E, or beta carotene on cardiovascular events among women at high risk for CVD.**

111

The Women's Antioxidant Cardiovascular Study (WACS) examined the effects of vitamins C and E and beta carotene, as well as their combinations, in a randomized factorial trial among women at increased risk of vascular events. There were no significant effects on the primary end point of total cardiovascular disease, suggesting that **widespread use of these agents for cardiovascular disease prevention does not appear warranted.**

Use of Supplements of Multivitamins, Vitamin C, and Vitamin E in Relation to Mortality (Pocobelli et al, 2007) (#77,719 subjects aged 50–76 years) Washington State residents aged 50–76 years who completed a mailed self-administered questionnaire in 2000–2002. **Multivitamin use was not related to total mortality.** However, **vitamin C and vitamin E use were associated with small decreases in risk.** In cause-specific analyses, use of multivitamins and use of vitamin E were associated with decreased risks of CVD mortality. In contrast, **vitamin C use was not associated with CVD mortality. Multivitamin and vitamin E use were not associated with cancer mortality.** Some of the associations we observed were small and may have been due to unmeasured healthy behaviors that were more common in supplement users.

Health Professionals Follow-up Study (2007): Effect of vitamins C, E, A and carotenoids and the occurrence of oral pre-malignant lesions (Maserejian et al, 2007) (#42,340 men enrolled in the Health Professionals Follow-up Study) (#207 found with oral premalignant lesions); researchers found no clear relationship with beta-carotene, lycopene, or lutein/zeaxanthin. **A trend for *increased risk of oral pre-malignant lesions was observed with vitamin E, especially among current smokers and with vitamin E supplements. Beta-carotene also increased the risk among current smokers.* However, dietary vitamin C was significantly associated with a reduced risk of oral premalignant lesions:** those with the highest intake had a 50 percent reduction in risk compared to those with the lowest intake.

Antioxidant meta-analysis for the treatment of macular degeneration (2007) (Chong et al, 2007) (#149,203 subjects); Investigators looked at 11 studies which included **149,203 people** - seven were prospective studies and three were randomized controlled trials

and found that vitamins A and E, zinc, lutein, zeaxanthin, beta-carotene, beta-cryptoxanthin and lycopene have **either a very slight or no effect** on primary prevention of early age-related macular degeneration. The researchers concluded that **there is not enough evidence to support the role of dietary antioxidants, including the use of dietary antioxidant supplements, for the primary prevention of early AMD.**

Effect of *RRR*-α-tocopherol supplementation on carotid atherosclerosis in patients with stable coronary artery disease (CAD) (Devaraj et al, 2007) (#90 patients with CAD); **No significant difference was observed in the mean change in total carotid IMT in the placebo and α-tocopherol groups.** In addition, **no significant difference in cardiovascular events was observed. Conclusions:** High-dose *RRR*-α-tocopherol supplementation in patients with CAD was safe and significantly reduced plasma biomarkers of oxidative stress and inflammation but **had no significant effect on carotid IMT during 2 years.**

Overview of the Women's Antioxidant Cardiovascular Study (WACS) (2007) (Zaharris et al, 2007) (#8,171 women); ascorbic acid (500 mg/d), vitamin E (600 IU every other day), and beta carotene (50 mg every other day); **There was no overall effect of ascorbic acid, vitamin E, or beta carotene on the primary combined end point or on the individual secondary outcomes of myocardial infarction, stroke, coronary revascularization, or CVD death.** But those randomized to both active ascorbic acid and vitamin E experienced fewer strokes. **Conclusion: There were no overall effects of ascorbic acid, vitamin E, or beta carotene on cardiovascular events among women at high risk for CVD.**

Serum α-tocopherol, concurrent and past vitamin E intake, and mild cognitive impairment (Dunn et al, 2007) (#526 subjects) 526 participants in a single-site ancillary study to the Women's Health Initiative, the Cognitive Change in Women study; In bivariate analyses, neither past dietary vitamin E intake (<8 mg/day vs more) nor current vitamin E supplement use was associated with impairment. CONCLUSION: **There was weak or no evidence of a protective effect of previous vitamin E intake on cognitive function.**

The role of vitamin E in the prevention of cancer: a meta-analysis of randomized controlled trials.

(Alkhenizan and Hafez, 2007) (#167,025 subjects) There are conflicting results in published randomized controlled trials (RCTs) on the role of vitamin E in the prevention of cancer. We conducted a meta-analysis of RCTs to evaluate the role of vitamin E in the prevention of cancer in adults. METHODS: We included RCTs in which the outcomes of the intake of vitamin E supplement alone or with other supplements were compared to a control group. The primary outcomes were total mortality, cancer mortality, total incidence of cancer, and incidence of lung, stomach, esophageal, pancreatic, prostate, breast and thyroid cancers. All identified trials were reviewed independently by the two reviewers to determine whether trials should be included or excluded. The quality of all included studies was scored independently by the two reviewers. RESULTS: Twelve studies, which included **167,025 participants**, met the inclusion criteria. There were no statistically significant differences in total mortality among the different groups of patients included in this meta-analysis. **Vitamin E was associated with a significant reduction in the incidence of prostate cancer, but it did not reduce the incidence of any other types of cancer.** CONCLUSIONS: **Vitamin E supplementation was not associated with a reduction in total mortality, cancer incidence, or cancer mortality,** but it was associated with a statistically significant reduction in the incidence of prostate cancer. Vitamin E can be used in the prevention of prostate cancer in men who are at high risk of prostate cancer. **This recently published meta-analysis of 12 randomized controlled trials concluded that vitamin E supplementation was not associated with overall cancer incidence, cancer mortality, or total mortality.**

Chemoprevention of Primary Liver Cancer: A Randomized, Double-Blind Trial in Linxian, China.

(Qu et al, 2007) (#29,450 initially healthy adults) Primary liver cancer is a common malignancy with a dismal prognosis. New primary prevention strategies are needed to reduce mortality from this disease. They examined the effects of supplementation with four different combinations of vitamins and minerals on primary liver cancer mortality among **29,450** initially healthy adults from Linxian, China. Methods: Participants were randomly assigned to take either a vitamin–mineral combination ("factor") or a placebo daily for 5.25 years (March 1986–May 1991). Four factors (at doses one to two times the US Recommended Daily Allowance)—retinol and zinc (factor A); riboflavin and niacin (factor B); ascorbic acid and molybdenum (factor C); and beta-carotene, alpha-tocopherol, and selenium (factor D)—were tested in a partial factorial design. The study outcome was primary liver cancer death occurring from 1986 through 2001. Adjusted Cox proportional hazards models were used to calculate hazard ratios (HRs) and 95% confidence intervals (CIs) of liver cancer death with and without each factor. All *P* values are two-sided. Results: A total of 151 liver cancer deaths occurred during the analysis period. **No statistically significant differences in liver cancer mortality were found comparing the presence and absence of any of the four intervention factors.** However, **both factor A and factor B reduced liver cancer mortality in individuals younger than 55 years at randomization but not in older individuals.** Factor C reduced liver cancer death, albeit with only borderline statistical significance in males but not in females. Cumulative risks of liver cancer death were 6.0 per 1000 in the placebo arm, 5.4 per 1000 in the arms with two factors, and 2.4 per 1000 in the arm with all four factors. Conclusion: **None of the factors tested reduced overall liver cancer mortality**. However, three factors reduced liver cancer mortality in certain subgroups.

As of 2007, no study had yet provided conclusive evidence of the beneficial effect of antioxidant supplementation in critically ill patients. The clinical evidence provided so far showed that there are several factors which might determine the efficacy of antioxidant supplementation in critically ill patients. There may be a need for large multi-center prospective randomized control trials to assess the effects of different types and doses of antioxidant supplementation in selected groups of patients with different types of critical illness. In critical illness, overwhelming inflammatory mediator response to infective or non-infective stimuli results in excessive production of free radicals (Mishra, 2007).

Risk of Mortality with Vitamin E Supplements: The Cache County Study. (Hayden et al, 2007) A recent meta-analysis reported increased mortality in clinical trial participants randomized to high-dose vitamin E. We sought to determine whether these mortality risks with vitamin E reflect adverse consequences of its use in the presence of cardiovascular disease. Methods: In a defined population aged 65 years or older, baseline interviews captured self- or proxy-reported history of cardiovascular illness. A medicine cabinet inventory verified nutritional

supplement and medication use. Three sources identified subsequent deaths. Cox proportional hazards methods examined the association between vitamin E use and mortality. Results: After adjustment for age and sex, there was no association in this population between vitamin E use and mortality. Predictably, deaths were more frequent with a history of diabetes, stroke, coronary artery bypass graft surgery, or myocardial infarction, and with the use of warfarin, nitrates, or diuretics. None of these conditions or treatments altered the null main effect with vitamin E, but *mortality was increased in vitamin E users who had a history of stroke, coronary bypass graft surgery, or myocardial infarction and, independently, in those taking nitrates, warfarin, or diuretics.*

Although not definitive, a consistent trend toward reduced mortality was seen in vitamin E users without these conditions or treatments. Conclusions: In this population-based study, **vitamin E use was unrelated to mortality, but this apparently null finding seems to represent a combination of increased mortality in those with severe cardiovascular disease and a possible protective effect in those without.**

Multivitamin-multimineral supplements and eye disease: age-related macular degeneration and cataract. (Seddon, 2007)

This **Dietary Ancillary Study of the Eye Disease Case-Control Study (EDCCS)** was designed to evaluate the relation between nutrition and AMD. Conclusion: **a multivitamin-multimineral supplement with a combination of vitamin C, vitamin E, beta-carotene, and zinc (with cupric oxide) is recommended for age-related macular degeneration (AMD) but not cataract.** Observational studies for cataract provide only weak support for multivitamins or other vitamin supplements. The results of observational studies suggest that a healthy lifestyle with a diet containing foods rich in antioxidants, especially lutein and zeaxanthin, and n–3 fatty acids appears beneficial for AMD and possibly cataract.

As regarded multivitamins, investigators were becoming aware that **the influence that some dietary supplements, especially multivitamin-multimineral supplements, may have on the occurrence of chronic diseases was largely unknown, but there was a potential for adverse effects associated with their use** (Mulholland and Benford, 2007).

Antioxidant Supplementation Increases the Risk of Skin Cancers in Women but Not in Men.

(Hercberg et al, 2007) (#French adults, 7,876 women and 5,141 men. Total # = 13,017) This research aimed to test whether supplementation with a combination of antioxidant vitamins and minerals could reduce the risk of skin cancers (SC). It was performed within the framework of the **Supplementation in Vitamins and Mineral Antioxidants study, a randomized, double-blinded, placebo-controlled, primary prevention trial** testing the efficacy of nutritional doses of antioxidants in reducing incidence of cancer and ischemic heart disease in the general population. French adults (7876 women and 5141 men) were randomized to take an oral daily capsule of antioxidants (120 mg vitamin C, 30 mg vitamin E, 6 mg *ß*-carotene, 100 *µ*g selenium, and 20 mg zinc) or a matching placebo. The median time of follow-up was 7.5 y. A total of 157 cases of all types of SC were reported, from which 25 were melanomas. Because the effect of antioxidants on SC incidence varied according to gender, men and women were analyzed separately. *In women, the incidence of SC was higher in the antioxidant group* [adjusted hazard ratio (adjusted HR) = 1.68; *P* = 0.03]. **Conversely, in men, incidence did not differ between the 2 treatment groups.** Despite the small number of events, *the incidence of melanoma was also higher in the antioxidant group for women.* The incidence of nonmelanoma SC did not differ between the antioxidant and placebo groups. Our findings suggest that antioxidant supplementation affects the incidence of SC differentially in men and women. (Hercberg et al, 2007)

Antioxidant Vitamin Supplement Use and Risk of Dementia or Alzheimer's Disease in Older Adults

(Gray et al, 2007) (#2,969)

Investigators examined whether use of vitamins C or E alone or in combination was associated with lower incidence of dementia or Alzheimer's disease (AD). Prospective cohort study. SETTING: Group Health Cooperative, Seattle, Washington. PARTICIPANTS: **Two thousand nine hundred sixty-nine participants** aged 65 and older without cognitive impairment at baseline in the Adult Changes in Thought study. MEASUREMENTS: Participants were followed biennially to identify incident dementia and AD diagnosed according to standard criteria. Participants were considered to be users of vitamins C or E if they self-reported use for at least 1 week during the month before baseline.

RESULTS: Over a mean follow-up±standard deviation of 5.5±2.7 years, 405 subjects developed dementia (289 developed AD). The use of vitamin E was not associated with dementia or with AD. No association was found between vitamin C alone or concurrent use of vitamin C and E and either outcome. CONCLUSION: In this study, **the use of supplemental vitamin E and C, alone or in combination, did not reduce risk of AD or overall dementia over 5.5 years of follow-up.**

(Shelly L. Gray et al. Antioxidant Vitamin Supplement Use and Risk of Dementia or Alzheimer's Disease in Older Adults. Journal of the American Geriatric Society. 2007. Volume 56 Issue 2, Pages 291 - 295)

Circa 2008

Antioxidant supplements for prevention of mortality in healthy participants and patients with various diseases. (Bjelakovic, Nikolova, Gludd, Simonetti and Gludd, 2008 Apr) (#232,550 Cochrane Database Syst Rev.) OBJECTIVES: To assess the effect of antioxidant supplements on mortality in primary or secondary prevention randomized clinical trials. We included all primary and secondary prevention randomized clinical trials on antioxidant supplements (beta-carotene, vitamin A, vitamin C, vitamin E, and selenium) versus placebo or no intervention. Trials with adequate randomization, blinding, and follow-up were classified as having a low risk of bias. RESULTS: **Sixty-seven randomized trials** with **232,550 participants** were included. Forty-seven trials including 180,938 participants had low risk of bias. Twenty-one trials included 164,439 healthy participants. Forty-six trials included 68,111 participants with various diseases (gastrointestinal, cardiovascular, neurological, ocular, dermatological, rheumatoid, renal, endocrinological, or unspecified). **Overall, the antioxidant supplements had no significant effect on mortality in a random-effects meta-analysis,** but *significantly increased mortality in a fixed-effect model.* **In the trials with a low risk of bias, the antioxidant supplements significantly increased mortality.** When the different antioxidants were assessed separately, analyses including trials with a low risk of bias and excluding selenium trials found *significantly increased mortality by vitamin A, beta-carotene, and vitamin E,* but **no significant detrimental effect of vitamin C.** Low-bias risk trials on

selenium found no significant effect on mortality. CONCLUSIONS: We found no evidence to support antioxidant supplements for primary or secondary prevention. **Vitamin A, beta-carotene, and vitamin E may increase mortality. Antioxidant supplements need to be considered medicinal products and should undergo sufficient evaluation before marketing.**

Systematic review: primary and secondary prevention of gastrointestinal cancers with antioxidant supplements. (Bjelakovic, Nikolova, Simonette and Gludd, 2008 Sept) (#211,818 participants) The evidence on whether antioxidant supplements prevent gastrointestinal cancers is contradictory. Using the Cochrane Collaboration methodology, we reviewed the randomized trials comparing antioxidant supplements with placebo or no intervention on the occurrence of gastrointestinal cancers. RESULTS:

We identified 20 randomized trials (211,818 participants) assessing beta-carotene, vitamin A, vitamin C, vitamin E, and selenium. **The antioxidant supplements were without a significant effect on the occurrence of gastrointestinal cancers.** *Antioxidant supplements had no significant effect on mortality in a random-effects model meta-analysis but significantly increased mortality in a fixed-effect model meta-analysis.* CONCLUSIONS: *There was no evidence that the studied antioxidant supplements prevented gastrointestinal cancers. On the contrary, they seem to increase overall mortality.*

Vitamins E and C in the prevention of cardiovascular disease in men: the Physicians' Health Study II randomized controlled trial (Sesso et al, 2008) (#14,641 US male physicians); a randomized, double-blind, placebo-controlled factorial trial of vitamin E and vitamin C that began in 1997 and continued until its scheduled completion on August 31, 2007. CONCLUSIONS: In this large, long-term trial of male physicians, **neither vitamin E nor vitamin C supplementation reduced the risk of major cardiovascular events. These data provide no support for the use of these supplements (vitamins E and C) for the prevention of cardiovascular disease in middle-aged and older men.**

Both {alpha}-and Beta-Carotene, but Not Tocopherols and Vitamin C, Are Inversely Related

to 15-Year Cardiovascular Mortality in Dutch Elderly Men (Buijsse et al, 2008) (#559 men (mean age ~72 y) free of chronic diseases); intake of different carotenoids, α- and ϒ-tocopherol, and vitamin C with 15-y CVD mortality in elderly men who participated in the Zutphen Elderly Study. **Carrots were the primary source of α- and** beta-carotene **and their consumption was related to a lower risk of death** from CVD. **Intakes of carotenoids other than α- and** beta-carotene **were not associated with CVD mortality, nor were vitamin C and α- and ϒ tocopherol.** CONCLUSION: **dietary intakes of α-carotene and** beta-carotene **are inversely associated with CVD mortality in elderly men. This study does not indicate an important role for other carotenoids, tocopherols, or vitamin C in lowering the risk of CVD death.**

Vitamin E and selenium supplementation and risk of prostate cancer in the Vitamins and lifestyle (VITAL) study cohort (Peters et al, 2008) (#35,242 men) RESULTS: **A 10-year average intake of supplemental vitamin E was not associated with a reduced prostate cancer risk overall.** CONCLUSIONS: In this prospective cohort, **long-term supplemental intake of vitamin E and selenium were not associated with prostate cancer risk overall**; however, risk of clinically relevant advanced disease was reduced with greater long-term vitamin E supplementation.

VITAL (VITamins And Lifestyle) study (2008)
(Slatore et al, 2008) (#77,721 men and women); explore the association of supplemental multivitamins, vitamin C, vitamin E, and folate with incident lung cancer; Prospective cohort; Cases were identified through the Seattle–Puget Sound **SEER (Surveillance, Epidemiology, and End Results)** cancer registry. **There was no inverse association with any supplement.** *Supplemental vitamin E was associated with a small increased risk of lung cancer.* This risk of supplemental vitamin E was largely confined to current smokers and was greatest for non–small cell lung cancer.

Conclusions: **Supplemental multivitamins, vitamin C, vitamin E, and folate were not associated with a decreased risk of lung cancer.** *Supplemental vitamin E was associated with a small increased risk.* Patients should be counseled against using these supplements to prevent lung cancer.

The Institute of Medicine states that most North American adults get enough vitamin E from their normal diets to meet current recommendations.

The recent announcement of early termination of the Selenium and Vitamin E Cancer Prevention Trial's (SELECT) interventions because of lack of efficacy and observation of possible adverse events (i.e., small and not statistically significant increases in type 2 diabetes in those receiving selenium alone and in prostate cancer incidence in the vitamin E (alone) group) should serve as a reminder that the unexpected can happen in these well-designed trials (Lippman et al, 2009).

Vitamin E for Alzheimers and mild cognitive impairment. Cochrane Database Syst Rev. (2008)

(Isaac et al, 2008) (#769 participants); assess the efficacy of Vitamin E in the treatment of Alzheimer's disease and prevention of progression of Mild Cognitive Impairment to Alzheimer's disease. *More participants taking Vitamin E suffered a fall.* There was no significant difference in the probability of progression from MCI to AD between the Vitamin E group and the placebo group. CONCLUSIONS: There is no evidence of efficacy of Vitamin E in the prevention or treatment of people with AD or MCI.

Efficacy of Antioxidant Supplementation in Reducing Primary Cancer Incidence and Mortality: Systematic Review and Meta-analysis

(Bardia et al, 2008) (#104,196 participants) Twelve eligible trials, 9 of high methodological quality, were identified (total subject population, 104,196). Antioxidant supplementation did not significantly reduce total cancer incidence or mortality or any site-specific cancer incidence. *Beta carotene supplementation was associated with an increase in the incidence of cancer among smokers and with a trend toward increased cancer mortality.* Selenium supplementation was associated with reduced cancer incidence in men but not in women and with reduced cancer mortality. Vitamin E supplementation had no apparent effect on overall cancer incidence or cancer mortality. CONCLUSION: Beta carotene supplementation appeared to increase cancer incidence and cancer mortality among smokers, whereas vitamin E supplementation had no effect. Selenium supplementation might have anticarcinogenic effects in men and thus requires further research.

Prof. Hon. Randolph M. Howes, M.D., Ph.D.

Carotenoids and the risk of developing lung cancer: a systematic review. (Gallicchio et al, 2008) (Six randomized clinical trials & 25 prospective observational studies)

Carotenoids are thought to have anti-cancer properties, but findings from population-based research have been inconsistent. OBJECTIVE: They aimed to conduct a systematic review of the associations between carotenoids and lung cancer. DESIGN: They searched electronic databases for articles published through September 2007. **Six randomized clinical trials examining the efficacy of beta-carotene supplements and 25 prospective observational studies** assessing the associations between carotenoids and lung cancer were analyzed by using random-effects meta-analysis. RESULTS: The pooled relative risk (RR) for the studies comparing beta-carotene supplements with placebo was 1.10. Among the observational studies that adjusted for smoking, the pooled RRs comparing highest and lowest categories of total carotenoid intake and of total carotenoid serum concentrations were 0.79 and 0.70, respectively. For beta-carotene, highest compared with lowest pooled RRs were 0.92 for dietary intake and 0.84 for serum concentrations. For other carotenoids, the RRs comparing highest and lowest categories of intake ranged from 0.80 for beta-cryptoxanthin to 0.89 for alpha-carotene and lutein-zeaxanthin; for serum concentrations, the RRs ranged from 0.71 for lycopene to 0.95 for lutein-zeaxanthin. CONCLUSIONS: **beta-Carotene supplementation is not associated with a decrease in the risk of developing lung cancer**. Findings from prospective cohort studies suggest inverse associations between carotenoids and lung cancer; however, **the decreases in risk are generally small and not statistically** significant. These inverse associations may be the result of carotenoid measurements' function as a marker of a healthier lifestyle (higher fruit and vegetable consumption) or of residual confounding by smoking.

Antioxidant enriched enteral nutrition and oxidative stress after major gastrointestinal tract surgery. (van Stijn et al, 2008) (#21 undergoing major upper gastrointestinal tract surgery)

Goal: To investigate the effects of an enteral supplement containing antioxidants on circulating levels of antioxidants and indicators of oxidative stress after major gastrointestinal surgery. METHODS: **Twenty-one patients** undergoing major upper gastrointestinal tract surgery were randomized in a single centre, open label study on the effect of postoperative enteral nutrition supplemented with antioxidants. The effect on circulating levels of antioxidants and indicators of oxidative stress, such as F2-isoprostane, was studied. RESULTS: The antioxidant enteral supplement showed no adverse effects and was well tolerated. After surgery a decrease in the circulating levels of antioxidant parameters was observed. Only selenium and glutamine levels were restored to pre-operative values one week after surgery. **F2-isoprostane increased in the first three postoperative days only in the antioxidant supplemented group**. Lipopolysaccharide binding protein (LBP) levels decreased faster in the antioxidant group after surgery. CONCLUSION: **Despite lower antioxidant levels there was no increase in the circulating markers of oxidative stress on the first day after major abdominal surgery.** The rise in F2-isoprostane in patients receiving the antioxidant supplement may be related to the conversion of antioxidants to oxidants which raises questions on antioxidant supplementation. Module AOX restored the postoperative decrease in selenium levels. The rapid decrease in LBP levels in the antioxidant group suggests a possible protective effect on gut wall integrity.

Vitamin E supplementation may transiently increase tuberculosis risk in males who smoke heavily and have high dietary vitamin C intake.

(Hemila and Kaprio, 2008 Oct) (#29,023 males aged 50-69 years, smoking at baseline, with no tuberculosis) Vitamin E and beta-carotene affect the immune function and might influence the predisposition of man to infections. To examine whether vitamin E or beta-carotene supplementation affects tuberculosis risk, we analysed data of the Alpha-Tocopherol Beta-Carotene Cancer Prevention (ATBC)Study, a randomised controlled trial which examined the effects of vitamin E (50 mg/d) and beta-carotene (20 mg/d) on lung cancer. The trial was conducted in the general community in Finland in 1985-93; the intervention lasted for 6.1 years (median). **The ATBC Study cohort consists of 29,023 males aged 50-69 years, smoking at baseline, with no tuberculosis diagnosis prior to randomization. Vitamin E supplementation had no overall effect on the incidence of tuberculosis nor had beta-carotene.** Nevertheless, **dietary vitamin C intake significantly modified the vitamin E effect.** *Among participants who obtained 90 mg/d or more of vitamin C in foods, vitamin E supplementation increased tuberculosis risk by 72%.* **This effect was restricted to participants who smoked heavily.** Finally, in participants not supplemented with vitamin E, dietary vitamin C had a negative association with tuberculosis risk so that the adjusted risk was 60 (95% CI 16, 81)% lower in the highest intake quartile compared with the lowest. *Our finding that vitamin E seemed to transiently increase the risk of tuberculosis in those who smoked heavily and had high dietary vitamin C intake should increase caution towards vitamin E supplementation for improving the immune system.*

Vitamin E supplementation and pneumonia risk in males who initiated smoking at an early age: effect modification by body weight and dietary vitamin C. (Hemila and Kaprio, 2008 Nov) (#21,657 ATBC Study participants who initiated smoking by the age of 20 years) *They had found a 14% higher incidence of pneumonia with vitamin E supplementation in a subgroup of the Alpha-Tocopherol Beta-Carotene Cancer Prevention (ATBC) Study cohort:* participants who had initiated smoking by the age of 20 years. In this study, they explored the modification of vitamin E effect by body weight, because the same dose could lead to a greater effect in participants with low body weight. METHODS: The ATBC Study recruited males aged 50-69 years who smoked at least 5 cigarettes per day at the baseline; it was conducted in southwestern Finland in 1985-1993. The current study was restricted to 21,657 ATBC Study participants who initiated smoking by the age of 20 years; the median follow-up time was 6.0 years. The hospital-diagnosed pneumonia cases were retrieved from the national hospital discharge register (701 cases). RESULTS: Vitamin E supplementation had no effect on the risk of pneumonia in participants with body weight in a range from 70 to 89 kg. *Vitamin E increased the risk of pneumonia in participants with body weight less than 60 kg, and in participants with body weight over 100 kg.* The harm of vitamin E supplementation was restricted to participants with dietary vitamin C intake above the median. CONCLUSION: **Vitamin E supplementation may cause harmful effects on health in certain groups of male smokers.** The dose of vitamin E used in the ATBC Study, 50 mg/day, is substantially smaller than conventional vitamin E doses that are considered safe. Our findings should increase caution towards taking vitamin E supplements.

Oral administration of vitamin C decreases muscle mitochondrial biogenesis and hampers

training-induced adaptations in endurance performance. (Gomez-Cabrera et al, 2008) (#14 men) Exercise

practitioners often take vitamin C supplements because **intense muscular contractile activity can result in oxidative stress,** as indicated by altered muscle and blood glutathione concentrations and increases in protein, DNA, and lipid peroxidation. There is, however, considerable debate regarding the beneficial health effects of vitamin C supplementation. OBJECTIVE: This study was designed to study the effect of vitamin C on training efficiency in rats and in humans. DESIGN: The human study was **double-blind and randomized. Fourteen men** (27-36 y old) were trained for 8 wk. Five of the men were supplemented daily with an oral dose of 1 g vitamin C. In the animal study, 24 male Wistar rats were exercised under 2 different protocols for 3 and 6 wk. Twelve of the rats were treated with a daily dose of vitamin C (0.24 mg/cm2 body surface area). RESULTS: *The administration of vitamin C significantly (P=0.014) hampered endurance capacity.* The adverse effects of vitamin C may result from its capacity to reduce the exercise-induced expression of key transcription factors involved in mitochondrial biogenesis. These factors are peroxisome proliferator-activated receptor co-activator 1, nuclear respiratory factor 1, and mitochondrial transcription factor A. **Vitamin C also prevented the exercise-induced expression of cytochrome C (a marker of mitochondrial content) and of the antioxidant enzymes superoxide dismutase and glutathione peroxidase.** CONCLUSION: **Vitamin C supplementation decreases training efficiency because it prevents some cellular adaptations to exercise.**

Antioxidant vitamin and mineral supplements for preventing age-related macular degeneration.

(Evans and Henshaw, 2008) (#23,099 participants) Some observational studies have suggested that people who eat a diet rich in antioxidant vitamins (carotenoids, vitamins C and E) or minerals (selenium and zinc) may be less likely to develop age-related macular degeneration (AMD). OBJECTIVES: The aim of this review was to examine the evidence as to whether or not taking vitamin or mineral supplements prevents the development of AMD. SEARCH STRATEGY: We searched the Cochrane Central Register of Controlled Trials (CENTRAL) (which contains the Cochrane Eyes and Vision Group Trials Register) in The Cochrane Library (2007, Issue 3), MEDLINE (1966 to August 2007), SIGLE (1980 to

2005/03), EMBASE (1980 to August 2007), National Research Register (2007, Issue 3), AMED (1985 to January 2006) and PubMed (on 24 January 2006 covering last 60 days), reference lists of identified reports and the Science Citation Index. We contacted investigators and experts in the field for details of unpublished studies. SELECTION: They included all randomized trials comparing an antioxidant vitamin and/ or mineral supplement (alone or in combination) to control. We included only studies where supplementation had been given for at least one year. DATA AND ANALYSIS: Both review authors independently extracted data and assessed trial quality. Data were pooled using a fixed-effect model. RESULTS: Three randomized controlled trials were included in this review (**23,099 people randomized**). These trials investigated **alpha-tocopherol and beta-carotene** supplements. **There was no evidence that antioxidant vitamin supplementation prevented or delayed the onset of AMD.** The pooled risk ratio for any age-related maculopathy (ARM) was 1.04, for AMD (late ARM) was 1.03. Similar results were seen when the analyses were restricted to beta-carotene and alpha-tocopherol. CONCLUSIONS: **There is no evidence to date that the general population should take antioxidant vitamin and mineral supplements to prevent or delay the onset of AMD.** There are several large ongoing trials. People with AMD should see the related Cochrane review "Antioxidant vitamin and mineral supplements for slowing the progression of age-related macular degeneration" written by the same author.

Dietary antioxidants and the long-term incidence of age-related macular degeneration: the Blue Mountains Eye Study. (Tan et al, 2008) (#2,454 Australian population-based cohort study)

PURPOSE: To assess the relationship between baseline dietary and supplement intakes of antioxidants and the long-term risk of incident age-related macular degeneration (AMD). DESIGN: Australian population-based cohort study. PARTICIPANTS: Of 3,654 baseline (1992-1994) participants initially 49 years of older, 2,454 were reexamined after 5 years, 10 years, or both. METHODS: Stereoscopic retinal photographs were graded using the Wisconsin Grading System. Data on potential risk factors were collected. Energy-adjusted intakes of alpha-carotene; beta-carotene; beta-cryptoxanthin; lutein and zeaxanthin; lycopene; vitamins A,

C, and E; and iron and zinc were the study factors. Discrete logistic models assessed AMD risk. Risk ratios (RRs) and 95% confidence intervals (CIs) were calculated after adjusting for age, gender, smoking, and other risk factors. MAIN OUTCOME MEASURES: Incident early, late, and any AMD. RESULTS: For dietary lutein and zeaxanthin, participants in the top tertile of intake had a reduced risk of incident neovascular AMD, and those with above median intakes had a reduced risk of indistinct soft or reticular drusen. For total zinc intake the RR comparing the top decile intake with the remaining population was 0.56 for any AMD and 0.54 for early AMD. The highest compared with the lowest tertile of total beta-carotene intake predicted incident neovascular AMD. Similarly, **beta-carotene intake from diet alone predicted neovascular AMD.** This association was evident in both ever and never smokers. **Higher intakes of total vitamin E predicted late AMD.** CONCLUSIONS: In this population-based cohort study, higher dietary lutein and zeaxanthin intake reduced the risk of long-term incident AMD. This study confirmed the Age-Related Eye Disease Study finding of protective influences from zinc against AMD. *Higher beta-carotene intake was associated with an increased risk of AMD.*

Multivitamin-multimineral supplement use and mammographic breast density. (Berube et al, 2008)

(#Premenopausal (777) and postmenopausal (783) women; total 1,560) The effect of multivitamin-multimineral supplements on the occurrence of chronic diseases, such as breast cancer, is unclear. Breast density is increasingly used as a biomarker of breast cancer risk. **Objective:** The present study evaluated the association of multivitamin-multimineral supplement use with breast density. **Design: Premenopausal (*n* = 777) and postmenopausal (*n* = 783) women** were recruited at the time of screening mammography. Diet and multivitamin-multimineral and individual vitamin and mineral supplement use were assessed with a self-administered food-frequency questionnaire. Breast density from screening mammograms was measured using a computer-assisted method. Crude and adjusted means in breast density were evaluated according to multivitamin-multimineral supplement use using generalized linear models. **Results: Current multivitamin-multimineral supplement use was reported by 21.7% of women** (20.7% and 22.6% of premenopausal and postmenopausal women, respectively). **Premenopausal women who were currently using multivitamin-multimineral supplements had higher adjusted mean breast density (45.5%) than past (42.9%) or never (40.2%) users**. Of the current users, breast density was not related to duration of multivitamin-multimineral supplement use. In postmenopausal women, multivitamin-multimineral supplement use was not associated with breast density. **Conclusion: *Regular use of multivitamin-multimineral supplements may be associated with higher mean breast density among premenopausal women.***

Mammographic breast density is increasingly used as a biomarker of breast cancer risk because of its strong positive relation to the risk of the disease (Pike, 2005).

Breast density has been hypothesized to reflect the quantity of breast tissue and the population of breast cells at risk of carcinogenic transformation (Boyd et al, 2005) (Trichopoulos, Lagiou and Adami, 2005).

Antioxidant supplements to prevent or slow down the progression of AMD: a systematic review and meta-analysis. (Evans, 2008) (#23,099 people

were randomized in three trials) The aim of this review was to examine the evidence as to whether antioxidant vitamin or mineral supplements prevent the development of AMD or slow down its progression. METHODS: Randomized trials comparing antioxidant vitamin and/ or mineral supplement to control were identified by systematic electronic searches (updated August 2007) and contact with investigators. Data were pooled after investigating clinical and statistical heterogeneity. RESULTS: **There was no evidence that antioxidant (vitamin E or beta-carotene) supplementation prevented AMD. A total of 23,099 people were randomized in three trials with treatment duration of 4-12 years.** There was evidence that antioxidant (beta-carotene, vitamin C, and vitamin E) and zinc supplementation slowed down the progression to advanced AMD and visual acuity loss in people with signs of the disease. The majority of people were randomized in one trial (AREDS, 3640 people randomized). There were seven other small trials (total randomized 525). CONCLUSIONS: **Current evidence does not support the use of antioxidant vitamin supplements to prevent AMD.** People with AMD, or early signs of the disease, may experience some benefit from taking supplements as used in the AREDS trial. *Potential harms of high-dose antioxidant supplementation must be considered. These may include an increased risk of lung cancer in smokers (beta-carotene), heart failure in people with vascular disease or diabetes (vitamin E) and hospitalization for genitourinary conditions (zinc).*

Circa 2009

Is there a role for supplemented antioxidants in the prevention of atherosclerosis? (Katsiki and Manes, 2009) (#22 trials (N=134,590 subjects) BACKGROUND: Oxidative stress is thought to play a substantial role in the pathogenesis of atherosclerosis. Supplementation of antioxidants has been studied as a strategy in the prevention of occurrence and progression of atherosclerosis. METHOD: We searched the MEDLINE and PubMed databases (up to February 2008) for **randomized, double-blind, placebo-controlled trials** of antioxidant (and in particular vitamins E, C and/or beta-carotene) supplementation, published in English. RESULTS: We identified **22 trials (N=134,590 subjects)** of antioxidant supplementation for the prevention of atherosclerosis (7 primary, 13 secondary and 2 both primary and secondary). Of these studies, 10 examined the effect of a single antioxidant supplementation on primary or secondary prevention of cardiovascular disease, while 12 the effect of a combination of antioxidants. CONCLUSION: **As the majority of studies included in this review does not support a possible role of antioxidant supplementation in reducing the risk of cardiovascular disease, no definite conclusion can be drawn to justify the use of antioxidant vitamin supplements for the prevention of atherosclerotic events.**

Plasma carotenoids, retinol, and tocopherols and postmenopausal breast cancer risk in the Multiethnic Cohort Study: a nested case-control study. (Epplein et al, 2009) (#286 incident postmenopausal breast cancer cases were matched to 535 controls)

Assessments by the handful of prospective studies of the association of serum antioxidants and breast cancer risk have yielded inconsistent results. This multiethnic nested case-control study sought to examine the association of plasma carotenoids, retinol, and tocopherols with postmenopausal breast cancer risk. Methods: From the biospecimen subcohort of the Multiethnic Cohort Study, **286 incident postmenopausal breast cancer cases were matched to 535 controls** on age, sex, ethnicity, study location (Hawaii or California), smoking status, date/time of collection and hours of fasting. We measured prediagnostic circulating levels of individual carotenoids, retinol, and tocopherols. Conditional logistic regression was used to compute odds ratios and 95% confidence intervals. **Results: Women with breast cancer tended to have lower levels of plasma carotenoids and tocopherols than matched controls, but the differences were not large or statistically significant and the trends were not monotonic. No association was seen with retinol.** A sensitivity analysis excluding cases diagnosed within 1 year after blood draw did not alter the findings. Conclusions: **The lack of significant associations in this multiethnic population is consistent with previously observed results from less racially-diverse cohorts and serves as further evidence against a causal link between plasma micronutrient concentrations and postmenopausal breast cancer risk.** Women with breast cancer tended to have lower levels of plasma carotenoids and tocopherols than matched controls, but the differences were not large or statistically significant and the trends were not monotonic.

Vitamins E and C in the prevention of prostate and total cancer in men: the Physicians' Health Study II randomized controlled trial (2009) (Gazziano et al, 2009) (#14,641 male physicians); evaluate whether long-term vitamin E or C supplementation decreases risk of prostate and total cancer events among men; a randomized, double-blind, placebo-controlled factorial trial of vitamins E and C that began in 1997 and continued until its scheduled completion on August 31, 2007. **Neither vitamin E nor vitamin C had a significant effect on prostate, colorectal, lung, or other site-specific cancers.** CONCLUSIONS: In this large, long-term trial of male physicians, neither vitamin E nor C supplementation reduced the risk of prostate or total cancer. These **data provide no support for the use of these supplements for the prevention of cancer in middle-aged and older men.**

Advertisers suggest that taking certain vitamin or mineral supplements can lower prostate cancer risk. While some studies have found that there might be a protective benefit from some supplements, recent **results from 2 large studies didn't find any.** (Lippman et al, 2009) (Gaziano et al, 2009)

In 2001, researchers from the National Cancer Institute (NCI) and the Southwest Oncology Group (SWOG) launched the massive **SELECT study (short for Selenium and Vitamin E Cancer Prevention Trial)** to find out whether taking <u>selenium</u> and <u>vitamin E</u> supplements could protect men from prostate cancer. **In October 2008, researchers halted the trial after early analysis showed the supplements weren't working, and in fact, in some cases, may have been doing more harm than good.**

In another large, long-term trial, called **the Physicians' Health Study II**, researchers from Brigham and Women's Hospital and Harvard Medical School studied whether taking vitamin E or vitamin C could reduce the risk of prostate cancer. Nearly **15,000 male doctors** participated in the trial. **After an average of 8 years, neither vitamin E nor vitamin C seemed to lower the risk of prostate cancer.**

Vitamin E, vitamin C, beta carotene, and cognitive function among women with or at risk of cardiovascular disease: The Women's Antioxidant and Cardiovascular Study (2009) (Kang et al, 2009)

(#2,824 participants); Vitamin E supplementation and beta carotene supplementation were not associated with slower rates of cognitive change. Although vitamin C supplementation was associated with better performance at the last assessment, it was not associated with cognitive change over time. CONCLUSIONS: **Antioxidant supplementation (vitamin E, C and beta carotene) did not slow cognitive change among women with preexisting cardiovascular disease or cardiovascular disease risk factors.**

Effects of vitamins C and E and beta-carotene on the risk of type 2 diabetes in women at high risk of cardiovascular disease: Women's Antioxidant Cardiovascular Study (2009) (Song et al, 2009) (#8,171

female health professionals); CONCLUSION: Our randomized trial data showed **no significant overall effects of vitamin C, vitamin E, and beta-carotene on risk of developing type 2 diabetes in women at high risk of CVD.**

Vitamins C and E and Beta Carotene Supplementation and Cancer Risk: Women's Antioxidant Cardiovascular Study (2009) (Lin et al, 2009) (#7,627 female health professionals); vitamin C (500 mg of ascorbic acid daily), natural-source vitamin E (600 IU of α-tocopherol every other day), and beta carotene (50 mg every other day). **There were no statistically significant effects of use of any antioxidant on total cancer incidence.** Conclusions: **Supplementation with vitamin C, vitamin E, or beta carotene offers no overall benefits in the primary prevention of total cancer incidence or cancer mortality.**

Effect of selenium and vitamin E on risk of prostate cancer and other cancers: the Selenium and Vitamin E Cancer Prevention Trial (SELECT) (2009) (Lippman et al, 2009) (#35,533 men) **There were statistically nonsignificant increased risks of prostate cancer in the vitamin E group** but not in the selenium + vitamin E group. CONCLUSION: **Selenium or vitamin E, alone or in combination at the doses and formulations used, did not prevent prostate cancer in this population of relatively healthy men.** *The trial was stopped ahead of its original 12 year deadline because of a lack of any noticeable benefit.*

"The largest prostate cancer prevention trial has found that **selenium is no more effective than a placebo**," said David Schardt, a senior nutritionist. "Bayer is ripping people off when it suggests otherwise in these dishonest ads."

Multivitamin Use and Risk of Cancer and Cardiovascular Disease in the Women's Health Initiative Cohorts (Neuhouser et al, 2009) (#161,808 postmenopausal women taking part in the Women's Health Initiative clinical trials); **Conclusion:** After a median follow-up of 8.0 and 7.9 years in the clinical trial and observational study cohorts, respectively, the Women's Health Initiative study provided convincing evidence that **multivitamin use has little or no influence on the risk of common cancers, CVD, or total mortality in postmenopausal women.**

There was no evidence that multivitamins confer meaningful benefit or harm in relation to cancer or cardiovascular disease. The risk for invasive cancers of the breast, colon/rectum, endometrium, lung, bladder, and ovary was no different among women who used multivitamin compared with those who did not use multivitamins. Similarly, risk of myocardial infarction, stroke, venous thrombosis, and death from any cause was no different for multivitamin users than for nonusers. **Multivitamins do not appear to be effective for the prevention of cancer or cardiovascular disease**.

Neuhouser said: "To our surprise, we found that multivitamins did not lower the risk of the most common cancers and also had no impact on heart disease."

Thus, the largest multivitamin study shows that they do nothing to protect against cancer. Marian L. Neuhouser, the lead author and a nutritional epidemiologist with the Fred Hutchinson Cancer Research Center in Seattle, said, "**Consumers spend money on dietary supplements with the thought that they are going to improve their health, but there's no evidence for this.** Buying more fruits and vegetables might be a better choice."

In a separate statement, Neuhouser said: "Dietary supplements are used by more than half of all Americans, who spend more than 20 billion dollars on these products each year. However, scientific data are lacking on the long-term health benefits of supplements." Neuhouser suggested that women concentrate on getting their nutrients from food rather than supplements.

Researchers found the 41.5% of women who regularly took multivitamins were no more likely to avoid a range of cancers, heart disease, stroke or blood clots than those who didn't. In short, this large US study of over 160,000 postmenopausal women that found no convincing evidence that long term use of multivitamins changed their risk of developing common cancers, cardiovascular disease or dying prematurely.

Effects of antioxidant supplements on cancer prevention: meta-analysis of randomized controlled trials (Myung et al, 2009) (#161,045 total subjects);

searched Medline (PubMed), Excerpta Medica database, and the Cochrane Review in October 2007; Among 3327 articles searched, 31 articles on 22 randomized controlled trials, which included 161,045 total subjects, 88,610 in antioxidant supplement groups and 72,435 in placebo or no-intervention groups, were included in the final analyses. **In a fixed-effects** meta-analysis of all 22 trials, antioxidant supplements were found to have no preventive effect on cancer. **Conclusions:** The meta-analysis of randomized controlled trials indicated that **there is no clinical evidence to support an overall primary and secondary preventive effect of antioxidant supplements on cancer.**

MULTIVITAMINS: There was no evidence that multivitamins confer meaningful benefit or harm in relation to cancer or cardiovascular disease. The risk for invasive cancers of the breast, colon/rectum, endometrium, lung, bladder, and ovary was no different among women who used multivitamin compared with those who did not use multivitamins. Similarly, risk of myocardial infarction, stroke, venous thrombosis, and death from any cause was no different for multivitamin users than for nonusers. Multivitamins do not appear to be effective for the prevention of cancer or cardiovascular disease.

Decision Analysis Supports the Paradigm That Indiscriminate Supplementation of Vitamin E Does More Harm than Good (Dotan et al, 2009) the **major randomized clinical trials have yielded disappointing results on the effects of vitamin E on both mortality and morbidity**. Recent meta-analyses have concluded that **vitamin E supplementation increases mortality.** This conclusion has raised much criticism, most of it relating to three issues: (1) the choice of clinical trials to be included in the meta-analyses; (2) the end point of these meta-analyses (only mortality); and (3) the heterogeneity of the analyzed clinical trials with respect to both population and treatment. Our goal was to bring this controversy to an end by using a Markov-model approach, which is free of most of the limitations involved in using meta-analyses. The researchers examined data from **more than 300,000 subjects in the US, Europe and Israel.** This "disappointing" study warns that **indiscriminate use of high-dose Vitamin E supplementation does more harm than good and that indiscriminate supplementation of high doses of vitamin E is not beneficial in preventing CVD.**

CONCLUSIONS: Their study demonstrated that in terms of QALY, **indiscriminate supplementation of high doses of vitamin E is not beneficial in preventing CVD.**

Their objective was to reassess the outcome of nondiscriminatory supplementation of vitamin E with respect to its effects on cardiovascular-related events and mortality. Their analysis, applying a Markov model, revealed that *supplementing the general public with vitamin E results in loss of quality-adjusted life years.*

Further, Dotan states, " **Unfortunately, major randomized clinical trials yielded disappointing results and recent meta-analyses concluded that indiscriminate, high dose vitamin E supplementation results in increased mortality.** Our major finding was that the average quality-adjusted life years (QALY) of vitamin E- supplemented individuals was 0.30 QALY less than that of untreated people. In our view, this supports the view that indiscriminate supplementation of high dose vitamin E can not be recommended to the general public. In short, we adopt the view that **vitamin E is a "double-edge sword" that should not be consumed until criteria are defined to predict who is likely to benefit from high dose supplementation of vitamin E."** (Dotan, Lichtenberg and Pinchuk, 2009)

Effects of long-term antioxidant supplementation and association of serum antioxidant concentrations with risk of metabolic syndrome in adults (SU. VI.MAX)

(Czernichow et al, 2009) (#5,220 adults) Adults (*n* = 5,220) participating in the SUpplementation en VItamines et Minéraux AntioXydants (SU.VI.MAX) primary prevention trial were randomly assigned to receive a supplement containing a combination of antioxidants (vitamins C and E, beta-carotene, zinc, and selenium) at nutritional doses or a placebo. **Antioxidant supplementation for 7.5 y did not affect the risk of metabolic syndrome (MetS);** *Baseline serum antioxidant concentrations of* beta-carotene *and vitamin C, however, were negatively associated with the risk of MetS*; the adjusted odds ratios, respectively. **Baseline serum zinc concentrations were positively associated with the risk of developing MetS. Conclusions: The experimental finding of no beneficial effects over seven-plus years of antioxidant supplementation** in a generally well-nourished population is **consistent with recent reports of a lack of efficacy of antioxidant supplements.**

Metabolic syndrome refers to a collection of risk factors for type 2 diabetes, heart disease and stroke -- including high blood pressure, abdominal obesity, low levels of "good" HDL cholesterol, elevated triglycerides and high blood sugar. The condition is diagnosed when a person has at least three of those risk factors.

In a study of nutrients in older American women (Women's Health Study cohort), for most nutrients, no decline in intake was observed, as might have been expected in an aging cohort. Instead, intake of many nutrients increased, primarily because of the rising use of dietary supplements. Use of dietary supplements by older individuals is of particular importance because of the potential risk to benefit ratio of synthetic supplement intake levels despite the possibility of declining food intake. However, possible risks from obtaining a large proportion of required nutrients from dietary supplements rather than deriving them from foods should be approached with caution (Park et al, 2009).

Total and Cancer Mortality After Supplementation With Vitamins and Minerals: 10 year Follow-up of the Linxian General Population Nutrition Intervention Trial. (Qiao et al, 2009) (#29,584

adult participants) The General Population Nutrition Intervention Trial was a randomized primary esophageal and gastric cancer prevention trial conducted from 1985 to 1991, in which **29, 584 adult participants** in Linxian, China, were given daily vitamin and mineral supplements. Treatment with "factor D," a combination of 50 μg selenium, 30 mg vitamin E, and 15 mg beta-carotene, led to decreased mortality from all causes, cancer overall, and gastric cancer. **Here, they present a 10-year follow-up after the end of active intervention.** Hazard ratios (HRs) and 95% confidence intervals (CIs) for the cumulative effects of four vitamin and mineral supplementation regimens were calculated using adjusted proportional hazards models. Results: **Participants who received factor D had lower overall mortality and gastric cancer mortality; reduction in cumulative gastric cancer mortality from 4.28% to 3.84%, than subjects who did not receive factor D.** Reductions were mostly attributable to benefits to subjects younger than 55 years. **Esophageal cancer deaths between those who did and did not receive factor D were not different overall**; however, decreased 17% among participants younger than 55 but *esophageal cancer deaths increased 14% among those aged 55 years or older. Vitamin A and zinc supplementation was associated with increased total and stroke mortality*; vitamin C and molybdenum supplementation, with decreased stroke mortality. Conclusion: The beneficial effects of selenium, vitamin E, and beta-carotene on mortality were still evident up to 10 years after the cessation of supplementation and were consistently greater in younger participants. Late effects of other supplementation regimens were also observed. **This study illustrates the confusion in the data, especially with the Linxian studies. They represent an exception to most of the other studies and should be viewed with caution.**

Vitamin A and retinol intakes and the risk of fractures among participants of the Women's Health Initiative Observational Study. (Caire-Juvera et al. 2009) (#75,747 women from the Women's Health Initiative Observational Study) Excessive intakes of vitamin A have been shown to have adverse skeletal effects in animals. High vitamin A intake may lead to an increased risk of fracture in humans. OBJECTIVE: The objective was to evaluate the relation between total vitamin A and retinol intakes and the risk of incident total and hip fracture in postmenopausal women. DESIGN: A total of **75,747 women from the Women's Health Initiative Observational Study** participated. The risk of hip and total fractures was determined using Cox proportional hazards models according to different intakes of vitamin A and retinol. RESULTS: In the analysis adjusted for some covariates, **the association between vitamin A intake and the risk of fracture was not statistically significant.** Analyses for retinol showed similar trends. When the interaction term was analyzed as categorical, the highest intake of retinol with vitamin D was significant (P = 0.033). **Women with lower vitamin D intake** (< or =11 microg/d) in the highest quintile of intake of both vitamin A **and retinol had a modest increased risk of total fracture.** CONCLUSIONS: No association between vitamin A or retinol intake and the risk of hip or total fractures was observed in postmenopausal women. **Only *a modest increase in total fracture risk with high vitamin A and retinol intakes was observed in the low vitamin D-intake group.***

Modification of the effect of vitamin E supplementation on the mortality of male smokers by age and dietary vitamin C. (Hemila and Kaprio, 2009 Apr) (#29,133) The Alpha-Tocopherol, Beta-Carotene Cancer Prevention (ATBC) Study (1985-1993) recruited **29,133 Finnish male cigarette smokers**, finding that vitamin E supplementation had no overall effect on mortality. The authors of this paper found that the effect of vitamin E on respiratory infections in ATBC Study participants was modified by age,

smoking, and dietary vitamin C intake; therefore, they examined whether the effect of vitamin E supplementation on mortality is modified by the same variables. During a median follow-up time of 6.1 years, 3,571 deaths occurred. Age and dietary vitamin C intake had a second-order interaction with vitamin E supplementation of 50 mg/day. *Among participants with a dietary vitamin C intake above the median of 90 mg/day, vitamin E increased mortality among those aged 50-62 years by 19%,* **whereas vitamin E decreased mortality among those aged 66-69 years by 41%. Vitamin E had no effect on participants who had a dietary vitamin C intake below the median.** Smoking quantity did not modify the effect of vitamin E. This study provides strong evidence that the effect of vitamin E supplementation on mortality varies between different population groups. Further study is needed to confirm this heterogeneity.

Vitamin E supplement use and the incidence of cardiovascular disease and all-cause mortality in the Framingham Heart Study: Does the underlying health status play a role?

(Dietrich et al, 2009) (#4,270 Framingham Study participants) Observational studies generally showed beneficial associations between supplemental vitamin E intake and cardiovascular disease (CVD) risk whereas intervention trials reported adverse effects of vitamin E supplements. We hypothesize that these discordant findings result from differing underlying health status of study participants in observational and intervention studies. Objective: Determine if the relation between supplemental vitamin E intake and CVD and all-cause mortality (ACM) depends on pre-existing CVD. Design: Proportional hazards regression to relate supplemental vitamin E intake to the 10-year incidence of CVD and ACM in **4,270 Framingham Study participants** stratified by baseline CVD status. Results: Eleven percent of participants used vitamin E supplements at baseline. In participants with pre-existing CVD, there were 28 (44%) and 20 (32%) incident cases of CVD and ACM in the vitamin E supplement users versus 249 (47%) and 202 (38%) in the non-users, respectively. In participants without pre-existing CVD, there were 51 (13%) and 47 (12%) cases of CVD and ACM in the vitamin E supplement group versus 428 (13%) and 342 (10%) in the non-vitamin E supplement group, respectively. Conclusion: **CVD status has no apparent influence on the association of supplemental vitamin E intake and risk for CVD and ACM in this**

large, community-based study. Further research is needed to clarify the basis for the discrepant results between intervention and observational studies of supplemental vitamin E intake.

Antioxidants prevent health-promoting effects of physical exercise in humans. (Ristow et al, 2009) (#39

healthy young men) **Exercise promotes longevity and ameliorates type 2 diabetes mellitus and insulin resistance.** However, **exercise also increases mitochondrial formation of presumably harmful reactive oxygen species** (ROS). They evaluated the effects of a combination **of vitamin C (1000 mg/day) and vitamin E (400 IU/ day)** on insulin sensitivity as measured by glucose infusion rates (GIR) during a hyperinsulinemic, euglycemic clamp in previously untrained (n = 19) and pretrained (n = 20) healthy young men. Before and after a 4 week intervention of physical exercise, GIR was determined, and muscle biopsies for gene expression analyses as well as plasma samples were obtained to compare changes over baseline and potential influences of vitamins on exercise effects. *Exercise increased parameters of insulin sensitivity (GIR and plasma adiponectin) only in the absence of antioxidants in both previously untrained (P < 0.001) and pretrained (P < 0.001) individuals.* This was **paralleled by increased expression of ROS-sensitive** transcriptional regulators of insulin sensitivity and ROS defense capacity, peroxisome-proliferator-activated receptor gamma (PPARgamma), and PPARgamma coactivators PGC1alpha and PGC1beta only in the absence of antioxidants (P < 0.001 for all). **Molecular mediators of endogenous ROS defense (superoxide dismutases 1 and 2; glutathione peroxidase) were also induced by exercise, and this effect too was blocked by antioxidant supplementation.** Consistent with the concept of mitohormesis, exercise-induced oxidative stress ameliorates insulin resistance and causes an adaptive response promoting endogenous antioxidant defense capacity. **Supplementation with antioxidants may preclude these health-promoting effects of exercise in humans.**

Long-term use of beta-carotene, retinol, lycopene, and lutein supplements and lung cancer risk: results from the VITamins And Lifestyle

(VITAL) study. (Satia et al, 2009) (#77,126 (VITAL) cohort
Study in Washington State) **High-dose beta-carotene supplementation
in high-risk persons has been linked to increased lung cancer risk
in clinical trials**; whether effects are similar in the general population is
unclear. The authors examined associations of supplemental beta-carotene,
retinol, vitamin A, lutein, and lycopene with lung cancer risk among
participants, aged 50-76 years, in the VITamins And Lifestyle (VITAL)
cohort Study in Washington State. In 2000-2002, eligible persons (n =
77,126) completed a 24-page baseline questionnaire, including detailed
questions about supplement use (duration, frequency, dose) during the
previous 10 years from multivitamins and individual supplements/mixtures.
Incident lung cancers (n = 521) through December 2005 were identified
by linkage to the Surveillance, Epidemiology, and End Results cancer
registry. *Longer duration of use of individual beta-carotene, retinol,
and lutein supplements (but not total 10-year average dose) was associated
with statistically significantly elevated risk of total lung cancer and
histologic cell types.* There was little evidence for effect modification by
gender or smoking status. **Long-term use of individual beta-carotene,
retinol, and lutein supplements should not be recommended for lung
cancer prevention, particularly among smokers.**

Although this book is primarily about multivitamins and antioxidant
vitamins, current discussions center around the antioxidant potential of
lycopene. The following abstract makes a key observation concerning any
contribution of lycopene as an effective antioxidant:

**Are the health attributes of lycopene related to
its antioxidant function?** (Erdman, Ford and Lindshield, 2009)
A variety of epidemiological trials have suggested that higher intake of
lycopene-containing foods (primarily tomato products) or blood lycopene
concentrations are associated with decreased cardiovascular disease
and prostate cancer risk. Of the carotenoids tested, lycopene has been
demonstrated to be the most potent in vitro antioxidant leading many
researchers to conclude that the antioxidant properties of lycopene are
responsible for disease prevention. In our review of human and animal
trials with lycopene, or lycopene-containing extracts, **there is limited
support for the in vivo antioxidant function for lycopene. Moreover,
tissue levels of lycopene appear to be too low to play a meaningful
antioxidant role. We conclude that there is an overall shortage of
supportive evidence for the "antioxidant hypothesis" as lycopene's**

major in vivo mechanism of action. Our laboratory has postulated that metabolic products of lycopene, the lycopenoids, may be responsible for some of lycopene's reported bioactivity.

Circa 2010

Vitamin C supplements and the risk of age-related cataract: a population-based prospective cohort study in women. (Rautiainen et al, 2010) (#24,593 women) Experimental animal studies have shown adverse effects of high-dose vitamin C supplements on age-related cataract. **Objective:** We examined whether **vitamin C supplements (≈1000 mg) and multivitamins containing vitamin C (≈60 mg)** are associated with the incidence of age-related cataract extraction in a population-based, prospective cohort of women. **Design:** Our study included **24,593 women** aged 49–83 y from the Swedish Mammography Cohort (follow-up from September 1997 to October 2005). We collected information on dietary supplement use and lifestyle factors with the use of a self-administrated questionnaire. Cataract extraction cases were identified by linkage to the cataract extraction registers in the geographical study area. **Results:** During the **8.2 y of follow-up** (184,698 person-years), we identified 2497 cataract extraction cases. The multivariable hazard ratio (HR) for vitamin C supplement users compared with that for nonusers was 1.25 (95% CI: 1.05, 1.50). The HR for the duration of >10 y of use before baseline was 1.46 (95% CI: 0.93, 2.31). The HR for the use of multivitamins containing vitamin C was 1.09 (95% CI: 0.94, 1.25). *Among women aged ≥65 y, vitamin C supplement use increased the risk of cataract by 38% (95% CI: 12%, 69%). Vitamin C use among hormone replacement therapy users compared with that among nonusers of supplements or of hormone replacement therapy was associated with a 56% increased risk of cataract* (95% CI: 20%, 102%). Vitamin C use among corticosteroid users compared with that among nonusers of supplements and corticosteroids was associated with an HR of 1.97 (95% CI: 1.35, 2.88). **Conclusion:** Our results indicate that *the use of vitamin C supplements may be associated with higher risk of age-related cataract among women*.

The harmful effects with the antioxidant vitamins raises the possibility the antioxidant enzymes may also be harmful. The following paper by Delcourt et al demonstrates an association between high levels of superoxide dismutase and glutathione peroxidase and an increased risk of cataract formation.

Associations of cataract with antioxidant enzymes and other risk factors: the French Age-Related Eye Diseases (POLA) Prospective Study.

(Delcourt et al, 2003) (#1,947 survivors)

PURPOSE: To determine the association of potential risk factors, including antioxidant enzymes, with the incidence of cataract. DESIGN: Cohort study. PARTICIPANTS: At baseline, the Age-Related Eye Diseases (Pathologies Oculaires Liées à l'Age, POLA) Study included **2,584 residents** of Sète (southern France) aged 60 years or older. From September 1998 to May 2000, **a 3-year follow-up examination was performed on 1947 of the 2436 surviving participants** (79.9%). METHODS: Cataract classification was based on a standardized lens examination at the slit lamp, according to Lens Opacities Classification System III. Biologic measurements were performed at baseline from fasting blood samples. MAIN OUTCOME MEASURES: At baseline and follow-up, the presence of cataract was defined as: NC or nuclear opalescence (NO) > or = 4 for nuclear cataract, C > or = 4 for cortical cataract, and P > or = 2 for posterior cataract (PSC) opacities, using opacity grades corrected for interobserver variability. Incidence rates were assessed separately for right and left eyes and for each type of cataract. RESULTS: In the multivariate model, **the incidence of cortical cataract was increased in subjects with high red blood cell superoxide dismutase activity. The incidence of PSC cataract was increased in subjects with a high level of plasma glutathione peroxidase. In addition to age, gender, and opacities at baseline, significant risk factors for incident cataract were: long-duration diabetes and lifetime heavy smoking**. CONCLUSIONS: Consistent with the baseline analysis, the results of this prospective study suggest that **antioxidant enzymes might be implicated in the etiology of cataract**. This supports my contention that cataracts are due to an EMOD insufficiency, as is the large group of coexistent diseases, such as cancer, heart disease, stroke, arthritis, diabetes, and cataract formation.

Micronutrient concentrations and subclinical atherosclerosis in adults with HIV. (Falcone et al, 2010)

(#298 Nutrition for Healthy Living participants) Extremes in micronutrient intakes are common in HIV-infected patients in developed countries and may affect the progression of atherosclerosis in this population. **Objective:** They completed a cross-sectional study examining the association between serum micronutrient concentrations and surrogate markers of atherosclerosis in a cohort of HIV-infected adults. **Design: They measured serum selenium, zinc, vitamin A, and vitamin E concentrations as well as carotid intima-media thickness (c-IMT) and coronary artery calcium (CAC) in 298 Nutrition for Healthy Living participants.** They performed multivariate regression of c-IMT and CAC with each micronutrient with adjustment for HIV-related and cardiovascular disease risk factors. **Results:** In the multivariate analysis, **the highest tertile of serum vitamin E concentration was associated with higher common and internal c-IMT and CAC scores. Participants with higher vitamin E concentrations were more likely to have detectable CAC and common c-IMT >0.8 mm.** Other than vitamin E, micronutrients had no association with markers of atherosclerosis. **Conclusions:** Our study showed that *elevated serum vitamin E concentrations are associated with abnormal markers of atherosclerosis and may increase the risk of cardiovascular complications in HIV-infected adults.*

Multivitamin use and breast cancer incidence in a prospective cohort of Swedish women. (Larsson et al, 2010) (#35,329 cancer-free women) Many women use multivitamins in the belief that these supplements will prevent chronic diseases such as cancer and cardiovascular disease. However, whether the use of multivitamins affects the risk of breast cancer is unclear. **Objective:** They prospectively examined the association between multivitamin use and the incidence of invasive breast cancer in the **Swedish Mammography Cohort. Design:** In 1997, **35,329 cancer-free women** completed a self-administered questionnaire that solicited information on multivitamin use as well as other breast cancer risk factors. Relative risks (RRs) and 95% CIs were calculated by using Cox proportional hazard models and adjusted for breast cancer risk factors. **Results:** During a mean follow-up of 9.5 y, 974 women were diagnosed with incident breast cancer. *Multivitamin use was associated with a statistically significant increased risk of breast cancer.* The association did not differ significantly by hormone receptor status of the breast tumor. **Conclusions:** These results suggest that *multivitamin use is associated with an increased risk of breast cancer. Use of multivitamins was linked to a statistically significant*

19 per cent increased risk of breast cancer (after adjusting for lifestyle and risk factors like weight, diet, smoking, exercise, and family history of breast cancer.

Women and men use multivitamins in the belief that they will protect them from chronic diseases like cancer and heart disease but that is not proven. Please remember that in **February 2009, the *Archives of Internal Medicine* published details of a large US study of over 160,000 postmenopausal women that found no convincing evidence that long term use of multivitamins changed their risk of developing common cancers, cardiovascular disease or dying prematurely.**

Other research has found that women who take multivitamins have increased breast density, which is linked to a relatively higher risk of breast cancer (Berube et al, 2008). **The widespread use of multiviamins points out an important public health concern.**

Vitamins C and E to prevent complications of pregnancy-associated hypertension (Roberts et al, 2010)

(#10,154) Oxidative stress has been proposed as a mechanism linking the poor placental perfusion characteristic of preeclampsia with the clinical manifestations of the disorder. We assessed the effects of **antioxidant supplementation with vitamins C and E**, initiated early in pregnancy, on the risk of serious adverse maternal, fetal, and neonatal outcomes related to pregnancy-associated hypertension. METHODS: They conducted a multicenter, **randomized, double-blind trial** involving nulliparous women who were at low risk for preeclampsia. Women were randomly assigned to begin daily supplementation with **1000 mg of vitamin C and 400 IU of vitamin E or matching placebo between the 9th and 16th weeks of pregnancy.** The primary outcome was severe pregnancy-associated hypertension alone or severe or mild hypertension with elevated liver-enzyme levels, thrombocytopenia, elevated serum creatinine levels, eclamptic seizure, medically indicated preterm birth, fetal-growth restriction, or perinatal death. RESULTS: A total of **10,154 women** underwent randomization. The two groups were similar with respect to baseline characteristics and adherence to the study drug. Outcome data were available for 9,969 women. **There was no significant difference between the vitamin and placebo groups in the rates of the primary outcome or in the rates of preeclampsia. Rates of adverse perinatal outcomes did not differ significantly between the groups.** CONCLUSIONS: **Vitamin C and E supplementation initiated in the 9th to 16th week of**

pregnancy in an unselected cohort of low-risk, nulliparous women did not reduce the rate of adverse maternal or perinatal outcomes related to pregnancy-associated hypertension.

Nutritional authority, Alice Lichenstein writes of a "Heart breaking story." Observational data have identified associations between carotenoids, folic acid, and vitamin E, or metabolites altered by these nutrients, and cardiovascular disease (CVD) risk. **Despite biological plausibility, for the most part, data derived from nutrient supplement trials using moderate to high doses of single nutrients or nutrient combinations (exceeding amounts to avoid nutrient deficiency) have been disappointing.** (There is that "disappointing" word again. In other words, the nutrients supplements have failed to live up to exalted their overstated expectations or the rosy predictions of the free radical theory.)

There is some evidence that use of nutrient supplements intended to decrease CVD risk has **resulted in unanticipated adverse consequences**. Potential discrepancies between observational and interventional data include concerns of residual confounding by diet and lifestyle patterns, publication bias against studies with null or negative outcomes, reliance on secondary rather than primary prevention trials, and unaccounted for contribution of genotypic variations. **At this time (2009) there are insufficient data to recommend the routine use of nutrient supplements to prevent or treat CVD** (Lichtenstein, 2009).

Given the widespread use of antioxidant vitamins and MVMs in our society and because of unexplained adverse effects of relatively high-dose single-agent supplementation of antioxidants and MVMs, it does not seem advisable to recommend either at this time. Benefits and risks from single antioxidant vitamin studies have shown few clear effects on chronic disease. Given the widespread use of antioxidant vitamins and MVMs in our society, risk to overall public health seems realistic and the hope of chronic disease prevention or cure seems remote.

Caveats from the Linus Pauling Institute, such as "the intake levels most likely to promote optimum health remain to be determined" and from others, such as "further research continues to be necessary" or "further studies are needed," emphasize our current state of ignorance. The discrepancy between the impressive observational data and clinical trials may be related to varying factors, such as identity, type, and form of antioxidant; particular antioxidant combinations; trial design issues; outcome measures; length; populations under study; etc. The fact that the antioxidant trials are based on the flawed free radical theory may be important in explaining the lack of agreement between the predicted positive benefits and the "disappointing" results of the clinical trials conducted to date.

Exuberant use of antioxidant vitamin supplements should be tempered somewhat by the above findings, which likely separates fact from factitious. Confusing and contradictory results are the norm for antioxidant vitamin studies. These results should be considered cautiously but they clearly serve as a refutation of the free radical theory.

In 2010, the popular Reader's Digest published an article by Christie Aschwanden entitled, "5 Vitamin truths and Lies," which acknowledged widespread misconceptions about vitamins and antioxidants. The lead paragraph stated, "Once upon a time, you believed in the tooth fairy. And you figured that taking vitamins was good for you. Oh, it's painful when another myth gets shattered. Recent research suggests that a daily multi is a waste of money for most people--and there's growing evidence that some other old standbys may even hurt your health."

SUMMARY

This is a selective systematic over view of 181 **interventional initial or follow up studies**, showing either marginal effect, negligible effects, no effects at all. Sixty of these studies showed harmful effects of the antioxidant vitamins A (beta carotene), C (ascorbic acid) or E (alpha tocopherol) or combinations thereof. Studies with multivitamins, which contain the antioxidant vitamins, were also included. Total number of participants for all of the above studies is over **8,600,000 subjects**, some of which may have been repeats in follow up or parallel studies.

Jeffrey Blumberg, an antioxidant researcher from Tufts University, has voiced a starkly opposing biased view of the vitamin facts. He said, "It makes sense to cast the net wider for more reliable vitamin facts. We need to look at in vitro studies, animal-model studies, observational studies of individual patients in clinics or large scale populations within or between countries."

Actually, this is the very approach that misled and misguided investigators in the first place. Been there, done that!

Blumberg went on to say that the important thing to remember about randomized clinical trials of antioxidant vitamins is that they may not mimic real-world usage in several ways:

- The specific form of the vitamin used may be inferior. "In vitamin E studies, almost all of them have been done with the synthetic form of vitamin E, which is different from the natural source forms," he said.
- Studies often fail to find the truly susceptible population, which means the "controls" fare as well as the vitamin takers.
- The study may look too early or too late in the stage of the disease to find a benefit.
- There may be synergistic co-factors that were not included in the experiment. "Remember that clinical trials look at one dose, usually of only one antioxidant. In some of the most sophisticated trials, they use two antioxidants, and in one or two cases, three - vitamin C, vitamin E and beta carotene," Blumberg said.
- The dosage used may not be optimal.

- There may have been insufficient follow-up. "If you are trying to show that you can prevent cancer in a three or four year study, that's a real limitation."
- Poor compliance. In many of the studies, members of the placebo group began taking vitamins on their own, "reducing the difference between the two groups."
- Poor screening. Some subjects in, say, a vitamin E study might have natively high blood plasma levels of E because of diet, genetics or some other factor, he said. A well designed study would balance such people between the experimental and control groups. But in no study that Blumberg has evaluated has there been any prior screening of blood plasma vitamin concentrations.

Because of all of this, Blumberg said, it is far too soon to conclude that "antioxidant vitamins don't work."

Dr. Andrew Weil, integrative medicine guru, agreed. He said, "The value of antioxidant vitamins has, in my view, been scientifically demonstrated **beyond any reasonable doubt**. Everyone should take a high-quality multivitamin daily."

All I will say here is "Follow the money." Check out Dr. Weil's website and the wide array of antioxidants he is selling. If **181** studies (reports), containing over 8.6 million participants does not raise "any reasonable doubt," in Dr. Weil's myopic mind, nothing ever will.

CHAPTER SIX:

60 Studies Showing Harmful Effects

SUMMARY OF 60 STUDIES/REPORTS

SHOWING ADVERSE, HARMFUL EFFECTS
R.M. Howes M.D., Ph.D.

Isotretinoin-Basal Cell Carcinoma Study Group
(Tangrea et al, 1992) (#981) randomly assigned; low-dose regimen of
isotretinoin; *associated with significant adverse systemic effects.*
(adverse mucocutaneous effects and serum triglyceride elevations)

**Prospective Study of the Intake of Vitamins C,
E, and A and the Risk of Breast Cancer** (Hunter et al,
1993) (#89,494 women); *A low intake of vitamin A may increase the
risk of this disease.*

**A randomized trial of vitamin A and vitamin
E supplementation for retinitis pigmentosa.** (Berson,
1993) (#601) While not statistically significant, similar trends were observed
for rates of decline of visual field area. Visual acuity declined about 1 letter
per year in all groups. Conclusions. These results support a beneficial effect
of 15 000 IU/d of vitamin A and suggest an adverse effect of 400 IU/d of

vitamin E on the course of retinitis pigmentosa. *Supplementation with 400 IU/day of vitamin E has been found to accelerate the progression of retinitis pigmentosa that is not associated with vitamin E deficiency.*

Alpha-Tocopherol, Beta Carotene Cancer Prevention Study (ATBC study) (Heinonen et al, 1994)

(#29,133); **E had no reduction in fatal heart attacks.** *50% increase in hemorrhagic stroke deaths* among vitamin E group; *11% increase in ischemic heart disease deaths among* beta-carotene *group; 18% increase in lung cancer among* beta-carotene *group.* **The incidence of lung cancer was 18% higher among men who took the beta-carotene supplement** and *eight percent more men in this group died, as compared to those receiving other treatments or placebo.*

The Beta-Carotene and Retinol Efficacy Trial (CARET) (Omenn et al, 1996) (#14,254 heavy smokers and 4,060

asbestos workers) (total #18,314); *28% increase in lung cancer; 26% increase in CVD (nonsignificant); 17% increase in total mortality among treatment group. Women had a higher risk of death from cardiovascular disease or from any cause than men. In addition, the incidence of lung cancer and deaths from all causes decreased but did not disappear completely after the supplementation ceased.*

Cambridge Heart Antioxidant Study (CHAOS)

(Stephens et al., 1996) (#2,002); alpha-tocopherol treatment substantially reduces the rate of non-fatal MI, with beneficial effects apparent after 1 year of treatment (**77% decrease in risk of subsequent nonfatal MI); no benefit on cardiovascular mortality,** *even though paralleled by a not significant 22% increase in all deaths.*

ATBC Sub-Study Shows Increased CVD Deaths

(Rapola et al, 1997) (#1,862 men, with prior myocardial infarction); *significantly more deaths from fatal coronary heart disease in the beta-carotene and combined alpha-tocopherol and beta-carotene groups than in the placebo group. The risk of fatal coronary heart disease increased in the groups that received either beta-carotene or the combination of alpha-tocopherol and beta-carotene.*

The Multivitamins and Probucol Study (Tardif et

al, 1997) (#317); (Beta carotene 30 000 IU, vitamin C 500 mg and E 700

IU); ***Probucol has been pulled off the market due harmful effects and the likelihood of cardiac arrhythmias.***

A study by Jacobs et al in the Nov. 2004 issue of American Journal of Clinical Nutrition, found that ***such supplements may actually promote the clogging of arteries.*** They evaluated cardiovascular disease in **1,923 post-menopausal women with diabetes,** part of the **Iowa Women's Health Study,** which collected data in 1986 about diets and vitamin C consumption in nearly **35,000 recruits.** The researchers found that **women with diabetes consuming at least 300 milligrams of vitamin C per day faced** ***2.3 times the risk of death from stroke and 2 times the risk of dying from coronary artery disease*** as did diabetic women who took in less of the vitamin C.

A recent study showed ***that mega-doses of vitamin C might actually speed up hardening of the arteries.*** Researchers from the University of Southern California studied **573** outwardly healthy middle-aged men and women. About 30% of them regularly took various vitamins. The study found no clear-cut sign that getting lots of vitamin C from food or a daily multivitamin does any harm. But ***those taking vitamin C pills had accelerated thickening of the walls of the big arteries in their necks. The more they took, the faster the buildup.***

Supplementation of healthy volunteers with *vitamin E decreased platelet function* whereas supplementation with vitamin c or beta-carotene had no significant effects. (Calzada et al, 1997)

Familial hypercholesterolemia, intima-to-media thickness (FH IMT study) (Raal et al, 1999)

(#15 with homozygous familial hypercholesterolemia); ***homozygous familial hypercholesterolemia, intima-to-media thickness (FH IMT study) increased with vitamin E supplements (400 mg/day) for 2 years,*** but decreased when subjects received statin therapy. **Vitamin E supplementation fails to slow (or inhibit) the progression of intima-to-media thickness in healthy men and women at low risk for cardiovascular disease.**

Antioxidant supplementation in vitro does not improve human sperm motility (Donnelly et al, Fertil Steril.

1999) (#60 patients) Percoll density centrifugation in **media supplemented with ascorbate or alpha-tocopherol to different concentrations within physiologic levels. The production of reactive oxygen species by sperm** was reduced by supplementation in vitro with ascorbate and alpha-tocopherol. However, *progressive motility, average path velocity, curvilinear velocity, straight-line velocity, and linearity were decreased significantly, with the greatest inhibition observed with the highest concentrations of antioxidants.* Supplementation of preparation media with ascorbate and alpha-tocopherol, either singly or in combination, is not beneficial to sperm motility. In short, *sperm motility was significantly decreased by antioxidants vitamin C and alpha-tocopherol.*

The effect of ascorbate and alpha-tocopherol supplementation in vitro on DNA integrity and hydrogen peroxide-induced DNA damage in human spermatozoa (Donnelly et al, Mutagenesis. 1999)

Addition of *both ascorbate and alpha-tocopherol in combination to sperm preparation medium actually induced DNA damage and intensified the damage induced by H_2O_2.*

The secondary prevention HDL Atherosclerosis Treatment study (HATS) (Brown et al., 2001) (#160 patients

with coronary disease); *when used in combination with simvastatin/niacin, antioxidants negated the benefit of the latter on plasma lipid profile and stenosis progression.*

Randomized Trial of Supplemental ß-Carotene to Prevent Second Head and Neck Cancer (Mayne et

al, 2001) (#264 patients who had been curatively treated for a recent early-stage squamous cell carcinoma of the oral cavity, pharynx, or larynx.); the *point estimates suggested a possible decrease in second head and neck cancer risk but a possible increase in lung cancer risk.*

HDL Atherosclerosis Treatment study (HATS)

(Brown et al, 2001) (#160); an antioxidant cocktail (vitamin E, ß-carotene, vitamin C, and selenium); *antioxidant supplements may have interfered with the efficacy of statin-plus-niacin therapy.*

Women's Angiographic Vitamin and Estrogen (WAVE) Trial (Waters et al, 2002) (#423 postmenopausal women,

with at least one 15% to 75% coronary stenosis); *postmenopausal women with coronary disease on hormone replacement therapy given vitamin E plus vitamin C had an unexpected significantly higher all-cause mortality rate and a trend for an increased cardiovascular mortality rate* compared with the vitamin placebo women.

Mega-dose vitamins and minerals in the treatment of non-metastatic breast cancer: an historical cohort study (Lesperance et al, 2002) (#90 patients)

Breast cancer–specific survival (i.e., patients censored only at death from breast cancer) and *disease-free survival were shorter in the nutrient-supplemented group* than in the non-supplemented group, but the differences were not statistically significant. Investigators stated that, "**It is troubling that both** (Lesperance et al, 2002 and Ferreira et al, 2004) **reported results suggesting poorer survival with concurrent administration of antioxidants and cytotoxic therapy.**"

Retinol intake and bone mineral density in the elderly: the Rancho Bernardo Study. (Promislow, 2002) (#570 women and 388 men)

the associations of log retinol with BMD and BMD change were negative for supplement users and positive for nonusers at the hip, femoral neck, and spine. At the femoral neck, for every unit increase in log retinol intake, supplement users had 0.02 g/cm² lower BMD and 0.23% greater annual bone loss, and nonusers had 0.02 g/cm² (p = 0.04) greater BMD and 0.22% greater bone retention. In both sexes, *increasing retinol became negatively associated with skeletal health at intakes not far beyond the recommended daily allowance (RDA), intakes reached predominately by supplement users.* This study suggests **there is a delicate balance between ensuring that the elderly consume sufficient vitamin A and simultaneously cautioning against excessive retinol supplementation.**

Vitamin A intake and hip fractures among postmenopausal women. (Feskanich, 2002) (#72,337 postmenopausal women) After controlling for confounding factors, *women in the highest quintile of total vitamin A intake (≥3000 µg/d of retinol equivalents [RE]) had a significantly elevated relative risk (RR) of*

hip fracture compared with women in the lowest quintile of intake. *This increased risk was attributable primarily to retinol. Long-term intake of a diet high in retinol may promote the development of osteoporotic hip fractures in women.*

Serum retinol levels and the risk of fracture.

(Michealsson, 2003) (#2,322 men) *The risk of fracture was highest among men with the highest levels of serum retinol.* Multivariate analysis of the risk of fracture in the highest quintile for serum retinol as compared with the middle quintile showed that the rate ratio was 1.64 for any fracture and 2.47 for hip fracture. *The risk of fracture was further increased within the highest quintile for serum retinol. Men with retinol levels in the 99th percentile had an overall risk of fracture that exceeded the risk among men with lower levels by a factor of seven.* Conclusions: Current levels of vitamin A supplementation and food fortification in many Western countries may need to be reassessed.

Vitamins E & A fail to reduce incidence or mortality of lung cancer: Cochrane Database Syst Rev. 2003. (Caraballoso et al., 2003) (#109,394 participants) increased risk of lung cancer incidence and mortality.

Use of antioxidant vitamins for the prevention of cardiovascular disease: meta-analysis of randomized trials. (Vivekananthan et al., 2003) (The vitamin E trials involved a total of #81,788 patients, and the beta-carotene trials involved #138,113); *Beta carotene led to small but statistically significant increase in all-cause mortality and a slight increase in cardiovascular death.*

Neoplastic and Antineoplastic Effects of Beta Carotene on Colorectal Adenoma Recurrence: Results of a Randomized Trial (Baron et al, 2003) (#864 subjects who had had an adenoma removed and were polyp-free); *For participants who smoked cigarettes and also drank more than one alcoholic drink per day, beta carotene doubled the risk of adenoma recurrence.*

Supplemental vitamin C increase cardiovascular disease risk in women with diabetes (Lee et al, 2004)

(#1,923 postmenopausal women who reported being diabetic) When dietary and supplemental vitamin C were analyzed separately, only supplemental vitamin C showed a positive association with mortality endpoints. CONCLUSION: *A high vitamin C intake from supplements is associated with an increased risk of cardiovascular disease mortality in postmenopausal women with diabetes.*

Cochrane Database Syst Rev. 2004: Vitamins E & A fail to reduce incidence or mortality of gastrointestinal cancer. (Cochrane Database Syst Rev. G.

Bjelakovic et al, 2004) (#170,525 participants); **the fixed effect unlike the random effects meta-analysis showed that** *antioxidant supplements significantly increased mortality. Beta-carotene and vitamin A and beta-carotene and vitamin E significantly increased mortality,* while beta-carotene alone only tended to do so. **When the selenium trials were excluded, both analyses showed a statistically significant increase in mortality, which was particularly strong in patients taking beta carotene and vitamin A.**

ATBC 6-year followup study (2004) (Thornwall et al., 2004) (#29,133 male smokers); *β-Carotene seemed to increase the post-trial risk of first-ever non-fatal MI.*

Meta-analysis: high-dosage vitamin E supplementation may increase all-cause mortality

(Miller et al., 2004) (#135,967); *high doses of vitamin E increased mortality.*

Vitamin C worsens coronary atherosclerosis in those with two copies of the haptoglobin 2 gene.

(Levy, 2004) (#299); **The relative benefit or harm of vitamin therapy on the progression of coronary artery stenoses in women in the WAVE study was dependent on haptoglobin type. Antioxidant therapy (1,000 mg/day of vitamin C + 800 IU/day of vitamin E) was associated with improvement of coronary** <u>atherosclerosis</u> **in diabetic women with two copies of the haptoglobin 1 gene but** *worsening of coronary atherosclerosis in those with two copies of the haptoglobin 2 gene.*

Use of multivitamins and prostate cancer mortality in a large cohort of US men. (Stevens et al, 2005) (#475,726 men who were cancer-free) Investigators assessed the association between the use of multivitamins and prostate cancer mortality. *The death rate from prostate cancer was marginally higher among men who took multivitamins regularly* (> or =15 times/month) **compared to non-users; this risk was statistically significant only for those multivitamin users who used no additional (vitamin A, C, or E) supplements.** In addition, risk was greatest during the initial four years of follow-up. CONCLUSIONS: *Regular multivitamin use was associated with a small increase in prostate cancer death rates.*

HOPE-TOO Extension (Lonn et al, 2005) (#3,994); *Another subgroup finding in HOPE-TOO was a vitamin E–associated increased risk of heart failure incidence that appeared in a secondary end point analysis in the 4.5-year report and persisted in the 7-year extended follow-up, as did the risk of hospitalization for heart failure. Patients in the vitamin E group had a higher risk of heart failure and hospitalization for heart failure.* In the HOPE-TOO trial, **there were no differences in cancer incidence, cancer deaths, and major cardiovascular events, but** *higher rates of heart failure and hospitalizations for heart failure.*

A randomized trial of antioxidant vitamins to prevent second primary cancers in head and neck cancer patients (Bairati et al, 2005 Apr 6) (#540), *patients receiving alpha-tocopherol supplements had a higher rate of second primary cancers during the supplementation period* but a lower rate after supplementation was discontinued. Similarly, *the rate of having a recurrence or second primary cancer was higher during* but a lower rate after supplementation was discontinued. Similarly, *the rate of having a recurrence or second primary cancer was higher during* but lower after supplementation with alpha-tocopherol. The proportion of participants free of second primary cancer overall after 8 years of follow-up was similar in both arms. CONCLUSIONS: *alpha-Tocopherol supplementation produced unexpected adverse effects on the occurrence of second primary cancers and on cancer-free survival.*

Randomized trial of antioxidant vitamins to prevent acute adverse effects of radiation therapy in head and neck cancer patients (Bairati et al, 2005 Aug 20) (#540) *supplementation with beta-carotene was discontinued because of ethical concerns.* Quality of life was not improved by the supplementation. *The rate of local recurrence of the head and neck tumor tended to be higher in the supplement arm (beta carotene and Vitamin E).*

Vitamin A Supplementation for Reducing the Risk of Mother-to-child Transmission of HIV Infection: Cochrane systematic review 2005.

(Wiysonge et al, 2005) (#3,033) Mother-to-child transmission (MTCT) of HIV is the dominant mode of acquisition of HIV infection for children, currently resulting in more than 2000 new pediatric HIV infections each day worldwide. However, there was evidence of heterogeneity between the three trials with information on MTCT of HIV. **While the trials conducted in South Africa and Malawi did not find evidence that the effect of Vitamin A supplementation was different from that of placebo,** *the trial in Tanzania found evidence that vitamin A supplementation increased the risk of MTCT of HIV* **compared with placebo and multivitamins (excluding vitamin A).**

Australian Collaborative Trial of Supplements (ACTS) (Rumbold et al, 2006) (#1,877); Supplementation with vitamin C (1,000 mg) and vitamin E (400 IU) This is **the second major report in a month to find no apparent benefit for the supplements in preventing pre-eclampsia**. These results followed closely similar findings reported in the March 30, 2006 issue of *The Lancet* by researchers at Kings College London. In that **randomized study of high-risk women not only did these vitamins fail to reduce the pre-eclampsia risk,** but *the rate of low-birth-weight babies was higher and the rate for gestational hypertension was higher for women in the vitamin group.*

Women in the vitamin group had an increased risk of being hospitalized antenatally for hypertension and having to take antihypertensive medication. In addition, a subgroup of women in the vitamin group had a higher frequency of abnormal liver-function tests.

Vitamins in Pre-eclampsia (VIP) Trial Consortium (Poston et al., 2006) (#2,410 women at increased risk for preeclampsia, analyzed 2,395) 1000 mg of vitamin C and 400 IU vitamin E; Concomitant supplementation with vitamin C and vitamin E does not prevent pre-eclampsia in women at risk, but does *increase the rate of babies born with a low birth weight.*

The Melbourne Atherosclerosis Vitamin E Trial (MAVET): a study of high dose vitamin E in smokers. (Magliano et al, 2006) (#409 male and female smokers) The Melbourne Atherosclerosis Vitamin E Trial (MAVET) was **a randomized, double-blind, placebo-controlled trial** in which **409 male and female smokers** aged 55 years and over were randomized to receive 500 IU per day of natural vitamin E or placebo. Results: *The mean increase in intima-media thickness over time in the vitamin E group was 0.0041 mm/year faster than placebo in smokers.*

Mortality in Randomized Trials of Antioxidant Supplements for Primary and Secondary Prevention; Systematic Review and Meta-analysis (Bjelakovic et al, 2007) (#with 232,606 participants); Conservatively, *the supplements increase the likelihood of dying by about 5 percent. When looked at separately, they found that Vitamin A increased death risk by 16 per cent, beta carotene by 7 per cent and Vitamin E by 4 per cent.*

Vitamin C gave contradictory results, but when given singly or in combination with other vitamins in good-quality trials, increased the death rate by 6 per cent.

Multivitamin Use and Risk of Prostate Cancer in the National Institutes of Health–AARP Diet and Health Study (Lawson et al, 2007) (#295,344 men); *use of multivitamins more than seven times per week, when compared with never use, was associated with a doubling in the risk of fatal prostate cancer.*

Health Professionals Follow-up Study (2007): Effect of vitamins C, E, A and carotenoids and the

occurrence of oral pre-malignant lesions (Maserejian et al, 2007) (#42,340 men enrolled in the Health Professionals Follow-up Study); **A trend for** *increased risk of oral pre-malignant lesions was observed with vitamin E, especially among current smokers and with vitamin E supplements. Beta-carotene also increased the risk among current smokers.*

Risk of Mortality with Vitamin E Supplements: The Cache County Study. (Hayden et al, 2007) Predictably,

deaths were more frequent with a history of diabetes, stroke, coronary artery bypass graft surgery, or myocardial infarction, and with the use of warfarin, nitrates, or diuretics. None of these conditions or treatments altered the null main effect with vitamin E, but *mortality was increased in vitamin E users who had a history of stroke, coronary bypass graft surgery, or myocardial infarction and, independently, in those taking nitrates, warfarin, or diuretics.*

Antioxidant Supplementation Increases the Risk of Skin Cancers in Women but Not in Men. (Hercberg

et al, 2007) (#French adults, 7,876 women and 5,141 men. Total # = 13,017) It was performed within the framework of the **Supplementation in Vitamins and Mineral Antioxidants study, a randomized, double-blinded, placebo-controlled, primary prevention trial** testing the efficacy of nutritional doses of antioxidants in reducing incidence of cancer and ischemic heart disease in the general population. French adults (7,876 women and 5,141 men) were randomized to take an oral daily capsule of antioxidants (120 mg vitamin C, 30 mg vitamin E, 6 mg β-carotene, 100 μg selenium, and 20 mg zinc) or a matching placebo. The median time of follow-up was 7.5 y. *In women, the incidence of SC was higher in the antioxidant group.* **Conversely, in men, incidence did not differ between the 2 treatment groups.** Despite the small number of events, *the incidence of melanoma was also higher in the antioxidant group for women.* The incidence of nonmelanoma SC did not differ between the antioxidant and placebo groups. Our findings suggest that antioxidant supplementation affects the incidence of SC differentially in men and women. (Hercberg et al, 2007)

Antioxidant supplements for prevention of mortality in healthy participants and patients

with various diseases. (Bjelakovic, Nikolova, Gludd, Simonetti and Gludd, 2008 Apr) (#232,550 Cochrane Database Syst Rev.) **Overall, the antioxidant supplements had no significant effect on mortality in a random-effects meta-analysis**, but *significantly increased mortality in a fixed-effect model.* **In the trials with a low risk of bias, the antioxidant supplements significantly increased mortality.** When the different antioxidants were assessed separately, analyses including trials with a low risk of bias and excluding *selenium trials found* **significantly increased mortality by vitamin A, beta-carotene, and vitamin E**, but **no significant detrimental effect of vitamin C.** We found no evidence to support antioxidant supplements for primary or secondary prevention. *Vitamin A, beta-carotene, and vitamin E may increase mortality.* **Antioxidant supplements need to be considered medicinal products and should undergo sufficient evaluation before marketing.**

Systematic review: primary and secondary prevention of gastrointestinal cancers with antioxidant supplements. (Bjelakovic, Nikolova, Simonette and Gludd, 2008) (#211,818) 20 randomized trials (211,818 participants) assessing beta-carotene, vitamin A, vitamin C, vitamin E, and selenium. **The antioxidant supplements were without a significant effect on the occurrence of gastrointestinal cancers.** *Antioxidant supplements had no significant effect on mortality in a random-effects model meta-analysis but significantly increased mortality in a fixed-effect model meta-analysis.* CONCLUSIONS: *There was no evidence that the studied antioxidant supplements prevented gastrointestinal cancers. On the contrary, they seem to increase overall mortality.*

VITAL (VITamins And Lifestyle) study (2008)
(Slatore et al, 2008) (#77,721 men and women); *Supplemental vitamin E was associated with a small increased risk of lung cancer.*

Vitamin E for Alzheimers and mild cognitive impairment. Cochrane Database Syst Rev. (2008)
(Isaac et al, 2008) (#769 participants); *More participants taking Vitamin E suffered a fall.*

Efficacy of Antioxidant Supplementation in Reducing Primary Cancer Incidence and Mortality:

Systematic Review and Meta-analysis (Bardia et al, 2008) (#104,196) *Beta carotene supplementation was associated with an increase in the incidence of cancer among smokers and with a trend toward increased cancer mortality.*

Vitamin E supplementation may transiently increase tuberculosis risk in males who smoke heavily and have high dietary vitamin C intake. (Hemila and Kaprio, 2008 Oct) (#29,023) The ATBC Study cohort consists of 29,023 males aged 50-69 years, smoking at baseline, with no tuberculosis diagnosis prior to randomization. Vitamin E supplementation had no overall effect on the incidence of tuberculosis nor had beta-carotene. Nevertheless, **dietary vitamin C intake significantly modified the vitamin E effect.** *Among participants who obtained 90 mg/d or more of vitamin C in foods, vitamin E supplementation increased tuberculosis risk by 72%.* This effect was restricted to participants who smoked heavily. *Our finding that vitamin E seemed to transiently increase the risk of tuberculosis in those who smoked heavily and had high dietary vitamin C intake should increase caution towards vitamin E supplementation for improving the immune system.*

Vitamin E supplementation and pneumonia risk in males who initiated smoking at an early age: effect modification by body weight and dietary vitamin C. (Hemila and Kaprio, 2008 Nov) (#21,657) *They had found a 14% higher incidence of pneumonia with vitamin E supplementation in a subgroup of the Alpha-Tocopherol Beta-Carotene Cancer Prevention (ATBC) Study cohort:* participants who had initiated smoking by the age of 20 years. **Vitamin E supplementation had no effect on the risk of pneumonia in participants with body weight in a range from 70 to 89 kg.** *Vitamin E increased the risk of pneumonia in participants with body weight less than 60 kg, and in participants with body weight over 100 kg. The harm of vitamin E supplementation was restricted to participants with dietary vitamin C intake above the median.* CONCLUSION: **Vitamin E supplementation may cause harmful effects on health in certain groups of male smokers.**

Oral administration of vitamin C decreases muscle mitochondrial biogenesis and hampers training-induced adaptations in endurance performance. (Gomez-Cabrera et al, 2008) (#14 men) Exercise practitioners often take vitamin C supplements because **intense muscular contractile activity can result in oxidative stress,** as indicated by altered muscle and blood glutathione concentrations and increases in protein, DNA, and lipid peroxidation. DESIGN: The human study was **double-blind and randomized. Fourteen men** (27-36 y old) were trained for 8 wk. Five of the men were supplemented daily with an oral dose of 1 g vitamin C. In the animal study, 24 male Wistar rats were exercised under 2 different protocols for 3 and 6 wk. Twelve of the rats were treated with a daily dose of vitamin C (0.24 mg/cm2 body surface area). RESULTS: *The administration of vitamin C significantly (P=0.014) hampered endurance capacity.* These factors are peroxisome proliferator-activated receptor co-activator 1, nuclear respiratory factor 1, and mitochondrial transcription factor A. **Vitamin C also prevented the exercise-induced expression of cytochrome C (a marker of mitochondrial content) and of the antioxidant enzymes superoxide dismutase and glutathione peroxidase.** CONCLUSION: **Vitamin C supplementation decreases training efficiency because it prevents some cellular adaptations to exercise.**

Dietary antioxidants and the long-term incidence of age-related macular degeneration: the Blue Mountains Eye Study. (Tan et al, 2008) (#2,454 Australian population-based cohort study)

PURPOSE: To assess the relationship between baseline dietary and supplement intakes of antioxidants and the long-term risk of incident age-related macular degeneration (AMD). DESIGN: Australian population-based cohort study. PARTICIPANTS: Of 3,654 baseline (1992-1994) participants initially 49 years of older, 2,454 were reexamined after 5 years, 10 years, or both. The highest compared with the lowest tertile of total beta-carotene intake predicted incident neovascular AMD. Similarly, **beta-carotene intake from diet alone predicted neovascular AMD.** This association was evident in both ever and never smokers. **Higher**

intakes of total vitamin E predicted late AMD. CONCLUSIONS: In this population-based cohort study, higher dietary lutein and zeaxanthin intake reduced the risk of long-term incident AMD. This study confirmed the Age-Related Eye Disease Study finding of protective influences from zinc against AMD. *Higher beta-carotene intake was associated with an increased risk of AMD.*

Multivitamin-multimineral supplement use and mammographic breast density. (Berube et al, 2008) (#Premenopausal (777) and postmenopausal (783) women; total 1,560)

The effect of multivitamin-multimineral supplements on the occurrence of chronic diseases, such as breast cancer, is unclear. Breast density is increasingly used as a biomarker of breast cancer risk. **Current multivitamin-multimineral supplement use was reported by 21.7% of women** (20.7% and 22.6% of premenopausal and postmenopausal women, respectively). **Premenopausal women who were currently using multivitamin-multimineral supplements had higher adjusted mean breast density (45.5%) than past (42.9%) or never (40.2%) users.** In postmenopausal women, multivitamin-multimineral supplement use was not associated with breast density. **Conclusion:** *Regular use of multivitamin-multimineral supplements may be associated with higher mean breast density among premenopausal women.*

Decision Analysis Supports the Paradigm That Indiscriminate Supplementation of Vitamin E Does More Harm than Good (Dotan et al, 2009)

applying a Markov model, revealed that *supplementing the general public with vitamin E results in loss of quality-adjusted life years (loss of about four months).*

Effects of long-term antioxidant supplementation and association of serum antioxidant concentrations with risk of metabolic syndrome in adults (SU.VI.MAX)

(Czernichow et al, 2009) (#5,220) *Baseline serum zinc concentrations were positively associated with the risk of developing metabolic syndrome (MetS).*

Total and Cancer Mortality After Supplementation With Vitamins and Minerals: 10 year Follow-up of the Linxian General Population Nutrition Intervention Trial. (Qiao et al, 2009) (#29,584)

Treatment with "factor D," a combination of 50 μg selenium, 30 mg vitamin E, and 15 mg beta-carotene, led to *esophageal cancer deaths increased 14% among those aged 55 years or older. Vitamin A and zinc supplementation was associated with increased total and stroke mortality.*

Vitamin A and retinol intakes and the risk of fractures among participants of the Women's Health Initiative Observational Study. (Caire-Juvera

et al. 2009) (#75,747) **the association between vitamin A intake and the risk of fracture was not statistically significant.** *Women with lower vitamin D intake and retinol had a modest increased risk of total fracture.* **Only a modest increase in total fracture risk with high vitamin A and retinol intakes was observed in the low vitamin D-intake group.**

Modification of the effect of vitamin E supplementation on the mortality of male smokers by age and dietary vitamin C. (Hemila and Kaprio, 2009)

(#29,133) The Alpha-Tocopherol, Beta-Carotene Cancer Prevention (ATBC) Study (1985-1993) recruited **29,133 Finnish male cigarette smokers**, finding that vitamin E supplementation had no overall effect on mortality. The authors of this paper found that the effect of vitamin E on respiratory infections in ATBC Study participants was modified by age, smoking, and dietary vitamin C intake; therefore, they examined whether the effect of vitamin E supplementation on mortality is modified by the same variables. *Among participants with a dietary vitamin C intake above the median of 90 mg/day, vitamin E increased mortality among those aged 50-62 years by 19%, whereas vitamin E decreased mortality among those aged 66-69 years by 41%. Vitamin E had no effect on participants who had a dietary vitamin C intake below the median.*

Antioxidants prevent health-promoting effects of physical exercise in humans. (Ristow et al, 2009) (#39 healthy young men)

Exercise promotes longevity and ameliorates type 2 diabetes mellitus and insulin resistance. However, **exercise also increases mitochondrial formation of presumably harmful reactive oxygen species** (ROS). The evaluated the effects of a combination **of vitamin C (1000 mg/day) and vitamin E (400 IU/day)** on insulin sensitivity as measured by glucose infusion rates (GIR) during a hyperinsulinemic, euglycemic clamp in previously untrained (n = 19) and pretrained (n = 20) healthy young men. *Exercise increased parameters of insulin sensitivity (GIR and plasma adiponectin) only in the absence of antioxidants in both previously untrained and pretrained individuals.* **Molecular mediators of endogenous ROS defense (superoxide dismutases 1 and 2; glutathione peroxidase) were also induced by exercise, and this effect too was blocked by antioxidant supplementation.** Consistent with the concept of mitohormesis, exercise-induced oxidative stress ameliorates insulin resistance and causes an adaptive response promoting endogenous antioxidant defense capacity. **Supplementation with antioxidants may preclude these health-promoting effects of exercise in humans.**

Long-term use of beta-carotene, retinol, lycopene, and lutein supplements and lung cancer risk: results from the VITamins And Lifestyle (VITAL) study. (Satia et al, 2009) (#77,126 (VITAL) cohort Study in Washington State) **High-dose beta-carotene supplementation in high-risk persons has been linked to increased lung cancer risk in clinical trials**; whether effects are similar in the general population is unclear. The authors examined associations of supplemental beta-carotene, retinol, vitamin A, lutein, and lycopene with lung cancer risk among participants, aged 50-76 years, in the VITamins And Lifestyle (VITAL) cohort Study in Washington State. In 2000-2002, eligible persons (n = **77,126**) completed a 24-page baseline questionnaire, including detailed questions about supplement use (duration, frequency, dose) during the previous 10 years from multivitamins and individual supplements/mixtures.

Incident lung cancers (n = 521) through December 2005 were identified by linkage to the Surveillance, Epidemiology, and End Results cancer registry. *Longer duration of use of individual beta-carotene, retinol, and lutein supplements (but not total 10-year average dose) was associated with statistically significantly elevated risk of total lung cancer and histologic cell types.* There was little evidence for effect modification by gender or smoking status. **Long-term use of individual beta-carotene, retinol, and lutein supplements should not be recommended for lung cancer prevention, particularly among smokers.**

Vitamin C supplements and the risk of age-related cataract: a population-based prospective cohort study in women.

(Rautiainen et al, 2010) (#24,593 women) Experimental animal studies have shown adverse effects of high-dose vitamin C supplements on age-related cataract. **Objective:** We examined whether **vitamin C supplements ($\approx$1000 mg) and multivitamins containing vitamin C ($\approx$60 mg)** are associated with the incidence of age-related cataract extraction in a population-based, prospective cohort of women. **Design:** Our study included **24,593 women** aged 49–83 y from the **Swedish Mammography Cohort** (follow-up from September 1997 to October 2005). **Results:** During the **8.2 y of follow-up** (184,698 person-years), we identified 2497 cataract extraction cases. The multivariable hazard ratio (HR) for vitamin C supplement users compared with that for nonusers was 1.25. The HR for the duration of >10 y of use before baseline was 1.46. The HR for the use of multivitamins containing vitamin C was 1.09. *Among women aged $\geq$ 65 y, vitamin C supplement use increased the risk of cataract by 38%. Vitamin C use among hormone replacement therapy users compared with that among nonusers of supplements or of hormone replacement therapy was associated with a 56% increased risk of cataract.* Vitamin C use among corticosteroid users compared with that among nonusers of supplements and corticosteroids was associated with an HR of 1.97. **Conclusion:** Our results indicate that *the use of vitamin C supplements may be associated with higher risk of age-related cataract among women.*

Micronutrient concentrations and subclinical atherosclerosis in adults with HIV.

(Falcone et al, 2010) (#298 Nutrition for Healthy Living participants) Extremes in micronutrient intakes are common in HIV-infected patients in developed countries and may affect the progression of atherosclerosis in this population. **Objective:** They completed a cross-sectional study examining the association between serum micronutrient concentrations and surrogate markers of atherosclerosis in a cohort of HIV-infected adults. **Design:** They measured serum selenium, zinc, vitamin A, and vitamin E concentrations as well as carotid intima-media thickness (c-IMT) and coronary artery calcium (CAC) in **298 Nutrition for Healthy Living participants.** They performed multivariate regression of c-IMT and CAC with each micronutrient with adjustment for HIV-related and cardiovascular disease risk factors. **Results:** In the multivariate analysis, **the highest tertile of serum vitamin E concentration was associated with higher common and internal c-IMT and CAC scores. Participants with higher vitamin E concentrations were more likely to have detectable CAC and common c-IMT** >0.8 mm. Other than vitamin E, micronutrients had no association with markers of atherosclerosis. **Conclusions:** Our study showed that *elevated serum vitamin E concentrations are associated with abnormal markers of atherosclerosis and may increase the risk of cardiovascular complications in HIV-infected adults.*

(Falcone et al, 2010)

Multivitamin use and breast cancer incidence in a prospective cohort of Swedish women. (Larsson et al, 2010) (#35,329 cancer-free women) Many women use multivitamins in the belief that these supplements will prevent chronic diseases such as cancer and cardiovascular disease. However, whether the use of multivitamins affects the risk of breast cancer is unclear. **Objective:** They prospectively examined the association between multivitamin use and the incidence of invasive breast cancer in the **Swedish Mammography Cohort. Design:** In 1997, **35,329 cancer-free women** completed a self-administered questionnaire that solicited information on multivitamin use as well as other breast cancer risk factors. Relative risks (RRs) and 95% CIs were calculated by using Cox proportional hazard models and adjusted for breast cancer risk factors. **Results:** During a mean follow-up of 9.5 y, 974 women were diagnosed with incident breast cancer. *Multivitamin use was associated with a statistically significant increased risk of breast cancer.* The association did not differ significantly by hormone receptor status of the breast tumor. **Conclusions:** These results suggest that *multivitamin use is associated with an increased risk of breast cancer. Use of multivitamins was linked to a statistically significant 19 per cent increased risk of*

breast cancer. **Given the widespread use of multivitamins, there is an important public health message in this study.**

Thus, sixty studies have shown possible harmful endpoints to antioxidant vitamin use.

Total human participants = over 2,600,000

On the Question of Mortality and Vitamin E

We have seen data analysis, re-analysis, meta-analysis and now, re-analysis of the meta-analysis. Gerss and Kopcke have reviewed the issue of studies showing an increased mortality associated with vitamin E and have concluded as follows:

"In the meta analysis 19 clinical trials comprising a total of **135,967 participants** were included. The dosages of vitamin E supplementation ranged from 16.5 to 2000 IU/d. In the present paper this data source was augmented and 10 additional trials were included (**2,495 additional participants** receiving vitamin E doses from 136 to 5000 IU/d). Moreover in 2 of the originally included trials updated results of mortality at longer periods of follow-up were available. The present paper yields contradictory results regarding the association of vitamin E supplementation and mortality. **Hierarchical logistic regression analyses confirm the former results showing an increased mortality of patients receiving high dose vitamin E.** Furthermore a traditional methodological approach of meta-regression was applied to the same data source. Contrary to the former result it showed that the increased mortality odds ratio in certain trials is not due to the higher dose of vitamin E supplementation. Rather it can be explained by a higher proportion of male patients that were included in these trials compared to other trials. **The causal relationship of vitamin E supplementation and increased mortality is questionable.** Different methodological approaches of meta analysis yield contradictory results. Thus, none of these results can be regarded to supply evidence in a statistical sense. In particular, high dose vitamin E supplementation can not be regarded proved to increase mortality." (Gerss and Kopcke, 2009)

Now that is totally confusing. Please try to "see through the fuzzy math" and look for common sense trends. The overall conclusion is that there is no clear cut benefit from the antioxidant vitamins and there is the potential for significant harm. That's about it in a nutshell.

CHAPTER SEVEN:

Where Are The Dead Bodies?

Here are the dead bodies

Adverse consequences of antioxidant vitamins and increased risk of death

Any agent which causes an increased risk of the following can contribute to the number of dead bodies. They need repeating.

Antioxidant vitamins can lead to increased risk of:
- lung cancer, 18%, 28%;
- lung cancer incidence and mortality;
- breast cancer;
- prostate cancer;
- multivitamins doubled risk of fatal prostate cancer
- head and neck cancer;
- skin cancer;
- melanoma;
- oral pre-malignant lesions, especially in smokers;

- total mortality, 17%;

- likelihood of dying by about 5%;

- esophageal cancer deaths 14%;

- doubled adenoma (polyp) recurrence in smokers and drinkers;

- had a higher rate of second primary cancers during the supplementation period

- hemorrhagic stroke deaths, 50%;

- increased total and stroke mortality;

- supplements increase the likelihood of dying by about 5%

- vitamin A increased death risk by 16%, beta carotene by 7%, vitamin E by 4 %;

- significant increase in all-cause mortality and a slight increase in cardiovascular death;

- mortality was increased in vitamin E users who had a history of stroke, coronary bypass graft surgery, or myocardial infarction and, independently, in those taking nitrates, warfarin, or diuretics;

- participants with a dietary vitamin C intake above the median of 90 mg/day, vitamin E increased mortality among those aged 50-62 years by 19%

- increased post-trial risk of first-ever non-fatal Myocardial Infarction (heart   attack);

- ischemic heart disease deaths, 11%;

- significantly more deaths from fatal coronary heart disease;

- 2.3 times risk of death from stroke and 2 times risk of dying from coronary artery disease in diabetic postmenopausal women;

- higher rates of heart failure and hospitalizations for heart failure

- total fracture;

- hip fracture;

- osteoporotic hip fractures in men and women;

- accelerate the progression of retinitis pigmentosa (eye disease);

- increased risk of age-related macular degeneration;

- higher risk of age-related cataract among women;

- among women aged ≥65 y, vitamin C supplement use increased the risk of cataract by 38%;

- vitamin C use among hormone replacement therapy users was associated with a 56% increased risk of cataract

- increased risk of Mother-to-child transmission of HIV;

- increased rate of low-birth-weight babies;

- increased rate for gestational hypertension;

- increased in having to take antihypertensive medication antenatally (after birth)

- suffered falling more often;

- E supplementation increased tuberculosis 72% and pneumonia risk 14%;

- vitamin E results in loss of quality-adjusted life years

- increase in the incidence of cancer among smokers and increased cancer mortality

- Multivitamin/Minerals associated with doubling in the risk of fatal prostate cancer

- increase in intima-media thickness over time in smokers

- rate of local recurrence of the head and neck tumor tended to be higher

- higher rate of second primary head and neck cancers

- worsening of coronary atherosclerosis in those with two copies of the haptoglobin 2   gene

- promote the clogging of arteries;

- accelerated thickening of the walls

- higher mortality rate in men

- adverse mucocutaneous effects and serum triglyceride elevations

- cardiac arrhythmias (probucol)

- negated the benefit of cholesterol lowering drugs (statin plus niacin)

- negatively associated with skeletal health

- 2 studies suggested poorer survival with concurrent administration of antioxidants and cytotoxic therapy in non-metastatic breast cancer

- C hampered endurance capacity

- multivitamins associated with higher mean breast density in premenopausal women

- multivitamins statistically significant increased risk 19 % of breast cancer

- supplementing the general public with vitamin E results in loss of quality-adjusted life years (loss of about four months)

- decreased sperm motility

- induced sperm DNA damage

Expansion of the Lawson et al study on Multivitamins

Any increase in cancer rates is going to lead to increased deaths. An article by Crystal Phend at MedPage Today (http://www.medpagetoday.com/Urology/ProstateCancer/5654. Accessed 4-19-10) was so impressive that I decided to excerpt the article as follows:

Men who take multi-vitamin supplements more than once a day are twice as likely to die of prostate cancer as men who never take supplements, researchers confirmed.

They were also at elevated risk of advanced prostate cancer compared with never users, reported Karla A. Lawson, Ph.D., of the National Cancer Institute here, and colleagues. The researchers reported the outcomes of the National Institutes of Health -- AARP Diet and Health Study in the **May 16, 2007 issue of the *Journal of the National Cancer Institute.***

The large, prospective investigation adds credence to the possibility of harm from antioxidant supplements as found in prior systematic reviews and meta-analyses, according to an accompanying editorial. The findings "underscore the possibility that antioxidant supplements could have unintended consequences for our health," wrote Goran

Bjelakovic, M.D., of the University of Nis, Serbia, and Christian Gluud, M.D., of the Copenhagen University Hospital.

The few previous prospective studies had suggested that multivitamin use may protect men from developing prostate cancer but speed its progression once begun, Dr. Lawson and colleagues wrote. **Because more than a third of American adults take vitamins, the researchers noted, "any association between intake of multivitamin supplements and the risk or severity of prostate cancer would have important consequences for public health."**

The prospective study included **295,344 men aged 50 to 71 and free of cancer** at enrollment in 1995 and 1996. Their multivitamin use was assessed at baseline using a self-administered, food-frequency questionnaire. Five percent used multivitamins more than seven times a week; 36% took a multivitamin daily.

Among the participants, 41% reported using a one-a-day type supplement, 12% reported using a theragran type (vitamins plus iron) supplement, and 6% reported use of a stress-tab type supplement (primarily B vitamins). Half of the supplements used were multivitamins. Outcomes were followed using subsequent questionnaires, Social Security Administration death records, and state cancer registries.

Over five years of follow-up, 10,241 developed incident prostate cancer. These cases included 8,765 localized and 1,476 advanced cancers. A separate mortality analysis found 179 cases of fatal prostate cancer over six years of follow-up.

Among the findings in a multivariate adjusted analysis, the researchers reported (more than daily use versus never users):

- **No association between multivitamin use and risk of prostate cancer overall (relative risk 1.06, 95% confidence interval 0.97 to 1.17).**
- **No association between multivitamin use and risk of localized prostate cancer (RR 1.02, 95% CI 0.92 to 1.14).**
- **Increased risk of advanced prostate cancer (RR 1.32, 95% CI 1.04 to 1.67).**
- **Elevated risk of fatal prostate cancers (RR 1.98, 95% CI 1.07 to 3.66).**
- **Higher incidence rates for advanced prostate cancer (143.8 versus 113.4 per 100,000 person-years).**
- **Higher incidence rates for fatal prostate cancer (18.9 versus 11.4 per 100,000 person-years).**

The associations were strongest in men with a family history of prostate cancer or those who took selenium, beta-carotene, **or zinc.** "Thus, excessive intake of certain individual micronutrients that are used in combination with multivitamins may be the underlying factor that is related to risk and not the multivitamins themselves," the researchers wrote.

Among men with prostate cancer in the family, **heavy multivitamin use (more than seven times per week) more than doubled advanced prostate cancer risk and fatal prostate cancer risk. Heavy use of selenium yielded a 37% increased risk of localized prostate cancer** ($P=0.008$ for interaction) Although based on a small sample, those who took more than seven multivitamins a week and were also taking a selenium supplement were at 5.8-fold higher risk of fatal prostate cancer than those not taking a selenium supplement ($P=0.037$ for interaction). The association between heavy multivitamin use and advanced prostate cancer was somewhat modified by beta-carotene use ($P=0.036$ for trend).

Men who used a zinc supplement in addition to heavy multivitamin use were at significantly elevated risk of fatal prostate cancer. This "could be due to nonessential, potentially harmful trace elements contained in zinc supplements, such as cadmium, a known carcinogen," the researchers said.

They noted that their study was limited by lack of information on duration of multivitamin use. Also, they said, heavy multivitamin users were more likely to have prostate cancer screening using prostate specific antigen.

While this could have biased diagnosis of localized prostate cancer, "increased multivitamin use due to early symptoms of prostate cancer cannot account for the increased risk of fatal prostate cancer among heavy multivitamin users because the association persisted and even strengthened when we disregarded those diagnosed in the initial years of follow-up," the researchers noted. Regardless, they concluded, "the possibility that men taking high levels of multivitamins along with other supplements have increased risk of advanced and fatal prostate cancers is of concern and merits further evaluation."

The reason why dietary intake of vitamins has been shown beneficial with mixed or negative results for supplements, editorialists Drs. Bjelakovic and Gluud suggested, **may be because of differences between natural and synthetic vitamins.**

"Antioxidant supplements in pills are synthetic, factory processed, and may not be safe compared with their naturally occurring counterparts," they wrote. Or, they added, it could be that the populations they have been tested in already get their full daily requirement of vitamins and trace elements from diet. **They pointed out that the American diet provides 120% of the recommended dietary allowances for beta-carotene, vitamin A, and vitamin C, and that dietary vitamin E deficiency has never been reported in the United States.**

They also suggested a possible mechanism for the negative findings: **"Reactive oxygen species in moderate concentrations are essential mediators of reactions by which the body gets rid of unwanted cells. Thus, if administration of antioxidant supplements decreases free radicals, it may interfere with essential defensive mechanisms for ridding the organism of damaged cells, including those that are precancerous and cancerous."**

I believe that just as there can be a dangerous build up of natural antioxidants, such as urate or bilirubin, this same condition could possible occur with synthetic antioxidants (even those contained in multivitamins), such as vitamins A, beta carotene, ascorbate and vitamin E (tocopherol). Their effects may be augmented by the build up of common synthetic food antioxidants, such as BHT and BHA.

Since supplement manufacturers have not provided the public with adequate safety information, I believe that it is time for a class action law suit to control and regulate the supplement industry, as it relates to antioxidants. Adequate scienfitic data is in, the conclusions are becoming clear and it is time to act on behalf of the people. **Marketing has placed antioxidants in products ranging from pizza dough to cake mix, from water to energy drinks, from doughnuts to dog food and from bread to bubble gum.**

Genetic engineers are mutating foods to create fruits and vegetables which contain mega-loads of antioxidants, effectively bringing us into the age of "fortified Franken-foods." These antioxidants have been and will be incorported into the general food supply, even though individuals may not want to ingest higher levels of these questionable and potentially dangerous antioxidants.

It would also appear that the insidious influence of antioxidant vitamins would be difficult to verify on autopsy, because it is so widespread and at the heart of energy production. However, certain cases of antioxidant doses have clearly resulted in "dead bodies."

The Antioxidant Killer, Uric Acid (urate)

First, consider the lethal potential of common natural antioxidants, such as uric acid, bilirubin and estrogen.

Hyperuricemia has been associated with increased morbidity in patients with hypertension and is associated with increased mortality in women and elderly persons. Hyperuricemia is clearly a powerful predictive factor for ischemic cardiovascular disease (CVD; and poor outcomes in these conditions), as recently reviewed. **The recently published National Health and Nutrition Examination Survey I (NHANES I) study of 5926 subjects concluded that increased uric acid is independently and significantly associated with cardiovascular mortality. In univariate Cox proportional hazard analyses, serum urate concentration was associated with CVD mortality. Uric acid levels also tended to be associated with death from any cause during follow-up.** (Niskanen et al, 2004).

Hyperuricemia has a strong association with the relative risks of death in all causes, coronary heart disease, stroke, hepatic disease and renal failure, and indicated that serum uric acid seems to be a considerable risk factor for reduced life expectancy (Tomita et al, 2000).

Men with hyperuricemic gout have a higher risk of death from all causes. Among men without preexisting CHD, the increased mortality risk is primarily a result of an elevated risk of CVD death, particularly from CHD (Choi and Curhan, 2007).

The Antioxidant Killer, Bilirubin

Free bilirubin is the most toxic substance produced by the human body. In normal adults, however, the bilirubin is conjugated in the liver, i.e. converted to a nontoxic form known as bilirubin-glucuronide.

Several reports have emphasized the antioxidant role **of bilirubin, which in human neonatal plasma seems to have a greater antioxidant capacity than urates, α-tocopherol, or ascorbates** (Miller et al, 1993).

Hyperbilirubinemia frequently occurs in the first five days of life of a newborn baby and may clear up within seven to fourteen days. This condition known as "physiological jaundice of newborns" or "neonatal jaundice" is due to incomplete development of certain mechanisms of the body resulting in a decreased ability to conjugate bilirubin with glucronic acid. Specifically, the key enzyme, UDP-glucuronyl transferase, is not present in the newborn, requiring several weeks to be fully induced. As a result, the bilirubin cannot be conjugated and is retained in the body for some time. The hyperbilirubinemia may be severe, lasting longer, and resulting in kernicterus.

Kernicterus can result in severe neurological deficits, mental retardation, loss of IQ and death. **The most popular treatment for neonatal juandice is phototherapy, which ironically generates large amounts of EMODs, especially excited singlet oxygen.** The light penetrates the skin, generates singlet oxygen and converts bilirubin to a less toxic substance, which is eliminated through the urine. In short, the lethal antioxidant hyperbilirubinemia death sentence is revoked and given a pardon by an EMOD, singlet oxygen.

In adults, hyperbilirubinemia, commonly referred to as "Gilbert's Disease", frequently results in death and the study appeared in the Oct. 30, 2008 *New England Journal of Medicine* (Morris et al, 2008). It is indeed ironic that the highly maligned EMODs must come to the rescue in the treatment of antioxidant induced lethal kernicterus.

The Antioxidant Killer, Estrogen

Long-term estrogen administration to post-menopausal women appears to have deleterious effects on rates of cardiovascular events such as myocardial infarction, strokes or venous thromboembolism (HERS) (Hulley et al, 1998) and Women's Health Initiative, **WHI** (WHI, 2002). **I believe that it must be kept in mind that estrogen is considered to be an antioxidant. Thus, I am not surprised by the fact that it actually increases the risk of developing EMOD insufficiency syndrome diseases.**

Older women who take hormone pills that combine estrogen and testosterone more than double their risk of breast cancer, according to a study of more than **70,000 nurses.** "This type of hormone therapy may help with mood, libido and bone mineral density, but the possible risk of breast cancer may outweigh these benefits," said study co-author Rulla Tamimi of Harvard Medical School. The findings, published in 7/24/06 issue of Archives of Internal Medicine, add to the evidence that **certain types of hormone supplements, such as estrogen-progestin pills, increase women's risk of breast cancer, strokes and heart attacks.**

Earlier research **also found a greater breast cancer risk in women with higher natural levels of testosterone.**

Tragic deaths of 38 infants by lethal IV antioxidant vitamin E

A fatal syndrome characterized by progressive clinical deterioration with unexplained thrombocytopenia, renal dysfunction, cholestasis, and ascites developed in certain infants throughout the United States who had received E-Ferol, an intravenous vitamin E supplement. (THE TRAGIC CASE HISTORY OF INTRAVENOUS VITAMIN E (The New York Times) May 27, 1984

By PHILIP M. BOFFEY)

Prolonged exposure to E-Ferol was associated with progressive intralobular cholestasis, inflammation of hepatic venules, and extensive sinusoidal veno-occlusion by fibrosis. E-Ferol, contained 25 units per milliliter of dl-alpha-tocopheryl acetate solubilized with 9% polysorbate 80 and 1% polysorbate 20. They proposed that vasculocentric hepatotoxicity is the basis for the observed clinical syndrome that represents the cumulative effect of one or more of the constituents of E-Ferol (Bove et al, 1985).

All affected infants received E-Ferol; some affected infants received up to 1 ml or more daily. **Both outbreaks ceased shortly after use of E-Ferol was discontinued. Three were jailed for selling drug (vitamin E) that killed 38 babies.**

E-Ferol Aqueous Solution was the brainchild of James B. Madison, executive vice president of operations at O'Neal, Jones and Feldman (OJF), a drug distribution firm in St. Louis. Madison, with the permission of his boss, Larry K. Hiland, president of OJF, asked Ronald Carter of Carter-Glogau Laboratories, a drug manufacturer in Glendale, Ariz., to develop the formula. They believed their product was a nutritional supplement, not a drug. But because the product was labeled for treating a disease--retrolental fibroplasia--the solution was legally a drug.

By April 23, 1984, FDA had completed recall audits of all the wholesale distributors and the 159 hospitals that had received E-Ferol, ensuring that all of the product was off the market, as it remains today. **But by that time, the infant death toll attributable to E-Ferol had reached 38.**

On Sept. 30, 1988, after a seven-week trial, a jury returned guilty verdicts against Carter-Glogau, Ronald M. Carter, Sr., and Larry K. Hiland for distributing an unapproved and misbranded drug with the intent to defraud and mislead, and for participating in a conspiracy to market the drug without testing and without FDA approval. Hiland,

the former president of OJF, was also found guilty of mail fraud in connection with the promotion of E-Ferol and was sentenced to a federal prison.

The **Center for Drug Evaluation and Research, Food and Drug Administration, Rockville, Maryland, concluded that the use of E-Ferol in these neonatal intensive care units was associated with increased morbidity and mortality among exposed infants** (Arrowsmith et al, 1989).

Research has shown infants who received E-Ferol injections are at an increased lifetime risk for reproductive problems, cervical and vaginal cancer, and other health problems. The drug was never FDA approved, but the companies sold E-Ferol to hospitals anyway, allegedly saying that it didn't need approval because it was a supplement.

"The E-Ferol scandal is one of the most shocking examples of corporate crime in American history."

There are the bodies! **The studies (RCTs) on vitamin E and beta carotene also argue for their toxicity and increased mortality.** Please refer to the section on "Antioxidant intervention trials."

Vitamin E deficiency is rare, and may occur in people with intestinal absorption problems, malnutrition, very low-fat diets, several genetic conditions, very low birth weight premature infants, or infants taking unfortified formulas. Supplementation with vitamin E may be necessary in these conditions and should be under strict medical attention. Prolonged vitamin E deficiency may cause severe medical complications.

Nutrient Intoxication

Fortification of foods has been associated with overdoses. Nutrient intoxication has been reported after consumption of fortified foods, primarily in instances when mistakes were made in over-fortifying the food product (e.g., **superabundant amounts of niacin improperly added to pumpernickel bagels** and **over fortification of milk with vitamin D**) (Niacin intox, 1983) (Blank et al, 1995) (Jacobus et al, 1992). Thus, it is possible that nutrient intoxidcation could occur with the antioxidant vitamins, due to it frequent and common place use with fortified foods and due to genetic engineering to produce fruits and vegetables with higher natural content of these same antioxidants.

CHAPTER EIGHT:

Vitamin A And Its Beta Carotene Precursor

The **NHANES III survey (1988-1994)** found that most Americans consume recommended amounts of vitamin A. More recent NHANES data (1999-2000) show average adult intakes to be about 3,300 IU per day, which also suggests that **most Americans get enough vitamin A** (U.S. Dept HHS, 2004).

There is no RDA for beta-carotene or other provitamin A carotenoids. Vitamin A deficiency is common in developing countries but **rarely seen in the United States.**

Researchers are now examining a potential new risk factor for osteoporosis: an excess intake of vitamin A. Animal, human, and laboratory research suggests an association between greater vitamin A intake and weaker bones (Binkley and Krueger, 2000) (Forsyth et al, 1989).

The **Nurses Health Study** looked at the association between vitamin A intake and hip fractures in over **72,000 postmenopausal women. Women who consumed the most vitamin A in foods and supplements (3,000 mcg or more per day as retinol equivalents, which is over three times the recommended intake) had a significantly increased risk of experiencing a hip fracture as compared to those consuming the least amount** (less than 1,250 mcg/day). The effect was lessened by use of estrogens. These observations raise questions about the effect of retinol because retinol intakes greater than 2,000 mcg/day were associated with an increased risk of hip fracture as compared to intakes less than 500 mcg (Feskanich et al, 2002).

A longitudinal study in more than **2,000 Swedish men** compared blood levels of retinol to the incidence of fractures in men. The investigators found **that the risk of fractures was greatest in men with the highest blood levels of retinol** (more than 75 mcg per deciliter [dL]). Men with blood retinol levels in the 99th percentile (greater than 103 mcg per dL) had an overall risk of fracture that exceeded the risk among men with lower levels of retinol by a factor of seven (Michaelsson et al, 2003).

Hypervitaminosis A refers to high storage levels of vitamin A in the body that can lead to toxic symptoms. **There are four major adverse effects of hypervitaminosis A: birth defects, liver abnormalities, reduced bone mineral density that may result in osteoporosis (see the previous section), and central nervous system disorders** (Bendich and Langseth, 1992).

Toxic symptoms can also arise after consuming very large amounts of preformed vitamin A over a short period of time. **Signs of acute toxicity include nausea and vomiting, headache, dizziness, blurred vision, and muscular uncoordination** (Bendich and Langseth, 1992).

Although hypervitaminosis A can occur when large amounts of liver are regularly consumed, most cases result from taking excess amounts of the nutrient in supplements.

Worldwide, the highest incidence of osteoporosis occurs in northern Europe, a population with a high intake of vitamin A (Whiting and Lemke, et al, 1999).

Also, please remember that in 2002, a Finnish study of 29,000 male smokers found taking beta carotene, which is converted into vitamin A in the body, was linked to an **18% increased risk of developing lung cancer** (ATBC study).

The IOM states that "beta-carotene supplements are not advisable for the general population," although they also state that this advice "does not pertain to the possible use of supplemental beta-carotene as a provitamin A source for the prevention of vitamin A deficiency in populations with inadequate vitamin A.

In October of 2009, the Royal College of Obstetricians and Gynaecologists (RCOG) Scientific Advisory Committee released a new opinion paper on **vitamin supplementation during pregnancy.** The paper examines the evidence for vitamin supplementation and provides guidance for pregnant women in the UK. The committee considered the use of multivitamin preparations, as well as the use of high dose individual vitamins for the prevention of specific diseases. The recommendations of the paper are as follows:

Vitamin A

High dose vitamin A supplementation (intake greater than 700mcg/day) is **not recommended due to potential teratogenic effects.** Pregnant women should also avoid eating liver and liver products, as these may contain high levels of vitamin A.

Vitamin C and E

Vitamin C is an essential water-soluble vitamin found widely in fruits and vegetables. It plays important roles in collagen synthesis, wound healing, prevention of anemia and as an antioxidant. Vitamin C is particularly important for pregnant women who are at increased risk of iron deficiency anaemia. A low dose of vitamin C (<200mg) is commonly included in many multivitamin pregnancy preparations.

While there has been considerable interest in the potential use of vitamin C and E to prevent pre-eclampsia, preterm rupture of membranes and fetal growth restriction, recent **studies have shown no difference in risk for women given antioxidant supplementation (including vitamin C and E).** In the absence of further evidence, routine supplementation with higher dose vitamin C and E is not recommended.

Actual vitamin C deficiency in the USA

The actual percentage of individuals with a vitamin C deficiency was measured in the NHANES studies as follows in their abstract:

Serum vitamin C and the prevalence of vitamin C deficiency in the United States: 2003–2004 National Health and Nutrition Examination Survey (NHANES). (Schleicher et al, 2009) (#7,277) Vitamin C (ascorbic acid) may be the most important water-soluble antioxidant in human plasma. **In the third National Health and Nutrition Examination Survey (NHANES III, 1988–1994), ≈13% of the US population was vitamin C deficient** (serum concentrations <11.4 μmol/L). **Objective:** The aim was to determine the most current distribution of serum vitamin

C concentrations in the United States and the prevalence of deficiency in selected subgroups. **Design:** Serum concentrations of total vitamin C were measured in 7,277 noninstitutionalized civilians aged ≥6 y during the cross-sectional, nationally representative NHANES 2003–2004. The prevalence of deficiency was compared with results from NHANES III. **Results:** The overall age-adjusted mean from the square-root transformed (SM) concentration was 51.4 μmol/L. **The highest concentrations were found in children and older persons. Within each race-ethnic group, women had higher concentrations than did men.** Mean concentrations of adult smokers were one-third lower than those of nonsmokers. **The overall prevalence (±SE) of age-adjusted vitamin C deficiency was 7.1 ± 0.9%.** Mean vitamin C concentrations increased and **the prevalence of vitamin C deficiency decreased with increasing socioeconomic status.** Recent vitamin C supplement use or adequate dietary intake decreased the risk of vitamin C deficiency. **Conclusions:** In NHANES 2003–2004, vitamin C status improved, and the prevalence of vitamin C deficiency was significantly lower than that during NHANES III, but smokers and low-income persons were among those at increased risk of deficiency (Schleicher et al, 2009).

Selenium

In short, **the risk for selenium deficiency in the United States is negligible,** and **the use of selenium supplements in this country is unlikely to increase the antioxidant activity of glutathione peroxidases** (Bleys et al, 2007).

Don't Count on Selenium to Prevent Lung Cancer Recurrence

According to Dr. Daniel D. Karp, a professor in the department of thoracic/head and neck medical oncology at the University of Texas M.D. Anderson Cancer Center, taking **the popular mineral supplement selenium doesn't reduce the likelihood of lung cancer recurrence.** As lead author, he presented the findings on 6/5/10 at the American Society of Clinical Oncology annual meeting, in Chicago.

Early studies had suggested an approximate 30% reduction of prostate and lung cancers with the use of selenium. However, Karp's study found that **among more than 1,500 stage 1 (early) non-small cell lung cancer patients who had survived their initial bout with the disease, selenium offered no protection against recurrence or the onset of a new cancer or second primary cancer.** The patients were tracked from 2000 to 2009, after all had undergone surgery to remove their initial tumors and remained cancer-free for a minimum of six months post-treatment and half of the patients were placed on a regimen of **200 micrograms of selenium vs.** half taking a placebo.

While 78 percent taking the placebo stayed alive over that time frame, the rate was just 72 percent among the selenium group. And while 1.4 percent of the placebo group developed a second primary tumor within a year, that figure rose to 1.9 percent among the selenium group, *an observation that led the research team to halt the study earlier than planned.* **Thus, the placebo group had better survival rates five years later than those taking the selenium supplement.**

This selenium study is similar to and consistent with my collective study data on the antioxidant vitamins A, C and E.

CHAPTER NINE:

Confounding Factors:

BIAS, CHANCE & CAUSE

Epidemiology teaches that every statistical association has only 3 possible explanations: bias, chance, and cause. However, I impugn this statement and would add to this 1) partial fabrication of data, 2) unscrupulous, self-serving manipulation of data and 3) completely made up data, i.e., bald-faced liars.

The evaluation of redox data is made more difficult by the large number of variables, which can affect the interpretation of the results of the data. The following is a list which I have accumulated over the years and illustrates my point. There are more.

THIRTY VARIABLES IN ANTIOXIDANT & EMOD (REDOX) STUDIES:

Variables and co-variants

1) **multitude of dietary variances** *(total energy intake and fat, carbohydrates, protein, fiber, electrolyte intake)*, 2) **varying environmental factors** *(sunshine exposure, excessive cold, heat, radiation exposure or treatment, second hand smoke, inhalation of inorganic particles such as asbestos and silica, ozone inhalation, socioeconomic factors, etc.)*, 3) **exercise level per se or lack thereof,** 4) **overall physical activity** *(number of hours of television watched per week)*, 5) **degrees of obesity,** 6) **race,** 7) **sex,** 8) **education,** 9) **presence of fever,** 10) **smoking,** 11) **alcohol use,** 12) **oral contraceptive use,** 13) **synthetic hormone intake,** 14) **pregnancy history,** 15) **dietary antioxidant use,** 16) **herbal supplement use,** 17) **use of medications,** 18) **anthropometry** *(height, weight, BMI, etc.)*, 19) **varying antioxidant dosage levels,** 20) **varying antioxidant combinations** *(nutrient synergy)*, 21) **synthetic or natural vitamin sources** *(L vs. D forms, alpha vs. gamma forms)*, 22) **improperly combined study groups,** 23) **use of improper exclusion criteria,** 24) **flawed statistical methods,** 25) **over generalization of findings,** 26) **accuracy of dietary records and questionnaires etc.** 27) **questionable species of animal studied** *(primates, invertebrates, exposure to insecticides or herbicides, etc.)*, 28) **durations of treatments,** 29) **studies targeted at different diseases/conditions, and** 30) **bias of investigators.**

To further complicate matters, there are over 40 methods for measurement of oxidant stress or antioxidant capacity. All are subject to artifactual errors and have varying degrees of concordance and thus, remain problematic.

QUANTIFYING ANTIOXIDANT ACTIVITY

There are numerous discrepant, conflicting and inconsistent ways of attempting to quantify antioxidant activity using a range of lab based assays, including the ferric reducing ability of plasma (FRAP), the oxygen radical absorbance capacity (ORAC) and the Trolox equivalent antioxidant capacity (TEAC). Test tube studies may have little relevancy to the living/breathing cell.

Also, the redox capacity of a site will vary between cellular organelles, cell to cell, cell to tissue, organ to organ and organ to organism. Again, interpretation of data is extremely difficult and fraught with potential for mistaken conclusions. There now appears to be compartmentalization of redox potentials and their respective redox potential varies greatly.

Biomarkers Lack Concordance

OXIDATIVE STRESS MEASUREMENT (markers or biomarkers)

- measurement of lipid oxidation products such as conjugated dienes, 4-hydroxynonenal (4-HNE) levels, malondialdehyde or thiobarbituric acid reactive substances (TBARS) in tissue, blood or urine;

- modified DNA bases (8-hydroxydeoxyguanosine) 8-oxoguanine, 8-hydroxy-2'-deoxyguanosine and/or DNA adducts, DNA breaks in peripheral blood cells or urine;

- oxidized proteins; increased GSSG;

- vitamin E or vitamin C levels in blood fractions;

- catalase, Gpx or superoxide dismutase levels in blood fractions;

- volatile gases such as pentane or ethane in expired breath;

- total peroxyl radical trapping antioxidant power of serum (TRAP assay);

- auto-oxidative (non-cyclooxygenase-derived) eicosanoids and prostanoids, 8-epiprostaglandin F2a, increased 8-isoprostane in plasma;

- and the in vitro oxidation of blood fractions such as LDL;

- transient enhancement of heme oxygenase 1;

- ascorbate free radical, salicylate, glutathione antioxidant system, advanced oxidation protein products, ubiquino/ ubiquinone ratio; etc.

REFERENCES

(Albanes et al, 1996) (Albanes D, Heinonen OP, Taylor PR, Virtamo J, Edwards BK, Rautalahti M, Hartman AM, Palmgren J, Freedman LS, Haapakoski J, Barrett MJ, Pietinen P, Malila N, Tala E, Lippo K, Salomaa ER, Tangrea JA, Teppo L, Askin FB, Taskinen E, Erozan Y, Greenwald P, Huttunen JK. Alpha-tocopherol and beta-carotene supplement and lung cancer incidence in the alpha-tocopherol, beta-carotene cancer prevention study: Effects of base-line characteristics and study compliance. J Natl Cancer Inst 1996;88:1560-70).

(Alberts et al, 2000) (Alberts DS, Martinez ME, Roe DJ, et al, Phoenix Colon Cancer Prevention Physicians' Network. Lack of effect of a high-fiber cereal supplement on the recurrence of colorectal adenomas. N Engl J Med. 2000;342:1156-1162)

(Albright et al, 2003) (Albright, C. D., Salganik, R. I., Craciunescu, C. N., Mar, M. H. & Zeisel, S. H. (2003) Mitochondrial and microsomal derived reactive oxygen species mediate apoptosis induced by transforming growth factor-beta1 in immortalized rat hepatocytes. J. Cell Biochem. 89: 254–261)

(Alkhenizan and Al-Omran, 2004) (Alkhenizan AH, Al-Omran MA. The role of vitamin E in the prevention of coronary events and stroke. Meta-analysis of randomized controlled trials. Saudi Med J. 2004 Dec;25(12):1808-14)

(Alkhenizan and Hafez, 2007) (Alkhenizan A, Hafez K. The role of vitamin E in the prevention of cancer: a meta-analysis of randomized controlled trials. Ann Saudi Med. 2007 Nov-Dec;27(6):409-14)

(Appel et al, 1997) (Appel LJ, Moore TJ, Obarzanek E, et al, and the DASH Collaborative Research Group. A clinical trial of the effects of dietary patterns on blood pressure. N Engl J Med. 1997;336:1117-1124)

(AREDS, 2001) (A randomized, placebo-controlled, clinical trial of high-dose supplementation with vitamins C and E and beta carotene for age-related cataract and vision loss: AREDS report no. 9. Age-Related Eye Disease Study Research Group. Arch Ophthalmol. 2001 Oct;119(10):1439-5)

(Arrowsmith et al, 1989) (Morbidity and mortality among low birth weight infants exposed to an intravenous vitamin E product, E-Ferol. JB Arrowsmith et al. Pediatrics. 1989 Feb;83(2):244-9).

(Ascherio et al. 1999) (Ascherio A, Rimm EB, Hernan MA, Giovannucci E, Kawachi I, Stampfer MJ, Willett WC. Relation of consumption of vitamin E, vitamin C, and carotenoids to risk for stroke among men in the United States. Ann Intern Med. 1999 Jun 15;130(12):963-70)

(Bairati et al, 2005 Apr 6) (Bairati I, Meyer F, Gélinas M, Fortin A, Nabid A, Brochet F, Mercier JP, Têtu B, Harel F, Mâsse B, Vigneault E, Vass S, del Vecchio P, Roy J. A randomized trial of antioxidant vitamins to prevent second primary cancers in head and neck cancer patients. J Natl Cancer Inst. 2005 Apr 6;97(7):481-8)

(Bairati et al, 2005 Aug 20) (Bairati I, Meyer F, Gélinas M, Fortin A, Nabid A, Brochet F, Mercier JP, Têtu B, Harel F, Abdous B, Vigneault E, Vass S, Del Vecchio P, Roy J. Randomized trial of antioxidant vitamins to prevent acute adverse effects of radiation therapy in head and neck cancer patients. J Clin Oncol. 2005 Aug 20;23(24):5805-13)

(Balaban et al, 2005) (Balaban, R.S., Nemoto, S., Finkel, T., 2005. Mitochondria, oxidants, and aging. Cell 120, 483–495)

(Bardia et al, 2008) (Aditya Bardia, Imad M. Tleyjeh, James R. Cerhan, Amit K. Sood, Paul J. Limburg, Patricia J. Erwin and Victor M. Montori. Efficacy of Antioxidant Supplementation in Reducing Primary Cancer

Incidence and Mortality: Systematic Review and Meta-analysis. January 2008 vol. 83 no. 1 23-34)

(Baron et al, 2003) (John A. Baron, Bernard F. Cole, Leila Mott, Robert Haile, Maria Grau, Timothy R. Church, Gerald J. Beck, E. Robert Greenberg. Neoplastic and Antineoplastic Effects of Beta Carotene on Colorectal Adenoma Recurrence: Results of a Randomized Trial. JNCI Journal of the National Cancer Institute 2003 95(10):717-722)

(Batieha et al, 1993) (Batieha AM, Armenian HK, Norkus EP, Morris JS, Spate VE, Comstock GW. Serum micronutrients and the subsequent risk of cervical cancer in a population-based nested case-control study. Cancer Epidemiol Biomarkers Prev. 1993 Jul-Aug;2(4):335-9)

(Bazzano et al, 2002) (Bazzano LA, He J, Ogden LG, et al. Dietary intake of folate and risk of stroke in US men and women: NHANES I Epidemiologic Follow-up Study. Stroke. 2002;33:1183-1188)

(Beckman and Ames, 1998) (Beckman, K.B., Ames, B.N., 1998. The free radical theory of aging matures. Physiol. Rev. 78, 547–581)

(Bendich and Langseth, 1992) (Bendich A, Langseth L. Safety of vitamin A. Am J Clin Nutr 1989;49:358-71) (Udall JN, Greene HL. Vitamin update. Pediatr Rev 1992;13:185-94)

(Berson et al, 1993) (Berson EL, Rosner B, Sandberg MA, et al. A randomized trial of vitamin A and vitamin E supplementation for retinitis pigmentosa. Arch Ophthalmol. 1993;111(6):761-772)

(Berube et al, 2008) (Sylvie Bérubé, Caroline Diorio and Jacques Brisson. Multivitamin-multimineral supplement use and mammographic breast density. American Journal of Clinical Nutrition, Vol. 87, No. 5, 1400-1404, May 2008)

(Binkley and Krueger, 2000) (Binkley N, Krueger D. Hypervitaminosis A and bone. Nutr Rev 2000;58:138-44)

(Bjelakovic et al, Cochrane Database Syst Rev. 2004) (Bjelakovic G, Nikolova D, Simonetti RG, Gluud C. Antioxidant supplements for preventing gastrointestinal cancers. Cochrane Database Syst Rev (2004) (4):CD004183)

(Bjelakovic et al, Lancet. 2004) (Bjelakovic G, Nikolova D, Simonetti RG, Gluud C. Antioxidant supplements for prevention of gastrointestinal cancers: a systematic review and meta-analysis. Lancet (2004) 364:1219–28)

(Bjelakovic et al., 2006) (Bjelakovic G, Nagorni A, Nikolova D, et al. Meta-analysis: antioxidant supplements for primary and secondary prevention of colorectal adenoma. Aliment Pharmacol Ther. 2006;24:281-91)

(Bjelakovic et al, 2007) (Goran Bjelakovic, Dimitrinka Nikolova, Lise Lotte Gluud, Rosa G. Simonetti, and Christian Gluud. "Mortality in Randomized Trials of Antioxidant Supplements for Primary and Secondary Prevention; Systematic Review and Meta-analysis." JAMA 2007;297:842-857. Vol. 297 No. 8, February 28, 2007)

(Bjelakovic, Nikolova, Gludd, Simonetti and Gludd, 2008 Apr) (Bjelakovic G, Nikolova D, Gluud LL, Simonetti RG, Gluud C.. Antioxidant supplements for prevention of mortality in healthy participants and patients with various diseases. Cochrane Database Syst Rev. 2008 Apr 16;(2):CD007176)

(Bjelakovic, Nikolova, Simonette and Gludd, 2008 Sept) (Bjelakovic G, Nikolova D, Simonetti RG, Gluud C. Systematic review: primary and secondary prevention of gastrointestinal cancers with antioxidant supplements. Aliment Pharmacol Ther. 2008 Sep 15;28(6):689-703)

(Blank et al, 1995) (Blank S, Scanlon KS, Sinks TH, Lett S, Falk H. An outbreak of hypervitaminosis D associated with the over fortification of milk from a home-delivery dairy. Am J Public Health. 1995;85:656-659)

(Blendon et al, 2001) (Blendon RJ, DesRoches CM, Benson JM, Brodie M, Altman DE. Americans' views on the use and regulation of dietary supplements. Arch Intern Med. 2001;161:805-10)

(Bleys et al, 2006) (Vitamin-mineral supplementation and the progression of atherosclerosis: a meta-analysis of randomized controlled trials. Joachim Bleys, Edgar R Miller, III, Roberto Pastor-Barriuso, Lawrence J Appel and Eliseo Guallar. American Journal of Clinical Nutrition, Vol. 84, No. 4, 880-887, October 2006)

(Bleys et al, 2007) (Selenium and Diabetes: More Bad News for Supplements. Joachim Bleys, Ana Navas-Acien, and Eliseo Gualla. Ann Intern Med 2007; 147: 271-272)

(Blot et al, 1993) (Blot WJ, Li JY, Taylor PR, Guo W, Dawsey S, Wang GQ, et al. Nutrition intervention trials in Linxian, China: supplementation with specific vitamin/mineral combinations, cancer incidence, and disease-specific mortality in the general population. J Natl Cancer Inst 1993;85:1483-92)

(Bohlke et al, 1999) (K Bohlke, D Spiegelman, A Trichopoulou, K Katsouyanni and D Trichopoulos. Vitamins A, C and E and the risk of breast cancer: results from a case-control study in Greece. British Journal of Cancer (1999) 79, 23–29)

(Bolton-Smith et al, 1992) (Bolton-Smith C, Woodward M, Tunstall-Pedoe H. The Scottish Heart Health Study. Dietary intake by food frequency questionnaire and odds ratios for coronary heart disease risk. II. The antioxidant vitamins and fibre. Eur J Clin Nutr 1992;46(2):85-93)

(Boothby and Doering, 2005) (Boothby LA, Doering PL. Vitamin C and vitamin E for Alzheimer's disease. Ann Pharmacother. 2005 Dec;39(12):2073-80)

(Bostick et al, 1993) (Bostick RM, Potter JD, McKenzie DR, Sellers TA, Kushi LH, Steinmetz KA, Folsom AR. Reduced risk of colon cancer with high intakes of vitamin E: The Iowa Women's Health Study. Cancer Res 1993;15:4230-17)

(Bostom et al, 1995) (Bostom AG, Hume AL, Eaton CB, Laurino JP, Yanek LR, Regan MS, McQuade WH, Craig WY, Perrone G, Jacques PF. The effect of high-dose ascorbate supplementation on plasma lipoprotein(a) levels in patients with premature coronary heart disease. Pharmacotherapy 1995 Jul-Aug;15(4):458-64)

(Bove et al, 1985) (Vasculopathic hepatotoxicity associated with E-Ferol syndrome in low-birth-weight infants. K. E. Bove, N. Kosmetatos, K. E. Wedig, D. J. Frank, S. Whitlatch, V. Saldivar, J. Haas, C. Bodenstein and W. F. Balistreri. JAMA. Vol. 254. No. 17. November 1, 1985)

(Boyd et al, 2005) (Boyd NF, Rommens JM, Vogt K, et al. Mammographic breast density as an intermediate phenotype for breast cancer. Lancet Oncol 2005;6:798–808)

(Brown et al, 2001) (Brown BG, Zhao XQ, Chait A, Fisher LD, Cheung MC, Morse JS, Dowdy AA, Marino EK, Bolson EL, Alaupovic P, Frohlich J, Albers JJ. Simvastatin and niacin, antioxidant vitamins, or the combination for the prevention of coronary disease. N Engl J Med. 2001 Nov 29;345(22):1583-92)

(Brown et al. 2002) (Antioxidant Vitamins and Lipid Therapy. End of a Long Romance? B. Greg Brown; Marian C. Cheung; Andrew C. Lee; Xue-Qiao Zhao; Alan Chait. Arteriosclerosis, Thrombosis, and Vascular Biology. 2002;22:1535)

(Buijsse et al, 2008) (B. Buijsse, E. J. M. Feskens, L. Kwape, F. J. Kok, and D. Kromhout. Both {alpha}- and -Carotene, but Not Tocopherols and Vitamin C, Are Inversely Related to 15-Year Cardiovascular Mortality in Dutch Elderly Men. J. Nutr., February 1, 2008; 138(2): 344 – 350)

(Buring and Hennekens, 1992) (Buring JE, Hennekens CH. The women's health study: summary of the design. J Myocardial Ischemia 1992;4:27-9)

(Caire-Juvera et al, 2009) (Caire-Juvera G,, Ritenbaugh C, Wactawski-Wende J, Snetselaar LG, Chen Z. Vitamin A and retinol intakes and the risk of fractures among participants of the Women's Health Initiative Observational Study. Am J Clin Nutr. 2009 Jan;89(1):323-30)

(Calzada et al, 1997) (Calzada C, Bruckdorfer KR, Rice-Evans CA. The influence of antioxidant nutrients on platelet function in healthy volunteers. Atherosclerosis 1997 Jan 3;128(1):97-105)

(Caraballoso et al., 2003) (Drugs for preventing lung cancer in healthy people. M. Caraballoso et al. Cochrane Database Syst Rev. 2003;(2):CD002141)

(Chance et al, 1979) (Chance B, Sies, H, Boveris A. Hydroperoxide metabolism in mammalian organs. Physiol Rev 1979; 59: 527-605)

(Chasan-Taber et al, 1999) (Chasan-Taber L, Willett W C, Seddon J M. et al A prospective study of vitamin supplement intake and cataract extraction among US women. Epidemiology 1999. 10679–684)

(Chen et al, 2006) (Chen et al. High-dose oral vitamin C partially replenishes vitamin C levels in patients with Type 2 diabetes and low vitamin C levels but does not improve endothelial dysfunction or insulin resistance. Am. J. Physiol. Heart Circ. Physiol. 2006;290:H137-H145)

(Chertow, 2004) (Chertow B. Advances in diabetes for the millennium: vitamins and oxidant stress in diabetes and its complications. MedGenMed. 2004 Nov 1;6 (3 Suppl):4.)

(Chiabrando et al., 2002) (Long-term vitamin E supplementation fails to reduce lipid peroxidation in people at cardiovascular risk: analysis of underlying factors. Chiabrando C, Avanzini F, Rivalta C, Colombo F, Fanelli R, Palumbo G, Roncaglioni MC; PPP Collaborative Group on the antioxidant effect of vitamin E. Curr Control Trials Cardiovasc Med. 2002 Mar 19;3(1):5)

(Cho et al, 2006) (Cho E. et al. Intakes of vitamins A, C and E and folate and multivitamins and lung cancer: a pooled analysis of 8 prospective studies. Int J Cancer. 2006 Feb 15;118(4):970-8)

(Choi and Curhan, 2007) (Choi HK, Curhan G. Independent impact of gout on mortality and risk for coronary heart disease. Circulation. 2007 Aug 21;116(8):894-900)

(Chong et al, 2007) ("Dietary antioxidants and primary prevention of age related macular degeneration: systematic review and meta-analysis" Elaine W-T Chong, Tien Y Wong, Andreas J Kreis, Julie A Simpson, Robyn H Guymer. British Medical Journal (BMJ)., doi:10.1136/bmj.39350.500428.47 (published 8 October 2007)

(Christen et al, 2003) (Christen WG; Manson JE; Glynn RJ; Gaziano JM; Sperduto RD; Buring JE; Hennekens CH. A randomized trial of beta carotene and age-related cataract in US physicians. Arch Ophthalmol. 2003; 121(3):372-8)

(Chylack et al. 2002) (Chylack LT Jr, Brown NP, Bron A, Hurst M, Kopcke W, Thien U, Schalch W. The Roche European American Cataract Trial (REACT): a randomized clinical trial to investigate the efficacy of an oral antioxidant micronutrient mixture to slow progression of age-related cataract. Ophthalmic Epidemiol. 2002 Feb;9(1):49-80)

(Clark et al., 1996) (Effects of selenium supplementation for cancer prevention in patients with carcinoma of the skin. A randomized controlled trial. Nutritional Prevention of Cancer Study Group. Clark LC, Combs GF Jr, Turnbull BW, Slate EH, Chalker DK, Chow J, Davis LS, Glover RA, Graham GF, Gross EG, Krongrad A, Lesher JL Jr, Park HK, Sanders BB Jr, Smith CL, Taylor JR. JAMA. 1996 Dec 25;276(24):1957-63. Erratum in: JAMA 1997 May 21;277(19):1520)

(Comhaire et al, 2000) (Comhaire FH, Christophe AB, Zalata AA, Dhooge WS, Mahmoud AM, Depuydt CE. The effects of combined conventional treatment, oral antioxidants and essential fatty acids on sperm biology in subfertile men. Prostaglandins Leukot Essent Fatty Acids. 2000 Sep;63(3):159-65)

(Cook et al, 2007) (A Randomized Factorial Trial of Vitamins C and E and Beta Carotene in the Secondary Prevention of Cardiovascular Events in Women: Results From the Women's Antioxidant Cardiovascular Study. Nancy R. Cook, ScD; Christine M. Albert, MD; J. Michael Gaziano, MD; Elaine Zaharris, BA; Jean MacFadyen, BA; Eleanor Danielson, MIA; Julie E. Buring, ScD; JoAnn E. Manson, MD, DrPH. Arch Intern Med. 2007;167(15):1610-1618)

(Coulter et al, 2006) (Antioxidants Vitamin C and Vitamin E for the Prevention and Treatment of Cancer. Coulter, Ian D.; Hardy, Mary L.; Morton, Sally C.; Hilton, Lara G.; Tu, Wenli; Valentine, Di; Shekelle, Paul G. Journal of General Internal Medicine, Volume 21, Number 7, July 2006, pp. 735-744(10))

(Creagan et al, 1979) (Creagan ET, Moertel CG, O'Fallon JR, Schutt AJ, O'Connell MJ, Rubin J, Frytak S. Failure of high-dose vitamin C (ascorbic acid) therapy to benefit patients with advanced cancer. A controlled trial. N Engl J Med. 1979 Sep 27;301(13):687-90)

(Czernichow et al, 2006) (Antioxidant supplementation does not affect fasting plasma glucose in the Supplementation with Antioxidant Vitamins and Minerals (SU.VI.MAX) study in France: association with dietary intake and plasma concentrations. S. Czernichow, A. Couthouis, S.

Bertrais, A.-C. Vergnaud, L. Dauchet, P. Galan, and S. Hercberg. Am. J. Clinical Nutrition, August 1, 2006; 84(2): 395 - 399)

(Czernichow et al, 2009) (Czernichow, S. et al. Effects of long-term antioxidant supplementation and association of serum antioxidant concentrations with risk of metabolic syndrome in adults. Am. J. Clinical Nutrition, Vol. 90, No. 2, 329-335, August 2009)

(Dagenais etg al, 2000) (Dagenais GR, Marchioli R, Yusuf S, Tognoni G. Beta-carotene, vitamin C, and vitamin E and cardiovascular diseases. Curr Cardiol Rep. 2000 Jul;2(4):293-9)

(de Gaetano et al, 2001) (de Gaetano G, and the Collaborative Group of the Primary Prevention Project. Low-dose aspirin and vitamin E in people at cardiovascular risk: a randomised trial in general practice. Lancet. 2001;357:89-95)

(Delcourt et al, 2003) (Delcourt C, Carriere I, Delage M, Descomps B, Cristol JP, Papoz L. Associations of cataract with antioxidant enzymes and other risk factors: the French Age-Related Eye Diseases (POLA) Prospective Study. Ophthalmology. 2003. Dec;110(12):2318-26)

(Devaraj et al, 2007) (S. Devaraj, R. Tang, B. Adams-Huet, A. Harris, T. Seenivasan, J. A de Lemos, and I. Jialal. Effect of high-dose {alpha}-tocopherol supplementation on biomarkers of oxidative stress and inflammation and carotid atherosclerosis in patients with coronary artery disease. Am. J. Clinical Nutrition, November 1, 2007; 86(5): 1392 – 1398)

(Dietrich et al, 2009) (M. Dietrich, P. Jacques, M. Pencina, K. Lanier, M. Keyes, G. Kaur, P. Wolf, R. D'Agostino, R. Vasan. Vitamin E supplement use and the incidence of cardiovascular disease and all-cause mortality in the Framingham Heart Study: Does the underlying health status play a role? Atherosclerosis, 2009. Volume 205, Issue 2, Pages 549-553)

(Donnelly et al, Fertil Steril. 1999) (Donnelly ET, McClure N, Lewis SE. Antioxidant supplementation in vitro does not improve human sperm motility. Fertil Steril. 1999 Sep;72(3):484-95)

(Donnelly et al, Mutagenesis. 1999) (Donnelly ET, McClure N, Lewis SE. The effect of ascorbate and alpha-tocopherol supplementation in vitro on

DNA integrity and hydrogen peroxide-induced DNA damage in human spermatozoa. Mutagenesis. 1999 Sep;14(5):505-12)

(Dorgan et al, 1998) (Dorgan JF, Sowell A, Swanson CA, et al. Relationships of serum carotenoids, retinol, alpha-tocopherol, and selenium with breast cancer risk: results from a prospective study in Columbia, Missouri (United States). Cancer Causes Control. 1998;9(1):89-97)

(Dotan et al, 2009) (Dotan et al. Decision Analysis Supports the Paradigm That Indiscriminate Supplementation of Vitamin E Does More Harm than Good. Arterioscler. Thromb. Vasc. Bio. 2009;29:1304-1309)

(Dotan, Lichtenberg and Pinchuk, 2009) (Dotan Y, Lichtenberg D, Pinchuk I. No evidence supports vitamin E indiscriminate supplementation. Biofactors. 2009 Nov-Dec;35(6):469-73)

(Douglas et al, 2004) (Douglas RM, Hemila H, D'Souza R, Chalker EB, Treacy B. Vitamin C for preventing and treating the common cold. Cochrane Database Syst Rev. 2004(4):CD000980)

(Dunn et al, 2007) (Julie E. Dunn, Sandra Weintraub, Anne M. Stoddard and Sarah Banks. Serum α-tocopherol, concurrent and past vitamin E intake, and mild cognitive impairment. Neurology. 200768:670-676)

(Eidelman et al., 2004) (Eidelman RS, Hollar D, Hebert PR, Lamas GA, Hennekens CH. Randomized trials of vitamin E in the treatment and prevention of cardiovascular disease. Arch Intern Med. 2004;164:1552-1556)

(Engelhart et al, 2002) (Engelhart et al. Dietary intake of antioxidants and risk of Alzheimer disease. (2002) JAMA 287, 3223-3229)

(Enstrom et al, 1992) (Enstrom J.E., Kanim L.E., and Klein M.A. Vitamin C intake and mortality among a sample of the United States population. Epidemiology 3 (1992):194–202)

(Epplein, 2009) (Meira Epplein et al. Plasma carotenoids, retinol, and tocopherols and postmenopausal breast cancer risk in the Multiethnic Cohort Study: a nested case-control study. Breast Cancer Research. 2009, 11:R49)

(Erdman, Ford and Lindshield, 2009) (Erdman J W Jr, Ford NA, Lindshield BL. Are the health attributes of lycopene related to its antioxidant function? Arch Biochem Biophys. 2009 Mar 15;483(2):229-35)

(Evans, 2008) (Evans J. Antioxidant supplements to prevent or slow down the progression of AMD: a systematic review and meta-analysis. Eye (Lond). 2008 Jun;22(6):751-60)

(Evans and Henshaw, 2008) (Evans JR, Henshaw K. Antioxidant vitamin and mineral supplements for preventing age-related macular degeneration. Cochrane Database Syst Rev. 2008 Jan 23;(1):CD000253)

(Fairfield et al, 2001) (Fairfield KM, Hankinson SE, Rosner BA, Hunter DJ, Colditz GA, Willett WC. Risk of ovarian carcinoma and consumption of vitamins A, C, and E and specific carotenoids: a prospective analysis. Cancer. 2001 Nov 1;92(9):2318-26)

(Falcone et al, 2010) (E Liana Falcone, Alexandra Mangili, Alice M Tang, Clara Y Jones, Margo N Coods, Joseph F Polak and Christine A Wanke . Micronutrient concentrations and subclinical atherosclerosis in adults with HIV. Am J Clin Nutr 91: 1213-1219, 2010. Vol. 91, No. 5, 1213-1219, May 2010)

(Fantanarosa et al, 2003) (Phil B. Fantanarosa, Drummond Rennie, and Catherine D. DeAngelis. The Need for Regulation of Dietary Supplements—Lessons From Ephedra. JAMA. 2003;289(12):1568-1570)

(Ferreira et al, 2004) (Ferreira PR, Fleck JF, Diehl A, et al. Protective effect of alpha-tocopherol in head and neck cancer radiation-induced mucositis: a double-blind randomized trial. Head Neck (2004) 26(4):313–321)

(Feskanich et al, 2002) (Feskanich D, Singh F, Willett WC, Colditz GA. Vitamin A intake and hip fractures among postmenopausal women. J Am Med Assoc 2002;287:47-54)

(Fillenbaum et al, 2005) (Fillenbaum et al. Dementia and Alzheimer's Disease in Community-Dwelling Elders Taking Vitamin C and/or Vitamin E. The Annals of Pharmacotherapy: Vol. 39, No. 12, pp. 2009-2014)

(Finkel and Holbrook, 2000) (Finkel, T., Holbrook, N.J., 2000. Oxidants, oxidative stress and the biology of ageing. Nature 408, 239–247)

(Forsyth et al, 1989) (Forsyth KS, Watson RR, Gensler HL. Osteotoxicity after chronic dietary administration of 13-cis-retinoic acid, retinyl palmitate or selenium in mice exposed to tumor initiation and promotion. Life Sci 1989;45:2149-56)

(Gallicchio et al, 2008) (Gallicchio L. et al. Carotenoids and the risk of developing lung cancer: a systematic review. Am J Clin Nutr. 2008 Aug;88(2):372-83

(Gaziano et al, 2009) (Vitamins E and C in the prevention of prostate and total cancer in men: the Physicians' Health Study II randomized controlled trial. Gaziano, JM., JAMA. 2009 Jan 7;301(1):52-62. Epub 2008 Dec 9)

(Gerss and Kopcke, 2009) (Gerss J, Köpcke W. The questionable association of vitamin E supplementation and mortality--inconsistent results of different meta-analytic approaches. Cell Mol Biol (Noisy-le-grand). 2009 Feb 25;55 Suppl:OL1111-20)

(Geva et al, 1996) (Geva E, Bartoov B, Zabludovsky N, Lessing JB, Lerner-Geva L, Amit A. The effect of antioxidant treatment on human spermatozoa and fertilization rate in an in vitro fertilization program. Fertil Steril. 1996 Sep;66(3):430-4)

(Gey et al, 1991) (Gey KF, Puska P, Jordan P, et al. Inverse correlation between plasma vitamin E and mortality from ischemic heart disease in cross-cultural epidemiology. Am J Clin Nutr 1991;53(1 Suppl):326-345)

(Gibbons et al, 2003) (Gibbons RJ, Abrams J, Chatterjee K, et al. ACC/AHA 2002 guideline update for the management of patients with chronic stable angina—summary article: a report of the American College of Cardiology/American Heart Association Task Force on Practice Guidelines (Committee on the Management of Patients With Chronic Stable Angina). Circulation. 2003;107:149-158)

(Giovannucci, et al., 1998) (Giovannucci, E., M.J. Stampfer, G.A. Colditz, D.J. Hunter, C. Fuchs, B.A. Rosner, F.E. Speizer & W.C. Willett. 1998. Multivitamin use, folate, and colon cancer in women in the Nurses' Health Study. Ann. Intern. Med. 129(7):517-524)

(GISSI-Prevenzione Investigators;1999) (Dietary supplement with n-3 polyunsaturated acids and vitamin E after myocardial infarction: results of the GISSI-Prevention trial. Gruppo, Italiano per lo Studio Sopravvivenza nell'Infarto miocardico. Lancet, 1999; 354: 447-455)

(Gomez-Cabrera et al, 2008) (Gomez-Cabrera MC, Domenech E, Romagnoli M, Arduini A, Borras C, Pallardo FV, Sastre J, Viña J. Oral administration of vitamin C decreases muscle mitochondrial biogenesis and hampers training-induced adaptations in endurance performance. Am J Clin Nutr. 2008 Jan;87(1):142-9)

(Goodman et al, 2004) (Goodman GE, Thornquist MD, Balmes J, Cullen MR, Meyskens Jr. FL, Omenn GS, et al. The Beta-Carotene and Retinol Efficacy Trial: Incidence of Lung Cancer and Cardiovascular Disease Mortality During 6-Year Follow-up After Stopping Beta-Carotene and Retinol Supplements. J Natl Cancer Inst 2004;96:1743-50)

(Graham et al, 1992) (Graham S, Sielezny M, Marshall J, Priore R, Freudenheim J, Brasure J, Haughey B, Nasca P, Zdeb M. Diet in the epidemiology of Postmenopausal Breast Cancer in the New York State Cohort. Am J Epidemiol 1992;136:3127-37)

(Gray et al, 2007) (Gray SL et al. Antioxidant Vitamin Supplement Use and Risk of Dementia or Alzheimer's Disease in Older Adults. Journal of the American Geriatric Society. 2007. Volume 56 Issue 2, Pages 291 - 295)

(Greenberg et al, 1990) (Greenberg ER, Baron JA, Stukel TA, et al.: A clinical trial of beta carotene to prevent basal-cell and squamous-cell cancers of the skin. The Skin Cancer Prevention Study Group. N Engl J Med 323 (12): 789-95, 1990)

(Greenberg et al, 1994) (Greenberg ER, Baron JA, Tosteson TD, Freeman DH Jr, Beck GJ, Bond JH, Colacchio TA, Coller JA, Frankl HD, Haile RW, et al. A clinical trial of antioxidant vitamins to prevent colorectal adenoma. Polyp Prevention Study Group. N Engl J Med. 1994 Jul 21;331(3):141-7)

(Greenberg et al, 1996) (Greenberg ER, Baron JA, Karagas MR, Stukel TA, Nierenberg DW, Stevens MM, Mandel JS, Haile RW. Mortality associated with low plasma concentration of beta carotene and the effect of oral supplementation. JAMA. 1996; 275: 699-703)

(Greenberg, 2005) (Greenberg ER. Vitamin E supplements: good in theory, but is the theory good? Ann Intern Med. 2005;142:75–76)

(Green et al, 1999) (Green A, Williams G, Neale R, et al.: Daily sunscreen application and beta carotene supplementation in prevention of basal-cell and squamous-cell carcinomas of the skin: a randomised controlled trial. Lancet 354 (9180): 723-9, 1999)

(Gritz, 2006) (Gritz DC, Srinivasan M, Smith SD, et al. The Antioxidants in Prevention of Cataracts Study: effects of antioxidant supplements on cataract progression in South India. Br J Ophthalmol. 2006;90(7):847-851)

(Gullar et al, 2005) (Eliseo Gullar, Daniel F. Hanley and Edgar R. Miller III. An Editorial Update: Annus horribilis for Vitamin E. Ann Intern Med. July 19, 2005. 143-145)

(Harman, 1956) (Harman D. Aging: a theory based on free radical and radiation chemistry. J Gerontol 11: 298–300, 1956)

(Harman D, "The biological clock: the mitochondria?" J Am Geriatr Soc 1972; 20: 145-147).

(Harman, 1981) (Harman, D., 1981. The aging process. Proc. Natl Acad. Sci. USA 78, 7124–7128)

(Harman, 2000) (Harman D, Aging; overview. Ann NY Acad Sci 2000; 928:1-21)

(Hasanain and Mooradian, 2002) (Hasanain B, Mooradian AD. Antioxidant vitamins and their influence in diabetes mellitus. Curr Diab Rep. 2002 Oct;2 (5):448-56)

(Hayden et al, 2007) (K. Hayden, K. Welsh-Bohmer, H. Wengreen, P. Zandi, C. Lyketsos, J. Breitner. Risk of Mortality with Vitamin E Supplements: The Cache County Study. Am J Med. 2007 Feb;120(2):180-4)

(Heinonen et al, 1994) (Heinonen, O.P., J.K. Huttunen, D. Albanes & ATBC cancer prevention study group. 1994. The effect of vitamin E and beta carotene on the incidence of lung cancer and other cancers in male smokers. N. Engl. J. Med. 330:1029-1035)

(Hemila and Kaprio, 2008 Oct) (Hemilä H, Kaprio J. Vitamin E supplementation may transiently increase tuberculosis risk in males who smoke heavily and have high dietary vitamin C intake. Br J Nutr. 2008 Oct;100(4):896-902)

(Hemila and Kaprio, 2008 Nov) (Hemilä H, Kaprio J. Vitamin E supplementation and pneumonia risk in males who initiated smoking at an early age: effect modification by body weight and dietary vitamin C. Nutr J. 2008 Nov 19;7:33)

(Hemila and Kaprio, 2009 Apr) (Hemilä H, Kaprio J. Modification of the effect of vitamin E supplementation on the mortality of male smokers by age and dietary vitamin C. Am J Epidemiol. 2009 Apr 15;169(8):946-53)

(Hennekens et al, 1996) (Hennekens CH, Buring JE, Manson JE, et al. Lack of effect of long-term supplementation with beta carotene on the incidence of malignant neoplasms and cardiovascular disease. N Engl J Med. 1996;334:1145-1149)

(Herbert et al, 1990) (Herbert V, Subak-Sharpe GJ, Hammock D, eds. The Mount Sinai School of Medicine Complete Book of Nutrition. (1990) New York (NY): St Martin's Press)

(Herbert, 1994) Herbert V. The antioxidant supplement myth. Am J Clin Nutr (1994) 60:157–8)

(Herbert, 1997) (Herbert V. The value of antioxidant supplements vs their natural counterparts. J Am Diet Assoc (1997) 97:375–6)

(Hercberg et al, 2004) (Hercberg S, Galan P, Preziosi P, Bertrais S, Mennen L, Malvy D, Roussel A-M, Favier A, Briançon S. SU.VI.MAX Study. Arch Intern Med 2004;164:2335–42)

(Hercberg et al, 2007) (Serge Hercberg et al. Antioxidant Supplementation Increases the Risk of Skin Cancers in Women but Not in Men. American Society for Nutrition J. Nutr. 137:2098-2105, September 2007)

(Herrera et al, 2009) (Herrera E, Jiménez R, Aruoma OI, Hercberg S, Sánchez-García I, Fraga C. Aspects of antioxidant foods and supplements in health and disease. Nutr Rev. 2009 May;67 Suppl 1:S140-4)

(Hodis et al, 1995) (Hodis HN, Mack WJ, LaBree L, et al. Serial coronary angiographic evidence that antioxidant vitamin intake reduces progression of coronary artery atherosclerosis. JAMA 1995;273(23):1849-54)

(Hodis et al, 2002) (Hodis HN, Mack WJ, LaBree L, Mahrer PR, Sevanian A, Liu CR, Liu CH, Hwang J, Selzer RH, Azen SP; VEAPS Research Group. Alpha-tocopherol supplementation in healthy individuals reduces low-density lipoprotein oxidation but not atherosclerosis: the Vitamin E Atherosclerosis Prevention Study (VEAPS). Circulation. 2002; 106: 1453–1459)

(Howes, 2004) (Howes, R. M. U.T.O.P.I.A. - Unified Theory of Oxygen Participation in Aerobiosis. © 2004. Free Radical Publishing Co. Kentwood, LA, available at www.iwillfindthecure.org.)

(Howes, 2009) (Howes, R. M. Reactive Oxygen Species Insufficiency (ROSI) as the Basis for Disease Allowance and Coexistence. © 2009. Free Radical Publishing Co. Kentwood, LA, available at www.iwillfindthecure. org.)

(Howes, Philica. Feb 26, 2007) (Howes M.D., PhD., R. (2007). Cancer, Apoptosis and Reactive Oxygen Species: A New Paradigm. PHILICA. COM Article number 86. Published on 26th February, 2007)

(Howes, Philica. April 5, 2007) (Howes M.D., PhD., R. (2007). Antioxidant Vitamins A, C & E; Death in Small Doses and Legal Liability? PHILICA. COM Article number 89. Published April 5, 2007)

(Howes, Philica. Feb 7, 2009) (Howes M.D., PhD., R. (2009). Dangers of Antioxidants in Cancer Patients: A Review. PHILICA.COM Article number 153. Published 7th February, 2009)

(Howes, Am J Cos Surg. 2009) (Antioxidant Vitamins: A Review of Policy Statements and Recommendations. R.M. Howes. The American Journal of Cosmetic Surgery. Vol. 26, No. 2, pg. 63-78, 2009)

(Howes, 2010) (R. Howes : Hydrogen Peroxide: A review of a scientifically verifiable omnipresent ubiquitous essentiality of obligate, aerobic, carbon-based life forms. The Internet Journal of Plastic Surgery. 2010 Volume 7 Number 1)

(Hu et al, 2000) (Hu FB, Rimm EB, Stampfer MJ, Ascherio A, Spiegelman D, Willett WC. Prospective study of major dietary patterns and risk of coronary heart disease in men. Am J Clin Nutr. 2000;72:912-921)

(Huang et al, 2006 May) (Huang HY, Caballero B, Chang S, Alberg A, Semba R, Schneyer C, Wilson RF, Cheng TY, Prokopowicz G, Barnes GJ 2nd, Vassy J, Bass EB. Multivitamin/mineral supplements and prevention of chronic disease. Evid Rep Technol Assess (Full Rep). 2006 May;(139):1-117)

(Huang et al, 2006 Sept) (H. Huang et al. The Efficacy and Safety of Multivitamin and Mineral Supplement Use To Prevent Cancer and Chronic Disease in Adults: A Systematic Review for a National Institutes of Health State-of-the-Science Conference. September 5, 2006, Vol. 145. Issue 5. Pages 372-385)

(Hughes et al, 1998) (Hughes CM, Lewis SE, McKelvey-Martin VJ, Thompson W. The effects of antioxidant supplementation during Percoll preparation on human sperm DNA integrity. Hum Reprod. 1998 May;13(5):1240-7)

(Hulten, 2001) (Hulten K, Van Kappel AL, Winkvist A, et al. Carotenoids, alpha-tocopherols, and retinol in plasma and breast cancer risk in northern Sweden. Cancer Causes Control. 2001;12(6):529-537)

(Hunter et al, 1993) (A Prospective Study of the Intake of Vitamins C, E, and A and the Risk of Breast Cancer. David J. Hunter, JoAnn E. Manson, Graham A. Colditz, Meir J. Stampfer, Bernard Rosner, Charles H. Hennekens, Frank E. Speizer, and Walter C. Willett. The New England Journal of Medicine. Vol. 329:234-240. No. 4. July 22, 1993)

(Hulley et al, 1998) (Hulley S, Grady D, Bush T et al. Randomized trial of estrogen plus progestin for secondary prevention of coronary heart disease in postmenopausal women. Heart and Estrogen/Progestin Replacement Study (HERS) Research Group. JAMA1998; 280:605–613)

(Isaac et al, 2008) (Vitamin E for Alzheimers and mild cognitive impairment. Isaac MG, Quinn R, Tabet N. .Cochrane Database Syst Rev. 2008 Jul 16;(3):CD002854)

(Iribarren et al, 1997) (Iribarren C, Folsom AR, Jacobs DR Jr, Gross MD, Belcher JD, Eckfeldt JH. Association of serum vitamin levels, LDL susceptibility to oxidation, and autoantibodies against MDA-LDL with carotid atherosclerosis. A case-control study. Arterioscler Thromb Vasc Biol. 1997;17:1171–1177)

(Jacobs, 2001) (Jacobs EJ, Connell CJ, Patel AV, Chao A, Rodriguez C, Seymour J, McCullough ML, Calle EE, Thun MJ. Vitamin C and vitamin E supplement use and colorectal cancer mortality in a large American Cancer Society cohort. Cancer Epidemiol Biomarkers Prev. 2001 Jan;10(1):17-23)

(Jacobs et al., 2002) (Jacobs EJ, Henion AK, Briggs PJ, Connell CJ, McCullough ML, Jonas CR, Rodriguez C, Calle EE, Thun MJ. Vitamin C and vitamin E supplement use and bladder cancer mortality in a large cohort of US men and women. American Journal of Epidemiology 2002;156: 1002-10)

(Jacobs et al. Jan. 2002) (Jacobs EJ, Connell CJ, McCullough ML, Chao A, Jonas CR, Rodriguez C, Calle EE, Thun MJ. Vitamin C, vitamin E, and multivitamin supplement use and stomach cancer mortality in the Cancer Prevention Study II cohort. Cancer Epidemiol Biomarkers Prev. 2002 Jan;11(1):35-41)

(Jacobus et al, 1992) (Jacobus CH, Holick MF, Shao Q, et al. Hypervitaminosis D associated with drinking milk. N Engl J Med. 1992;326:1173-1177)

(Jaques et al, 1995) (Jacques PF, Sulsky SI, Perrone GE, Jenner J, Schaefer EJ Epidemiology Program, US Department of Agriculture Human Nutrition Research Center on Aging, Tufts University, Boston, MA 02111, USA. (Jacques PF, Sulsky SI, Perrone GE, Jenner J, Schaefer EJ. Effect of vitamin C supplementation on lipoprotein cholesterol, apolipoprotein, and triglyceride concentrations. Ann Epidemiol 1995 Jan;5(1):52-9)

(Johansen et al, 2005) (Oxidative stress and the use of antioxidants in diabetes: Linking basic science to clinical practice. Jeanette Schultz Johansen et al. Cardiovasc Diabetol. 2005; 4: 5)

(Kang et al., 2006) (A randomized trial of vitamin E supplementation and cognitive function in women. Kang JH, Cook N, Manson J, Buring JE, Grodstein F. Arch Intern Med. 2006 Dec 11-25;166(22):2462-8)

(Kang et al, 2009) (Vitamin E, vitamin C, beta carotene, and cognitive function among women with or at risk of cardiovascular disease: The Women's Antioxidant and Cardiovascular Study. Kang JH, Cook NR,

Manson JE, Buring JE, Albert CM, Grodstein F. Circulation. 2009 Jun 2;119(21):2772-80. Epub 2009 May 18)

(Katsiki and Manes, 2009) (Katsiki N, Manes C. Is there a role for supplemented antioxidants in the prevention of atherosclerosis? Clin Nutr. 2009 Feb;28(1):3-9)

(Katz et al, 2004) (D. L. Katz, M. A. Evans, W. Chan, H. Nawaz, B. P. Comerford, M. L. Hoxley, V. Y. Njike, and P. M. Sarrel. Oats, Antioxidants and Endothelial Function in Overweight, Dyslipidemic Adults. J. Am. Coll. Nutr., October 1, 2004; 23(5): 397 – 403)

(Kimura et al, 2005) (Kimura H, Sawada T, Oshima S, Kozawa K, Ishioka T, Kato M. Toxicity and roles of reactive oxygen species. Curr Drug Targets Inflamm Allergy. 2005;4:489-495)

(Kirsh et al, 2006) (Kirsh VA, Hayes RB, Mayne ST, Chatterjee N, Subar AF, Dixon LB, et al. Supplemental and Dietary Vitamin E, Beta-Carotene, and Vitamin C Intakes and Prostate Cancer Risk. PCLO. J Natl Cancer Inst 2006;98:245-254)

(Klipstein-Grobusch et al, 1999) (K. Klipstein-Grobusch, J. M Geleijnse, J. H den Breeijen, H. Boeing, A. Hofman, D. E Grobbee, and J. C. Witteman. Dietary antioxidants and risk of myocardial infarction in the elderly: the Rotterdam Study. Am. J. Clinical Nutrition, February 1, 1999; 69(2): 261 - 266)

(Knekt et al, 1994) (Knekt P, Reunanen A, Jarvinen R, et al. Antioxidant vitamin intake and coronary mortality in a longitudinal population study. Am J Epidemiol 1994;139(12):1180-9)

(Knekt et al, 2004) (P. Knekt, J. Ritz, M. A Pereira, E. J O'Reilly, K. Augustsson, G. E Fraser, U. Goldbourt, B. L Heitmann, G. Hallmans, S. Liu, et al. Antioxidant vitamins and coronary heart disease risk: a pooled analysis of 9 cohorts. Am. J. Clinical Nutrition, December 1, 2004; 80(6): 1508 - 1520)

(Kris-Etherton et al, 2004) (Kris-Etherton P, Lichtenstein AH, Howard B, et al. Antioxidant vitamin supplements and cardiovascular disease. Circulation. 2004;110:637-641)

(Kushi et al, 1996) (L. H. Kushi et al. Dietary Antioxidant Vitamins and Death from Coronary Heart Disease in Postmenopausal Women. New England Journal of Medicine. Vol. 334. No. 18. May 2, 1996. pp. 1156-1162)

(Larsson et al, 2010) (Susanna C Larsson, Agneta Åkesson, Leif Bergkvist, and Alicja Wolk. Multivitamin use and breast cancer incidence in a prospective cohort of Swedish women. Am J Clin Nutr Published online 24 March 2010. Am J Clin Nutr Vol. 91, No. 5, 1268-1272, May 2010)

(Laurin et al, 2002) (Laurin D, Foley DJ, Masaki KH, et al. Vitamin E and C supplements and risk of dementia. JAMA 2002;288:2266–8)

(Laurin et al, 2003)(Midlife Dietary Intake of Antioxidants and Risk of Late-Life Incident Dementia: The Honolulu-Asia Aging Study)

(Law and Morris, 1998) (Law MR, Morris JK. By how much does fruit and vegetable consumption reduce the risk of ischaemic heart disease? Eur J Clin Nutr. 1998;52:549-556)

(Lawson et al, 2007) (Lawson KA, Wright ME, Subar A, Mouw T, Schatzkin A, Leitzmann MF. Multivitamin use and risk of prostate cancer in the National Institutes of Health–AARP Diet and Health Study. J Natl Cancer Inst (2007) 99:754–64)

(Lee et al., 1999) (Lee IM, Cook NR, Manson JE, Buring JE, Hennekens CH. Beta-carotene supplementation and incidence of cancer and cardiovascular disease: the Women's Health Study. J Natl Cancer Inst. 1999 Dec 15;91(24):2102-6)

(Lee et al, 2004) (Duk-Hee Lee, Aaron R Folsom, Lisa Harnack, Barry Halliwell and David R Jacobs, Jr. Does supplemental vitamin C increase cardiovascular disease risk in women with diabetes? American Journal of Clinical Nutrition, Vol. 80, No. 5, 1194-1200, November 2004)

(Lee, Koo and Min, 2004) (Lee, J., Koo, N. and Min, D.B. Reactive oxygen species, aging and antioxidative neutraceuticals. Comprehensive Reviews in Food Science and Food Safety. 2004, Vol. 3, pp. 21-33)

(Lee et al, 2005) (Vitamin E in the primary prevention of cardiovascular disease and cancer: the Women's Health Study: a randomized controlled trial. Lee IM, Cook NR, Gaziano JM, Gordon D, Ridker PM, Manson JE, et al. JAMA. 2005;294:56–65)

(Lesperance et al, 2002) (Lesperance ML, Olivotto IA, Forde N, et al. Mega-dose vitamins and minerals in the treatment of non-metastatic breast cancer: an historical cohort study. Breast Cancer Res Treat (2002) 76(2):137–143)

(Levy, 2002) (Vitamin C, Infectious Diseases, and Toxins: Curing the Incurable, by Thomas E. Levy, M.D. Philadelphia: Xlibris Corporation, 2002)

(Levy et al, 2004) (Levy AP, Friedenberg P, Lotan R, et al. The effect of vitamin therapy on the progression of coronary artery atherosclerosis varies by haptoglobin type in postmenopausal women. Diabetes Care. 2004;27(4):925-930)

(Lichtenstein and Russell, 2005) (Alice H. Lichtenstein and Robert M. Russell. Essential Nutrients: Food or Supplements? JAMA. 2005;294:351-358)

(Lichtenstein, 2009) (A.H. Lichtenstein. Nutrient supplements and cardiovascular disease: a heartbreaking story. J. Lipid Res., April 1, 2009; 50(Supplement): S429 - S433)

(Lim et al, 2005) (Oxidative Damage in Mitochondrial DNA Is Not Extensive. K. S. Lim, K. J. Aseelan, M. Whiteman, A. Jenner and B. Halliwell. Ann. N.Y. Acad. Sci. 1042: 210–220 (2005)

(Lin et al, 2009) (Vitamins C and E and Beta Carotene Supplementation and Cancer Risk: A Randomized Controlled Trial. Jennifer Lin, Nancy R. Cook, Christine Albert, Elaine Zaharris, J. Michael Gaziano, Martin Van Denburgh, Julie E. Buring, JoAnn E. Manson. JNCI Journal of the National Cancer Institute 2009 101(1):14-23)

(Lippman et al, 2009) (Effect of selenium and vitamin E on risk of prostate cancer and other cancers: the Selenium and Vitamin E Cancer Prevention Trial (SELECT). Lippman, SM. JAMA. 2009 Jan 7;301(1):39-51. Epub 2008 Dec 9)

(Liu et al., 2006) (S. Liu, I-M. Lee, Y. Song, M. Van Denburgh, N. R. Cook, J. E. Manson, and J. E. Buring. Vitamin E and Risk of Type 2

Diabetes in the Women's Health Study Randomized Controlled Trial. Diabetes, October 1, 2006; 55(10): 2856 – 2862)

(Longnecker, 1997) (Longnecker MP, Newcomb PA, Mittendorf R, Greenberg ER, Willett WC. Intake of carrots, spinach, and supplements containing vitamin A in relation to risk of breast cancer. Cancer Epidemiol Biomarkers Prev. 1997;6(11):887-892)

(Lonn et al. 2002) (Eva Lonn et al. Effects of Vitamin E on Cardiovascular and Microvascular Outcomes in High-Risk Patients With Diabetes. Results of the HOPE Study and MICRO-HOPE Substudy. Diabetes Care 25:1919-1927, 2002)

(Lonn et al, 2005) (Effects of long-term vitamin E supplementation on cardiovascular events and cancer: a randomized controlled trial. E. Lonn et al. JAMA. 2005 Mar 16;293(11):1338-47)

(Lopez-Lazaro, 2010) (Miguel Lopez-Lazaro. A New View of Carcinogenesis and an Alternative Approach to Cancer Therapy. Mol Med 16(3-4) 144-153)

(Luchsinger et al, 2003) (Luchsinger et al. Antioxidant Vitamin Intake and Risk of Alzheimer Disease. Arch Neurol 2003;60:203-208)

(Luoma et al, 1995) (Luoma PV, Nayha S, Sikkila K, et al. High serum alpha-tocopherol, albumin, selenium and cholesterol, and low mortality from coronary heart disease in northern Finland. J Intern Med 1995;237(1):49-54)

(Magliano et al, 2006) (Magliano, Dianna; McNeil, John; Branley, Pauline; Shiel, Louise; Demos, Lisa; Wolfe, Rory; Kotsopoulos, Dimitra; McGrath, Barry. The Melbourne Atherosclerosis Vitamin E Trial (MAVET): a study of high dose vitamin E in smokers. European Journal of Cardiovascular Prevention & Rehabilitation. June 2006 - Volume 13 - Issue 3 - pp 341-347)

(Manda et al, 2009) (Gina Manda, Marina Tamara Nechifor and Teodora-Monica Neagu. Reactive Oxygen Species, Cancer and Anti-Cancer Therapies. Current Clinical Biology, 2009, 3, 342-366)

(Mann et al, 2004) (Effects of vitamin E on cardiovascular outcomes in people with mild-to-moderate renal insufficiency: results of the HOPE study. J.F. Mann et al. Kidney Int. 2004 Apr;65(4):1375-80)

(Marchioli and Valagussa, 2000) (Marchioli, R and Valagussa, F. The results of the GISSI-Prevenzione trial in the general framework of secondary prevention. Europ Heart J 2000; 21: 949-952)

(Matthan et al, 2003) (Matthan N.R. et al. Impact of simvastatin, niacin, and/or antioxidants on cholesterol metabolism in CAD patients with low HDL. Journal of Lipid Research, Vol. 44, 800-806, April 2003)

(Maserejian et al, 2007) (Maserejian NW, Giovanncci E, Rosner B, Joshipura K. Prospective Study of Vitamins C, E, A, and Carotenoids and Risk of Oral Premalignant Lesions in Men. International J of Cancer. 120(5):970-7; 2006)

(Mayer-Davis et al, 1997) (Mayer-Davis EJ, Monaco JH, Marshall JA, Rushing J, Juhaeri. Vitamin c intake and cardiovascular disease risk factors in persons with non-insulin-dependent diabetes mellitus. From the Insulin Resistanc Atherosclerosis Study and the San Luis Valley Diabetes Study. Prev Med 1997 May-Jun;26(3):277-83)

(Mayne et al, 2001) (Susan T. Mayne et al. Randomized Trial of Supplemental ß-Carotene to Prevent Second Head and Neck Cancer. Cancer Research 61, 1457-1463, February 15, 2001)

(Maxwell, 1999) (Maxwell SR. Antioxidant vitamin supplements: update of their potential benefits and possible risks. Drug Saf (1999) 21:253–66)

(McNeil et al, 2004) (McNeil JJ, Robman L, Tikellis G, Sinclair MI, McCarty CA, Taylor HR. Vitamin E supplementation and cataract: randomized controlled trial. Ophthalmology. 2004;111(1):75-84)

(McQuillan et al. 2001) (McQuillan BM, Hung J, Beilby JP, Nidorf M, Thompson PL. Antioxidant vitamins and the risk of carotid atherosclerosis. The Perth Carotid Ultrasound Disease Assessment study (CUDAS). J Am Coll Cardiol. 2001 Dec;38(7):1788-94)

(Medical letter, 1998) The Medical Letter (Vitamin supplements. The Medical Letter on Drugs and Therapeutics 40:75-77, 1998).

(Meagher et al. 2001) (Meagher EA, Barry OP, Lawson JA, et al. Effects of vitamin E on lipid peroxidation in healthy persons. JAMA. 2001;285:1178-1182)

(Michaelsson et al, 2003) (Michaelsson K, Lithell H, Vessby B, Mehus H. Serum retinol levels and the risk of fracture. N Engl J Med 2003;348:287-94)

(Michels, 2001) (Michels KB, Holmberg L, Bergkvist L, Ljung H, Bruce A, Wolk A. Dietary antioxidant vitamins, retinol, and breast cancer incidence in a cohort of Swedish women. Int J Cancer. 2001;91(4):563-567)

(Millen et al, 2004) (Millen AE, Dodd KW, Subar AF. Use of vitamin, mineral, nonvitamin, and nonmineral supplements in the United States: The 1987, 1992, and 2000 National Health Interview Survey results. J Am Diet Assoc. 2004;104:942-50)

(Miller et al, 1993) (Miller NJ, Rice-Evans C, Davies MJ, et al. A novel method for measuring antioxidant capacity and its application to monitoring the antioxidant status in premature neonates. Clin Sci 1993;84:407–12)

(Miller et al., 1997) (Miller, E.R. 3rd, L.J. Appel, O.A. Levander & D.M. Levine. 1997. The effect of antioxidant vitamin supplementation on traditional cardiovascular risk factors. J. Cardiovasc. Risk. 4(1):19-24)

(Miller et al., 2004) (Miller ER 3d, Pastor-Barriuso R, Dalal D, Riemersma RA, Appel LJ, Guallar E. Meta-analysis: high-dosage vitamin E supplementation may increase all-cause mortality. Ann Intern Med 2005;142:37-46)

(Mishra, 2007) (Mishra V. Oxidative stress and role of antioxidant supplementation in critical illness. in Lab. 2007;53(3-4):199-209)

(Moertel et al, 1985) (Moertel CG, Fleming TR, Creagan ET, Rubin J, O'Connell MJ, Ames MM. High-dose vitamin C versus placebo in the treatment of patients with advanced cancer who have had no prior chemotherapy. A randomized double-blind comparison. N Engl J Med. 1985 Jan 17;312(3):137-41)

(Moilanen and Hovatta, 1995) (Moilanen J, Hovatta O. Excretion of alpha-tocopherol into human seminal plasma after oral administration. Andrologia. 1995 May-Jun;27(3):133-6)

(Morris et al, 2008) (Morris, Brenda H et al. Aggressive vs. conservative phototherapy for infants with extremely low birth weight. The New England Journal of Medicine 2008;359(18):1885-96)

(Morris et al, 2002) (Morris et al. Dietary intake of antioxidant nutrients and the risk of incident Alzheimer disease in a biracial community study (2002) JAMA 287, 3230-3237)

(Morris and Carson, 2003) (Routine Vitamin Supplementation To Prevent Cardiovascular Disease: A Summary of the Evidence for the U.S. Preventive Services Task Force. Morris and Carson. ANN INTERN MED 2003;139:56-70. Review)

(Moyad, 2002) (Moyad et al, 2002) (M.A. Moyad. Selenium and vitamin E supplements for prostate cancer: evidence or embellishment? Urology. 2002 Apr;59(4 Suppl 1):9-19)

(MRC/BHF, 2002) (MRC/BHF Heart Protection Study of antioxidant vitamin supplementation in 20,536 high-risk individuals: a randomized placebo-controlled trial. Lancet. 2002 Jul 6;360(9326):23-33)

(Mulholland and Benford, 2007) (Mulholland CA, Benford DJ. What is known about the safety of multivitamin-multimineral supplements for the generally healthy population? Theoretical basis for harm. Am J Clin Nutr 2007;85(suppl):318S–22S)

(Muntwyler et al. 2002) (Muntwyler J, Hennekens CH, Manson JE, Buring JE, Gaziano JM. Vitamin supplement use in a low-risk population of US male physicians and subsequent cardiovascular mortality. Arch Intern Med. 2002 Jul 8;162(13):1472-6)

(Myung et al, 2009) (S.-K. Myung et al. Effects of antioxidant supplements on cancer prevention: meta-analysis of randomized controlled trials. Annals of Oncology Advance Access published online on July 21, 2009) (Myung, S.-K., Kim, Y., Ju, W., Choi, H. J., Bae, W. K. (2010). Effects of antioxidant supplements on cancer prevention: meta-analysis of randomized controlled trials. Ann Oncol 21: 166-179)

(Ness and Powles, 1997) (Ness AR, Powles JW. Fruit and vegetables, and cardiovascular disease: a review. Int J Epidemiol. 1997;26:1-13)

(Neuhouser et al, 2009) (Multivitamin Use and Risk of Cancer and Cardiovascular Disease in the Women's Health Initiative Cohorts. Marian L. Neuhouser et al. Arch Intern Med. 2009;169(3):294-304)

(Niacin intox, 1983) (Niacin intoxication from pumpernickel bagels: New York. MMWR Morb Mortal Wkly Rep. 1983;32:305)

(Niskanen et al, 2004) (Niskanen L, Laaksonen D, Nyyssonen K, et al.: Uric acid level as a risk factor for cardiovascular and all-cause mortality in middle-aged men. Arch Intern Med 2004, 164:1546–1551)

(Omenn et al., 1996) (Risk factors for lung cancer and for intervention effects in CARET, the Beta-Carotene and Retinol Efficacy Trial. G.S. Omenn et al. J Natl Cancer Inst. 1996 Nov 6;88(21):1550-9)

(Omenn et al, NEJM. 1996) (Omenn GS, Goodman GE, Thornquist MD, et al. Effects of a combination of beta carotene and vitamin A on lung cancer and cardiovascular disease. N Engl J Med. 1996;334:1150-1155)

(Ohtake et al, 2005) (Ohtake T, Kobayashi S, Negishi K, Moriya H. Supplement nephropathy due to long-term, high-dose ingestion of ascorbic acid, calcium lactate, vitamin D and laxatives. Clin Nephrol. 2005 Sep;64(3):236-40)

(Pani et al, 2000) (Pani, G., Colavitti, R., Bedogni, B., Anzevino, R., Borrello, S. and Galecotti, T. A redox signaling mechanism for density-dependent inhibition of cell growth. J Biol Chem 2000; 275: 38891-38899)

(Park et al, 2009) (K. Park, L. Harnack, and D. R. Jacobs Jr. Trends in Dietary Supplement Use in a Cohort of Postmenopausal Women From Iowa. Am. J. Epidemiol., April 1, 2009; 169(7): 887 - 892)

(Patterson et al, 2007) (Patterson RE, White E, Kristal AR, Neuhouser ML, Potter JD. Vitamin supplements and cancer risk: the epidemiologic evidence. Cancer Causes Control. 1997 Sep;8(5):786-802)

(Peters et al, 2008) (U. Peters et al. Vitamin E and selenium supplementation and risk of prostate cancer in the Vitamins and lifestyle (VITAL) study cohort. Cancer Causes Control. 2008 Feb;19(1):75-87)

(Pike, 2005) (Pike MC. The role of mammographic density in evaluating changes in breast cancer risk. Gynecol Endocrinol 2005;21(suppl 1):1–5)

(Pocobelli et al, 2007) (Gaia Pocobelli, Ulrike Peters, Alan R. Kristal and Emily White. Use of Supplements of Multivitamins, Vitamin C, and Vitamin E in Relation to Mortality. American Journal of Epidemiology 2009 170(4):472-483)

(Poston et al., 2006) (L. Poston et al. Vitamin C and vitamin E in pregnant women at risk for pre-eclampsia (VIP trial): randomised placebo-controlled trial. The Lancet, Volume 367, Issue 9517, Pages 1145 - 1154, 8 April 2006)

(Promislow et al, 2002) (Promislow JH, Goodman-Gruen D, Slymen DJ, Barrett-Connor E. Retinol intake and bone mineral density in the elderly: the Rancho Bernardo Study. J Bone Miner Res. 2002;17(8):1349-1358)

(Qiao et al, 2009) (Y.-L. Qiao, S. M. Dawsey, F. Kamangar, J.-H. Fan, C. C. Abnet, X.-D. Sun, L. L. Johnson, M. H. Gail, Z.-W. Dong, B. Yu, et al. Total and Cancer Mortality After Supplementation With Vitamins and Minerals: Follow-up of the Linxian General Population Nutrition Intervention Trial. J Natl Cancer Inst, April 1, 2009; 101(7): 507 - 518)

(Qu et al, 2007) (Chen-Xu Qu et al, Chemoprevention of Primary Liver Cancer: A Randomized, Double-Blind Trial in Linxian, China. Journal of the National Cancer Institute. Vol 99, Issue 16. August 15, 2007. pp. 1240-1247)

(Raal et al, 1999) (Efficacy of vitamin E compared with either simvastatin or atorvastatin in preventing the progression of atherosclerosis in homozygous familial hypercholesterolemia. Raal FJ, Pilcher GJ, Veller MG, Kotze MJ, Joffe BI. Am J Cardiol. 1999 Dec 1;84(11):1344-6, A7)

(Rapola et al, 1997) (Rapola, J.M., J. Virtamo, S. Ripatti, J.K. Huttunen, D. Albanes, P.R. Taylor & O. P. Heinonen. 1997. Randomized trial of alpha-tocopherol and beta-carotene supplements on incidence of major coronary events in men with previous myocardial infarction. Lancet. 349(9067):1715-1720)

(Rapola et al, 1998) (J M Rapola, J Virtamo, S Ripatti, J K Haukka, J K Huttunen, D Albanes, P R Taylor, and O P Heinonen. Effects of alpha tocopherol and beta carotene supplements on symptoms, progression, and prognosis of angina pectoris Heart, May 1, 1998; 79(5): 454 - 458)

(Rautiainen et al, 2010) (Susanne Rautiainen, Birgitta Ejdervik Lindblad, Ralf Morgenstern and Alicja Wolk. Vitamin C supplements and the risk of age-related cataract: a population-based prospective cohort study in women. Am J Clin Nutr 91: 487-493, 2010)

(Reaven, 1995) (Reaven PD, Herold DA, Barnett J, Edelman S. Effects of Vitamin E on susceptibility of low-density lipoprotein and low-density lipoprotein subfractions to oxidation and on protein glycation in NIDDM. Diabetes Care. 1995;18(6):807-816)

(Riemersma et al, 2000) (R. A Riemersma, K. F Carruthers, R. A Elton, and K. A. Fox. Vitamin C and the risk of acute myocardial infarction. Am. J. Clinical Nutrition, May 1, 2000; 71(5): 1181 - 1186)

(Rimm et al, 1993) (Rimm EB, Stampfer MJ, Ascherio A, et al. Vitamin E consumption and the risk of coronary heart disease in men. N Engl J Med 1993;328(20):1450-6)

(Ristow et al, 2009) (Ristow M, Zarse K, Oberbach A, Klöting N, Birringer M, Kiehntopf M, Stumvoll M, Kahn CR, Blüher M. Antioxidants prevent health-promoting effects of physical exercise in humans. Proc Natl Acad Sci U S A. 2009 May 26;106(21):8665-70)

(Roberts et al, 2010) (Roberts JM et al, Vitamins C and E to prevent complications of pregnancy-associated hypertension. N Engl J Med (2010) 362: 1282-91)

(Rogovik, Vohra and Goldman, 2010) (Alexander L. Rogovik, Sunita Vohra, and Ran D. Goldman. Safety considerations and Potential Interactions of Vitamins: Should Vitamins Be Considered Drugs? The Annals of Pharmacotherapy. Vol. 44, No. 2, pp. 311-324)

(Rolf et al, 1999) (Rolf C, Cooper TG, Yeung CH, Nieschlag E. Antioxidant treatment of patients with asthenozoospermia or moderate oligoasthenozoospermia with high-dose vitamin C and vitamin E: a randomized, placebo-controlled, double-blind study. Hum Reprod. 1999 Apr;14(4):1028-33)

(Rumbold et al, 2006) (Vitamins C and E and the Risks of Preeclampsia and Perinatal Complications Alice R. Rumbold, Ph.D., Caroline A. Crowther, Ross R. Haslam, Gustaaf A. Dekker, and Jeffrey S. Robinson, for the ACTS Study Group. N Engl J Med. 2006 Apr 27;354(17):1796-806)

(Sacks et al, 2001) (Sacks FM, Svetkey LP, Vollmer WM, et al. DASH-Sodium Collaborative Research Group: effects on blood pressure of reduced dietary sodium and the Dietary Approaches to Stop Hypertension (DASH) diet. N Engl J Med. 2001;344:3-10)

(Salganik et al, 2000, 2003) (Salganik, R. I., Albright, C. D., Rodgers, J., Kim, J., Zeisel, S. H., Sivashinskiy, M. S. & Van Dyke, T. A. (2000) Dietary antioxidant depletion: enhancement of tumor apoptosis and inhibition of brain tumor growth in transgenic mice. Carcinogenesis 21: 909–914)

(Salganik, 2001) (Salganik RI. The benefits and hazards of antioxidants: controlling apoptosis and other protective mechanisms in cancer patients and the human population. J Am Coll Nutr. 2001;20(suppl):464S-472S)

(Satia et al, 2009) (Satia JA, Littman A, Slatore CG, Galanko JA, White E. Long-term use of beta-carotene, retinol, lycopene, and lutein supplements and lung cancer risk: results from the VITamins And Lifestyle (VITAL) study. Am J Epidemiol. 2009 Apr 1;169(7):815-28)

(Schatzkin et al, 2000) (Schatzkin A, Lanza E, Corle D, et al, Polyp Prevention Trial Study Group. Lack of effect of a low-fat, high-fiber diet on the recurrence of colorectal adenomas. N Engl J Med. 2000;342:1149-1155)

(Schleicher et al, 2009) (#7,277) (Rosemary L Schleicher, Margaret D Carroll, Earl S Ford and David A Lacher. Serum vitamin C and the prevalence of vitamin C deficiency in the United States: 2003–2004 National Health and Nutrition Examination Survey (NHANES). Am J Clin Nutr 90: 1252-1263, 2009)

(Seddon, 2007) (Johanna M Seddon. Multivitamin-multimineral supplements and eye disease: age-related macular degeneration and cataract. American Journal of Clinical Nutrition, Vol. 85, No. 1, 304S-307S, January 2007)

(Seifried et al, 2003) (Seifried HE, McDonald SS, Anderson DE, Greenwald P, Milner JA. The antioxidant conundrum in cancer. Cancer Res (2003) 63:4295–8)

(Sesso et al, 2008) (Vitamins E and C in the prevention of cardiovascular disease in men: the Physicians' Health Study II randomized controlled trial. Sesso, HD. et al. JAMA. 2008 Nov 12;300(18):2123-33. Epub 2008 Nov 9)

(Shekelle et al, 2004) (Shekelle PG, Morton SC, Jungvig LK, et al. Effect of supplemental vitamin E for the prevention and treatment of cardiovascular disease. J Gen Intern Med 2004;19:380-389)

(Shenkin, 2006) (Shenkin A (2006). "The key role of micronutrients". Clin Nutr 25 (1): 1–13)

(Siekmeier and Marz, 2006) (Siekmeier R, Steffen C, März W. Can antioxidants prevent atherosclerosis? Bundesgesundheitsblatt Gesundheitsforschung Gesundheitsschutz. 2006 Oct;49(10):1034-49)

(Siekmeier and Marz, 2007) (Siekmeier R, Steffen C, März W. Role of oxidants and antioxidants in atherosclerosis: results of in vitro and in vivo investigations. J Cardiovasc Pharmacol Ther. 2007 Dec;12(4):265-82)

(Simon et al, 2000) (Simon HU, Haj-Yehia A, Levi-Schaffer F. Role of reactive oxygen species (ROS) in apoptosis induction. Apoptosis. 2000;5:415-418)

(Slatore et al, 2008) (Christopher G. Slatore, Alyson J. Littman, David H. Au, Jessie A. Satia, and Emily White Long-Term Use of Supplemental Multivitamins, Vitamin C, Vitamin E, and Folate Does Not Reduce the Risk of Lung Cancer. Am. J. Respir. Crit. Care Med. 177: 524-530. First published online Nov. 7, 2007 as doi:10.1164/rccm.200709-1398OC. Published in print March 1, 2008)

(Stampfer et al, 1993) (Stampfer MJ, Hennekens CH, Manson JE, et al. Vitamin E consumption and the risk of coronary disease in women. N Engl J Med 1993;328(20):1444-9)

(Stanner et al, 2004) (Stanner SA, Hughes J, Kelly CN, Buttriss J (2004). "A review of the epidemiological evidence for the 'antioxidant hypothesis'". Public Health Nutr 7 (3): 407–22)

(Steinmetz and Potter, 1996) (Steinmetz KA, Potter JD. Vegetables, fruit, and cancer prevention: a review. J Am Diet Assoc. 1996;96:1027-1039)

(Stephens et al., 1996) (Stephens, NG et al. Randomized controlled trial of vitamin E in patients with coronary artery disease: Cambridge Heart Antioxidant Study (CHAOS)," Lancet, March 23, 1996; 347:781-786.)

(Stevens et al, 2005) (Stevens VL, McCullough Ml, Diver WR, Rodriguez C, Jacobs EJ, thun MJ, Calle EE. Use of multivitamins andprostate cancer mortality in a large cohort of US men. Cancer Causes Control. 2005 Aug; 16(6):643-50)

(Stone et al, 2005) (Effect of intensive lipid lowering, with or without antioxidant vitamins, compared with moderate lipid lowering on myocardial ischemia in patients with stable coronary artery disease: the Vascular Basis for the Treatment of Myocardial Ischemia Study. P.H. Stone et al. Circulation. 2005 Apr 12;111(14):1747-55)

(Strandhgen et al, 2000) (Strandhagen E, Hansson PO, Bosaeus I, Isaksson B, Eriksson H. High fruit intake may reduce mortality among middle-aged and elderly men: the Study of Men Born in 1913. Eur J Clin Nutr. 2000;54:337-341)

(Tan et al, 2008) (Tan JS, Wang JJ, Flood V, Rochtchina E, Smith W, Mitchell P. Dietary antioxidants and the long-term incidence of age-related macular degeneration: the Blue Mountains Eye Study. Ophthalmology. 2008 Feb;115(2):334-41)

(Tangrea et al, 1992) (Tangrea JA, Edwards BK, Taylor PR, et al.: Long-term therapy with low-dose isotretinoin for prevention of basal cell carcinoma: a multicenter clinical trial. Isotretinoin-Basal Cell Carcinoma Study Group. J Natl Cancer Inst 84 (5): 328-32, 1992)

(Tangrea et al, 1993) (Tangrea JA, Adrianza E, Helsel WE, et al.: Clinical and laboratory adverse effects associated with long-term, low-dose isotretinoin: incidence and risk factors. The Isotretinoin-Basal Cell Carcinomas Study Group. Cancer Epidemiol Biomarkers Prev 2 (4): 375-80, 1993 Jul-Aug)

(Tardif et al, 1997) (Tardif, J.C., Cote, G and Lesperance, J., et al. Probucol and multivitamins in the prevention of restenosis after coronary angioplasty. Multivitamins and Probucol Study Group. N Engl J Med 1997; 337(6): 365-372)

(Tatsioni et al, 2007) (Persistence of Contradicted Claims in the Literature. Athina Tatsioni, MD; Nikolaos G. Bonitsis, MD; John P. A. Ioannidis, MD. JAMA 2007; 298:2517-2526)

(Teikari et al, 1997) (Teikari JM, Virtamo J, Rautalahti M, Palmgren J, Liesto K, Heinonen OP. Long-term supplementation with alpha-tocopherol and beta-carotene and age-related cataract. Acta Ophthalmol Scand 1997;75:634-40)

(Teikari et al, 1998) (Teikari JM, Rautalahti M, Haukka J, et al. Incidence of cataract operations in Finnish male smokers unaffected by alpha tocopherol or beta carotene supplements. J Epidemiol Community Health. 1998;52(7):468-472)

(Taylor et al, 2002) (Taylor HR, Tikellis G, Robman LD, McCarty CA, McNeil JJ. Vitamin E supplementation and macular degeneration: randomised controlled trial. BMJ. 2002 Jul 6;325(7354):11)

(Thannical and Fanburg, 2000) (Thannical VJ, Fanburg BL. Reactive oxygen species in cell signaling. Am J Physiol Lung Cell Mol Physiol 2000; 279: L1005-L1028)

(Tomita et al, 2000) (Tomita M. et al. Does hyperuricemia affect mortality? A prospective cohort study of Japanese male workers. J Epidemiol. 2000 Nov;10(6):403-9).

(Thörnwall et al., 2004) (Effect of α-tocopherol and ß-carotene supplementation on coronary heart disease during the 6-year post-trial follow-up in the ATBC study. Markareetta E. Törnwall et al. European Heart Journal 2004 25(13):1171-1178)

(Tran et al, 2001) (Thuan L. Tran, MD. Antioxidant supplements to prevent heart disease: Real hope or empty hype? Vol. 109. No.1. Jan. 2001. Postgraduate Medicine)

(Trichopoulos, Lagiou and Adami, 2005) (Trichopoulos D, Lagiou P, Adami HO. Towards an integrated model for breast cancer etiology: the crucial role of the number of mammary tissue-specific stem cells. Breast Cancer Res 2005;7:13–7)

(Trombo, 2005) (Paula R. Trumbo. The Level of Evidence for Permitting a Qualified Health Claim: FDA's Review of the Evidence for Selenium and Cancer and Vitamin E and Heart Disease. The American Society for Nutritional Sciences. J. Nutr. 135:354-356, February 2005)

(UNICEF, 2001) (UNICEF-sponsored program gone awry. India's National Magazine, The Hindu. 8-21 December, 2001, Issue 25)

(U.S. Dept HHS, 2004) (U.S. Department of Health and Human Services. Advance Data from Vital and Health Statistics. Dietary Intake of Selected Vitamins for the United States Population: 1999-2000. Centers for Disease Control and Prevention. National Center for Health Statistics. Number 339, 2004)

(van Stijn et al, 2008) (van Stijn MF, Ligthart-Melis GC, Boelens PG, Scheffer PG, Teerlink T, Twisk JW, Houdijk AP, van Leeuwen PA. Antioxidant enriched enteral nutrition and oxidative stress after major gastrointestinal tract surgery. World J Gastroenterol. 2008 Dec 7;14(45):6960-9)

(Vasquez et al., 1998) (The SUVIMAX (France) study: the role of antioxidants in the prevention of cancer and cardiovascular disease. Vasquez, Martínez C, Galán P, Preziosi P, Ribas L, Serra LL, Hercberg S. Rev Esp Salud Publica. 1998 May-Jun;72(3):173-83.)

(Verlangieri et al, 1985) (Verlangieri AJ, Kapeghian JC, el-Dean S, et al. Fruit and vegetable consumption and cardiovascular mortality. Med Hypotheses 1985;16(1):7-15)

(Virtamo et al, 1998) (Virtamo J, Rapola JM, Ripatti S, et al. Effect of vitamin E and beta carotene on the incidence of primary nonfatal myocardial infarction and fatal coronary heart disease. Arch Intern Med. 1998;158:668-675)

(Vivekananthan et al., 2003) (Vivekananthan DP, Penn MS, Sapp SK, Hsu A, Topol EJ. Use of antioxidant vitamins for the prevention of cardiovascular disease: meta-analysis of randomised trials 2003 Lancet 2003 June 14; 361: 2017–23)

(Waters et al, 2002) (Waters DD, Alderman EL, Hsia J, Howard BV, Cobb FR, Rogers WJ, Ouyang P, Thompson P, Tardif JC, Higginson L, Bittner V, Steffes M, Gordon DJ, Proschan M, Younes N, Verter JI. Effects of hormone replacement therapy and antioxidant vitamin supplements on coronary atherosclerosis in postmenopausal women: a randomized controlled trial. JAMA. 2002; 288: 2432–40)

(Westhuyzen et al, 1997) (Westhuyzen J, Cochrane AD, Tesar PJ, Mau T, Cross DB, Frenneaux MP, Khafagi FA, Fleming SJ. Effect of preoperative supplementation with alpha-tocopherol and ascorbic acid on myocardial injury in patients undergoing cardiac operations. J Thorac Cardiovasc Surg 1997 May;113(5):942-8)

(Wheeler, 2001) (A SCIENTIFIC LOOK AT ALTERNATIVE MEDICINE. Thomas J. Wheeler, PhD. Department of Biochemistry and Molecular Biology, University of Louisville School of Medicine, Louisville KY 40292 (tjwheeler@louisville.edu)

(WHI, 2002) (Risks and benefits of estrogen plus progestin in healthy postmenopausal women: principal results From the Women's Health Initiative randomized controlled trial. JAMA2002; 288:321–333)

(Whiting and Lemke, et al, 1999) (Whiting SJ, Lemke B. Excess retinol intake may explain the high incidence of osteoporosis in northern Europe. Nutr Rev 1999;57:249-50)

(Wiysonge et al, 2005) (Wiysonge CS, Shey MS, Sterne JA, Brocklehurst P. Vitamin A supplementation for reducing the risk of mother-to-child transmission of HIV infection. Cochrane Database Syst Rev. 2005;(4):CD003648)

(Woodside, et al. 1998) (Woodside JV, Yarnell JW, McMaster D, Young IS, Harmon DL, McCrum EE, Patterson CC, Gey KF, Whitehead AS, Evans A. Effect of B-group vitamins and antioxidant vitamins on hyperhomocysteinemia: a double-blind, randomized, factorial-design, controlled trial. Am J Clin Nutr. 1998 May;67(5):858-66).

(Wu et al, 2002) (Wu K, Willett WC, Chan JM, Fuchs CS, Colditz GA, Rimm EB, Giovannucci EL. A prospective study on supplemental vitamin E intake and risk of colon cancer in women and men. Cancer Epidemiol Biomarkers Prev 2002;11:1298-304)

(Yaffe et al, 2004) (Yaffe K, Clemons TE, McBee WL, Lindblad AS; Age-Related Eye Disease Study Research Group. Impact of antioxidants, zinc, and copper on cognition in the elderly: a randomized, controlled trial. Neurology. 2004 Nov 9;63(9):1705-7)

(Yusuf et al. 2000) (Yusuf, S., Dagenais, G., Progue, J. et al. Vitamin E supplementation and cardiovascular evens, in high-risk patients the Heart Outcomes Prevention Evaluation Study Investigators. N Engl J Med. 2000; 342; 154-160)

(Zaharris et al, 2007) (A Randomized Factorial Trial of Vitamins C and E and Beta Carotene in the Secondary Prevention of Cardiovascular Events in Women: Results From the Women's Antioxidant Cardiovascular Study. Zaharris, J. MacFadyen, E. Danielson, J. E. Buring, and J. E. Manson. Arch Intern Med, August 13, 2007; 167(15): 1610 – 1618)